AF834530

Allen R. Huang • Louise Mallet
Editors

Medication-Related Falls in Older People

Causative Factors and Management Strategies

Adis

Editors
Allen R. Huang
Head, Division of Geriatric Medicine
University of Ottawa and
The Ottawa Hospital

Associate Professor of Medicine
University of Ottawa

Adjunct Professor of Medicine
McGill University
Montréal, Québec
Canada

Louise Mallet
Head, Faculty of Pharmacy
Université de Montréal
Montréal, Québec
Canada

Clinical Pharmacist in Geriatrics
McGill University Health Centre
Montréal, Québec
Canada

ISBN 978-3-319-32302-2 ISBN 978-3-319-32304-6 (eBook)
DOI 10.1007/978-3-319-32304-6

Library of Congress Control Number: 2016944151

© Springer International Publishing Switzerland 2016
This work is subject to copyright. All rights are reserved by the Publisher, whether the whole or part of the material is concerned, specifically the rights of translation, reprinting, reuse of illustrations, recitation, broadcasting, reproduction on microfilms or in any other physical way, and transmission or information storage and retrieval, electronic adaptation, computer software, or by similar or dissimilar methodology now known or hereafter developed.
The use of general descriptive names, registered names, trademarks, service marks, etc. in this publication does not imply, even in the absence of a specific statement, that such names are exempt from the relevant protective laws and regulations and therefore free for general use.
The publisher, the authors and the editors are safe to assume that the advice and information in this book are believed to be true and accurate at the date of publication. Neither the publisher nor the authors or the editors give a warranty, express or implied, with respect to the material contained herein or for any errors or omissions that may have been made.

Printed on acid-free paper

This Adis imprint is published by Springer Nature
The registered company is Springer International Publishing AG Switzerland

Medication-Related Falls in Older People

Preface

The aging of the world population is highlighting the problems encountered by older people as they seek health care. Medication use is a double-edged sword: the beneficial effects of drug therapy must be balanced against potential and real side effects that drugs can cause in older patients. The situation is made more complex for individual patients because of the multiple factors involved, such as the physiologic changes in the body due to aging processes, the accumulation of comorbidities, and the use of drugs to manage various conditions and symptoms. Falls are a dreaded event in older people. It can affect a person biologically, resulting in soft tissue and bony trauma including fractures, psychologically resulting in fear of falling and mental health well-being resulting in depression. The identification of and reduction in fall risks in older people is a worldwide concern. Falls (or the reduction in their numbers) are a ubiquitous quality measure of health care delivery. Medication use is an important and potentially modifiable factor. This book serves as a repository of knowledge and scientific evidence concerning medications and their effects on falls risk. The book will inform readers of the complexity of the issue of medication-related falls in older people and provide strategies for its management. The target audience for this book includes (1) health professionals with an interest in researching and caring for older people, (2) managers of institutions or health systems, (3) policy-makers and health system funding decision-makers, and (4) the general public seeking high-quality information on this topic – especially those individuals with aging parents who have experienced falls or medication problems. This book will not be able to provide a single solution to this important clinical problem because of its complexity. Perhaps in the future, as a convergence of genomics, proteomics, and therapeutics occurs, health science may be able to optimize medication use in each individual person to minimize the risk of side effects and adverse events.

Ottawa, ON, Canada — Allen R. Huang
Montréal, QC, Canada — Louise Mallet

Contents

Part I
Background

Chapter 1
Introduction

Allen R. Huang and Louise Mallet

Abstract Every person will fall throughout their life. More than one-third of community-dwelling older adults fall every year. One of the important risk factors for falling is taking medications. The contents of this book will help the reader understand the various factors involved in increasing the risk for falls in older adults and the various medications that contribute to that risk. This book represents a repository of scientific evidence current at the time of its publication and can help students and researchers understand the problem. People involved in health policy-making may also be engaged to help address this global problem. Additionally anyone with an interest in this topic can learn about medications and falls.

> Books, in all their variety, offer the human intellect the means whereby civilisation may be carried triumphantly forward. (Winston Churchill, November 8, 1937, Statement for the National Book Fair)

The inspiration for this book came from the editor-in-chief of the journal *Drugs and Aging*, Professor David Williamson. The invitational e-mail message arrived in my inbox one morning, asking whether I would be interested in editing a book on the topic of medication-related falls in the elderly. This topic was the subject of a review article published in *Drugs and Aging* in 2012 that was among the top 10 downloaded articles from that journal and was frequently cited in other works. After reflecting for a few hundreds of milliseconds, accounting for my aging neurones, I replied "yes" and immediately consulted with my colleague and geriatric pharmacist Louise Mallet. The idea of producing a book in the era of digital data, 9-second

---

A.R. Huang, MDCM, FRCPC (✉)
Division of Geriatric Medicine, University of Ottawa and The Ottawa Hospital, Ottawa, ON, Canada

Adjunct Professor of Medicine, McGill University, Montréal, QC, Canada
e-mail: allenhuang@toh.ca

L. Mallet, BScPharm, PharmD, CGP, FESCP
Faculty of Pharmacy, Université de Montréal, Montréal, QC, Canada

Department of Pharmacy, McGill University Health Centre, Montréal, QC, Canada
e-mail: louise.mallet@umontreal.ca

© Springer International Publishing Switzerland 2016
A.R. Huang, L. Mallet (eds.), *Medication-related falls in older people*,
DOI 10.1007/978-3-319-32304-6_1

sound bites[1], and instant information where "google" is now a verb[2] initially seemed counter-intuitive. This book project reminds me of one of the original Star Trek television episodes, entitled "Court Martial" (season 1, episode 20, 1967) when Captain Kirk was accused of reckless behaviour during an ion storm, resulting in the ejection of a research pod in order to save the starship. His legal case was defended by attorney Samuel T. Cogley, who insisted on trusting his books and not relying on computer records. His case was won when the logician, Mr. Spock, observed that he was able to repeatedly win at computer chess, indicating that something had changed in the ship's computer and therefore also the logs. The episode came to the conclusion that computers are not infallible and that human intuition, logic, and understanding of out of range results are needed to arrive at the truth. Similarly, I feel that books lend a permanency to information and knowledge. Maybe it represents a subconscious comfort, reliving the time spent in the medical library, searching for information by poring through references in the huge tomes of Index Medicus. Although a published work may appear static, the words and writing it contains embody the deep knowledge and personalities of the authors. Therefore, a book lives and breathes. The words tell the reader about the knowledge and wisdom the author wishes the reader to understand.

Every person will fall throughout their life: as a toddler learning to walk, as a child and adolescent partaking in sporting activities, as an adult partaking in thrill-seeking activities and finally as an older adult. More than one-third of community-dwelling older adults fall every year. One of the important risk factors for falling is taking medications. Prescription medications are a double-edged sword: they help manage various medical conditions and they also have potential side effects that can affect an older person's blood pressure and neuromuscular control resulting in an increased risk for falling. The topic of medication-related falls in older people has many moving parts: physical and physiologic changes in the aging body, changes in the way the body handles medications and the effects of those medications, the puzzling presentation of illness in older people, the medication cascade, the need for health-care workers and professionals to think differently and health-care systems that need to better manage older patients. After all, we wish to improve the health-care system to look after ourselves when we grow old and need those services for ourselves.

We hope that this book will help health-care providers recognize the role of medications in increasing the risk of falls. With this awareness, more frequent review of medications and targeting of fall risk-increasing drugs and proactive interventions with the goal of fall prevention can occur. This book is divided into four parts. The Background section describes the scope of the global problem of falls and how to critically interpret the myriad published data on falls. Part 2, "Why Are Older People At Risk?" describes the various factors, both intrinsic to older people and extrinsic, that are modifiable which conspire to put older people at higher risk

[1] Ryfe and Kemmelmeier [1].

[2] The word "google" was added as a transitive verb to the *Oxford English Dictionary* on June 15, 2006.

for falls. Part 3 drills down into the details of various medication classes that have been identified as being associated with increased fall risk. Finally in Part 4, "Management of Medication-Related Falls" evidence supporting various strategies will be presented that clinicians can use to modify fall risk in older patients taking medications.

This work was designed to serve several purposes. Firstly, it represents a repository of scientific evidence concerning the topics discussed in each chapter. We had thought: "Wouldn't it be handy to have a single volume containing all the significant references so that future students, and investigators would have this information at their fingertips?" Secondly, a reader who wishes to skim the chapters and scan the abstracts or very important points (VIPs) boxes can get a good overview of this important clinical topic. Thirdly, people who are involved in policy-making can use this book and the knowledge and data embedded in its chapters to develop systems (environmental, social, health, education) which can help address this global problem. Finally, people who are sometimes patients can read and learn about medications and falls.

Although this book is destined to be available primarily in electronic format, we hope that it also finds a place on your bookshelf. For me a book is best embodied in its paper form. Paper is a universal operating system. It does not crash. Page corner turndowns become satisfying bookmarks. Touching a line of text with a highlighter pen or underlining with a pencil or pen somehow reinforces the understanding and memory of what was just read. Whatever your preference, Louise and I hope that this book will help you understand and appreciate the topic of medication-related falls in the elderly.

Acknowledgments Lastly, Louise and I wish to gratefully acknowledge and thank all the contributors who invested their time to write in order to communicate their knowledge within this book.

Reference

1. Ryfe DM, Kemmelmeier M (2011) Quoting practices, path dependency and the birth of modern journalism. J Stud 12:10–26

Chapter 2
The Aging Population and Falls: Consequences and Costs

Paula M. Horsley and Allen R. Huang

Abstract Adults 60 years of age and older are the fastest-growing group in the world. Falling is defined as "an event which results in a person coming to rest inadvertently on the ground or floor or other lower level" and is a common clinical and public health problem that affects many older adults. Approximately 5-10% of falls result in serious injury to the person. Bipedal locomotion that evolved as humans evolved places us at higher risk for falling. Perturbations to circulatory, respiratory, nervous, and musculoskeletal systems, along with impaired cognition and concentration, can increase fall risk. Falls are costly. Falls can also have a significant impact on the quality of life of older adults. Fall prevention is paramount. Strategies aimed at preventing falls need to be multifaceted and widespread to address the many different risk factors.

Adults over the age of 60 years are the fastest-growing group within the global population [28]. It is projected that this population group will increase in number from 841 million in 2013 to over 2 billion in 2050 [21]. This means that older adults, who currently make up 12% of the population, will more than double in size and make up 21.1 % of the population in the year 2050 [21]. By 2050 (or even a few years earlier), it is expected that older adults will outnumber children for the first time in the history of the world [21]. The growth of this population group is not expected to stop in 2050; in fact, the United Nations predicts that the number of older adults will continue to grow and will triple in number by the year 2100 [22, 23]. This tremendous increase in the global population of older adults will significantly impact society and our world as we know it.

P.M. Horsley (✉)
Faculty of Medicine, University of Ottawa, Ottawa, ON, Canada
e-mail: phors065@uottawa.ca

A.R. Huang, MDCM, FRCPC
Division of Geriatric Medicine, University of Ottawa and The Ottawa Hospital, Ottawa, ON, Canada

Adjunct Professor of Medicine, McGill University, Montréal, QC, Canada
e-mail: allenhuang@toh.ca

© Springer International Publishing Switzerland 2016

A.R. Huang, L. Mallet (eds.), *Medication-related falls in older people*,
DOI 10.1007/978-3-319-32304-6_2

Although older adults make up a large proportion of our global population, it is important to note that some regions within the world have a greater impact on these numbers than others [30]. Based on statistics taken by the World Health Organization in 2013, the Region of the Americas, the Western Pacific Region, and the European Region currently have the highest proportion of adults over the age of 60 years (14 %, 15 %, and 21 %, respectively) [30]. Older adults in the African Region, Eastern Mediterranean Region, and Southeast Asia Region make up a smaller proportion of their populations, ranging from 5 to 8 % [30]. Therefore, the impact that this growing global population group has on each country varies geographically. Particular attention has been placed on the cohort of people aged 85 years and older, since this cohort is expanding at the most rapid rate and life expectancy for males and females combined in Canada is projected to increase from 82.6 years to 92.2 years by the year 2100 [23].

Falling is a common clinical and public health problem that affects many older adults around the world [15, 17, 20, 28, 29]. The World Health Organization defines a fall as "an event which results in a person coming to rest inadvertently on the ground or floor or other lower level" [27, 29]. Falls are a significant concern for many older adults, as approximately one-third of older adults living in the community fall each year [3, 6, 24]. As one ages, there is an increased risk of falling and the falls are often of greater significance [14]. This risk continues to increase over time [24], as evidenced by fatal fall rates peaking in the 85-year-old and older category [28]. Although not every fall leads to a serious injury, approximately 5–10 % do [3]. A fall can lead to chronic pain, fear of future falls, decreased independence, and decreased quality of life [28], as well as immobility, morbidity, early long-term care placement, and even death [15]. In 2012 alone, 28,753 deaths in the United States were due to unintentional falls [13]. Globally, unintentional falls are the second leading cause of injury resulting in death and most commonly occur in adults over the age of 60 years [27, 29].

In order to understand why humans fall, it is important to consider many factors that increase one's risk of falling, starting with our desire to walk on two feet. The evolution of the human ability to walk upright occurred in a stepwise manner, as evidenced by differing physical features seen in our ancestors as we transitioned from quadrupeds to bipeds [26]. As a biped, the human body relies heavily on the musculoskeletal system and brain to continuously make adjustments to one's posture due to the lack of rigid fixation between our vertically stacked body parts [16]. This lack of fixation, combined with a constant force of gravity acting upon it, increases our risk of falling whenever we move and disturb this vertical alignment [16]. A high center of mass, as a result of our upright posture, and small surface area with which to balance on further contribute to our instability as bipeds [16].

The pathophysiology of a fall in older adults is complex and often involves a combination of many different factors [1, 12]. Adding to this complexity is the significant amount of diversity between older adults, which makes it even more difficult to determine an individual person's risk for falling [28]. The intricate interplay of many different systems, such as the coordinated interactions of the circulatory, respiratory, nervous, and musculoskeletal systems, along with functioning cognition and concentration, plays an important role in fall prevention [1, 15, 20]. With age, these systems start to become less efficient and effective, which increases one's risk for falling [1]. Older adults often have a more rigid and less coordinated gait than younger populations, which, in combination with decreased reflexes, muscle strength, and posture control, impairs their ability to maintain balance [15]. There are also many external factors that can increase an individual's risk for falling, such as environmental hazards [28, 29], individual behaviors (such as risk-taking and ethanol consumption) [28], pain [19], and a selection of associated medications [1, 4, 7, 9, 20, 24]. The subsequent chapter on "Age-Related Physical and Physiologic Changes and Co-morbidities in Older People: Association With Falls" will describe these factors in detail.

Falls are costly. Approximately 0.85–1.5 % of total health-care dollars in North America, Australia, the United Kingdom, and Europe are spent on costs relating to falls [8, 14]. Based on the data collected by Stevens and colleagues [18] and correcting for inflation, the Centers for Disease Control and Prevention estimated that the direct medical costs for falls in the elderly in 2013 in the United States were approximately US$ 34 billion [2]. The actual cost is likely higher, as estimates do not take into account the costs associated with disability, reliance on others, time lost from both in-home and out-of-home work, or decreased quality of life [2]. Current projections indicate a continued increase in the costs associated with falls, as the global population ages and more falls occur [2].

Not only are falls costly, but they can also have a significant impact on the life of older adults. The fear of falling is a common concern that affects many individuals, even in those who have no previous history of falling [11]. Sixty-three percent of seniors in long-term care and 26–55 % of community dwelling older adults are afraid of falling [10]. Older adults will often limit their activities, resulting in physical deconditioning and a decreased quality of life, due to fear of injuring themselves when mobilizing [10, 15]. In addition to concerns about injury, older adults often fear falling because they do not want to be embarrassed socially, lose their independence, or need to move out of their own home [28].

Fall prevention is paramount. Strategies aimed at preventing falls need to be multifaceted and widespread to address many different risk factors that play a role in falling [29]. As described by the World Health Organization in their recent age-friendly world initiative, proper community planning, such as ensuring that buildings are accessible, public transportation is safe, and social and leisure activities are abundant and available for older adults, is an essential component in fall prevention [31]. Assessing and modifying one's own home environment, particularly in high-risk fallers, to increase safety and minimize hazards have also been found to reduce the risk of falling in older adults [6]. Promoting healthy societal and individual attitudes, such as encouraging older adults to stay active, participate in social activities, and ask for help when needed, would help dispel the false belief that falling is a normal age-related change and would also help engage individuals in fall prevention precautions [25, 28, 31]. Physical activity has been shown to help prevent falls in the elderly [5, 6], including falls that would have resulted in severe injury [5]. Muscle strengthening, flexibility, and improving sense of balance have been shown to be cost-effective ways to address this multifaceted issue. Last but certainly not least, proper management of medications plays a key role in preventing falls [4, 7, 9, 24]. Polypharmacy is a common clinical challenge that must be reviewed and evaluated at each clinical encounter, as many medications, especially when taken improperly, increase one's risk for falling [4, 7, 9, 24]. Spending time to review medications can help ensure that patients are taking the correct medications, at the correct doses, and all unnecessary medications are deprescribed appropriately, in order to maximize benefit and minimize potential harm [4, 9]. Limiting the number and frequency of medications, educating patients about their medications, and organizing the medications for patients, such as in blister packs or dosette boxes, can help improve adherence and possibly decrease the risk for medication-related falls [7]. Details will follow in subsequent chapters in this book.

In summary, the global population is aging; projections suggest that the number of older adults will increase twofold by 2050 and threefold by 2100. Falls are a common health concern among older adults and have a significant impact on both the individual and the health-care system. A proactive approach to fall prevention needs to be implemented, as reactionary approaches have been shown to be more costly. Designing interventions that work at the individual, environmental, social, and governmental levels will ensure many different risk factors are targeted and outcomes are optimized. We invite the readers to explore the contents of this book in order to understand the opportunities that exist for improving this significant health-care problem.

References

1. Al-Aama T (2011) Falls in the elderly. Can Fam Physician 57:771–776
2. Centers for Disease Control and Prevention (2015) Cost of falls among older adults. Accessed on 18 Jan 2016. From http://www.cdc.gov/HomeandRecreationalSafety/Falls/fallcost.html
3. Deandrea S, Lucenteforte E, Bravi F, Foschi R, La Vecchia C, Negri E (2010) Risk factors for falls in community-dwelling older people: a systematic review and meta-analysis. Epidemiology 21(5):658–668
4. Dyks D, Sadowski CA (2015) Interventions to reduce medication-related falls. Can Geriatr Soc J Contin Med Educ 5(1):23–31
5. El-Khoury F, Cassou B, Charles MA, Dargent-Molina P (2013) The effect of fall prevention exercise programmes on fall induced injuries in community dwelling older adults: systematic review and meta-analysis of randomised controlled trials. Br Med J 347, F6234. doi: 10.1136/bmj.f6234 (Published 29 October 2013)
6. Gillespie LD, Robertson MC, Gillespie WJ, Sherrington C, Gates S, Clemson LM, Lamb SE (2012) Interventions for preventing falls in older people living in the community. Cochrane Database Syst Rev (9):CD007146. DOI: 10.1002/14651858.CD007146.pub3.
7. Hart M, Giancroce P (2015) Safer prescribing in elderly patients. Can Geriatr Soc J Contin Med Educ 5(1):16–22
8. Heinrich S, Rapp K, Rissmann U, Becker C, Konig HH (2010) Cost of falls in old age:a systemati review. Osteoporosis International 21(6):891–902
9. Huang AR, Mallet L, Rochefort CM, Eguale T, Buckeridge DL, Tamblyn R (2012) Medication-related falls in the elderly. Drugs Aging 29(5):360–376

10. Lach HW, Parsons JL (2013) Impact of fear of falling in long term care: an integrative review. J Am Med Dir Assoc 14(8):573–577
11. Liu JYW (2015) Fear of falling in robust community-dwelling older people: results of a cross-sectional study. J Clin Nurs 24:393–405. doi:10.1111/jocn.12613
12. López-Soto PJ, Manfredini R, Smolensky MH, Rodríguez-Borrego MA (2015) 24-hour pattern of falls in hospitalized and long-term care institutionalized elderly persons: a systematic review of the published literature. Chronobiol Int 32(4):548–556
13. Murphy SL, Kochanek KD, Xu J, Heron M (2015) Deaths: final data for 2012. Accessed on 18 Jan 2016. From http://www.cdc.gov/nchs/data/nvsr/nvsr63/nvsr63_09.pdf
14. Peel NM (2011) Epidemiology of falls in older age. Can J Aging/La Rev Can Vieillissement 30(01):7–19
15. Rubenstein LZ (2006) Falls in older people: epidemiology, risk factors and strategies for prevention. Age Ageing 35:ii37–ii41
16. Skoyles JR (2006) Human balance, the evolution of bipedalism and disequilibrium syndrome. Med Hypotheses 66:1060–1068
17. Speechley M (2011) Unintentional falls in older adults: a methodological historical review. Can J Aging/La Rev Can Vieillissement 30(01):21–32. doi:10.1017/S0714980810000735.
18. Stevens JA, Corso PS, Finkelstein EA, Miller TR (2006) The costs of fatal and non-fatal falls among older adults. Injury Prevention 12:290–295.
19. Stubbs B, Binnekade T, Eggermont L, Sepehry AA, Patchay S, Schofield P (2014) Pain and the risk for falls in community-dwelling older adults: systematic review and meta-analysis. Arch Phys Med Rehabil 95(1):175–187.e9
20. Tinetti ME, Speechley M, Ginter SF (1988) Risk factors for falls among elderly persons living in the community. N Engl J Med 319(26):1701–1707
21. United Nations (2013) World population ageing 2013. Accessed on 14 April 2016. From http://www.un.org/en/development/desa/population/publications/pdf/ageing/WorldPopulationAgeing2013.pdf
22. United Nations (2015) Word population projected to reach 9.7 billion by 2050. Accessed on 18 Jan 2016. From http://www.un.org/en/development/desa/news/population/2015-report.html
23. United Nations (2015) World population prospects: key findings and advance tables. Accessed on 14 April 2016. From http://esa.un.org/unpd/wpp/Publications/Files/Key_Findings_WPP_2015.pdf
24. Van Der Cammen TJM, Rajkumar C, Onder G, Sterke C, Petrovic M (2014) Drug cessation in complex older adults: time for action. Age Aging 43:20–25
25. Van Der Meulen E, Zijlstra GAR, Ambergen T, Kempen GIJM (2014) Effect of fall-related concerns on physical, mental, and social function in community-dwelling older adults: a prospective cohort study. J Am Geriatr Soc 62(12):2333–2338
26. Williams SA, Russo GA (2015) Evolution of the hominoid vertebral column: the long and the short of it. Evol Anthropol Issues News Rev 24(1):15–32
27. World Health Organization (n.d.) Falls. Accessed on 14 April 2016. From http://www.who.int/violence_injury_prevention/other_injury/falls/en/
28. World Health Organization (2007) WHO global report on falls prevention in older age. Accessed on 18 Jan 2016. From http://www.who.int/ageing/publications/Falls_prevention-7March.pdf?ua=1
29. World Health Organization (2012) Falls. Accessed on 14 April 2016. From http://www.who.int/mediacentre/factsheets/fs344/en/#
30. World Health Organization (2015) World health statistics 2015. Accessed on 14 April 2016. From http://apps.who.int/iris/bitstream/10665/170250/1/9789240694439_eng.pdf?u=1&ua=1
31. World Health Organization (2015) Age-friendly world. Accessed on 14 April 2016. From http://agefriendlyworld.org/en/

Chapter 3
Falls Count and Counting Falls: Making Sense of Data About Falls

Nancy E. Mayo and Sabrina M. Figueiredo

Abstract It is often challenging to make sense of research reports on falls. The choice of statistical method depends on whether the outcome is binary (faller: yes/no), a rate (falls per person-time in view), ordinal (number of falls per person) or time to fall (first). The most useful methods for analysing falls are those that estimate parameters as they provide an estimated value for risk associated with different levels of a factor or intervention. Less useful are statistics that simply provide a yes/no answer as to whether the factor or intervention affects risk (hypothesis testing). As falls are negative events, when parameters such as odds ratios (OR), incidence rate ratios (IRR), hazard ratios (HR), proportional odds ratios (POR) or cumulative odds ratios (COR) are greater than 1.0, they indicate that the factor is associated with a higher risk of falls; when <1.0, the factor or the intervention is associated with a lower risk of falls. All of these statistical parameters can be used to identify risk factors for falls or to evaluate effective interventions.

N.E. Mayo, BSc(PT), MSc, PhD (✉)
Center for Outcomes Research and Evaluation, McGill University Health Centre - Research Institute, Montreal, QC, Canada

Faculty of Medicine, Division of Clinical Epidemiology, McGill University, Montreal, QC, Canada

Faculty of Medicine, School of Physical and Occupational Therapy, McGill University, Montreal, QC, Canada
e-mail: nancy.mayo@mcgill.ca

S.M. Figueiredo, BSc(PT), MSc
Division of Clinical Epidemiology, McGill University, Montreal, QC, Canada

Faculty of Medicine, School of Physical and Occupational Therapy, McGill University, Montreal, QC, Canada
e-mail: sabrina.figueiredo@mcgill.ca

© Springer International Publishing Switzerland 2016

A.R. Huang, L. Mallet (eds.), *Medication-related falls in older people*,
DOI 10.1007/978-3-319-32304-6_3

Abbreviations

AR	Attributable risk
CI	Confidence interval
COR	Cumulative odds ratios
df	Degree of freedom
FRIDs	Fall risk-increasing drugs
GEE	Generalised estimating equations
HR	Hazard ratio
IRR	Incidence rate ratio
IR	Incidence rate
NNH	Number needed to harm
NNT	Number needed to treat
OBD	Occupied bed days
OR	Odds ratio
PAR	Population attributable risk
POR	Proportional odds ratios
RCT	Randomised controlled trial
RR	Rate ratio
SD	Standard deviation
VIP	Very important point

3.1 Falls Are an Important Health Concern

Falls are the leading cause of injury amongst seniors across Canada [1] resulting in disability, chronic pain, loss of independence, reduced quality of life and even death [2–5]. In 2012–2013, Canadian seniors experienced almost 85,000 fall-related hospitalizations; of those, 39 % involved a hip fracture and 8 % resulted in an in-hospital death [6].

In addition to physical disabilities, falls also lead to psychosocial consequences. Falls may result in fear of falling, which opens a vicious cycle of reduced confidence, reduced mobility and social participation, weakness and deconditioning, which then culminate with recurrent falls [7, 8].

Going beyond patients' perspective, falls also represent a financial burden to the health-care system [6]. According to the Public Health Agency of Canada [1], more than $2 billion is spent each year with fall-related expenses in the senior population. For instance, on average, patients admitted with a fall-related hospitalisation stayed 6 days longer than all other hospitalizations and 29 % of nonresidential care patients were transferred to residential care after a fall-related hospitalisation [9].

These physical, mental and economic implications are even more alarming due to the fact that the number of falls is expected to increase as seniors are the fastest-growing segment of the population [9, 10].

3.2 What Is a Fall?

It seems strange to have to define a fall but, as truth can be stranger than fiction, there are a number of ways that people end up on the ground. Clarity on definition is needed for purposes of clinical safety and research. Having studied falls on and off over several decades, what I find missing from these rather dry definitions is why the person has fallen. In my experience falls can be classified as fit falls, fluke falls or frail falls.

Fit falls are those that occur amongst skiers, skaters, bike riders, hikers and climbers, for example. Some of these fit people can be elderly, and the fall can be a tipping point against their continued thriving [11–14]. *Fluke falls* are those that occur in unusual circumstances such as tripping over the cat or when the dog wraps the leash around the legs; holes in the ground do not help, nor does inclement weather, snow banks or small children with or without scattered toys. While these kinds of falls pose a public health concern, they may not have been preventable except by heightened vigilance on the part of the 'fallee' when they are in these unusual circumstances. What is of clinical concern are frail falls. *Frail falls* occur amongst people who are challenged to maintain physical function against gravity, and, hence, even small perturbations can result in a fall. These falls are serious as they may herald further clinical deterioration, or they are the straw that breaks the camel's back and result in injury, hospitalisation and even death [15].

The aim is to prevent any of these falls by identifying risk factors and intervene to reduce risk. The risk factors for frail falls are likely quite different from risk factors for fit and fluke falls and, if all falls are grouped together, it may be very difficult to identify common risks. While it is likely that fit falls will be excluded from a fall study, many studies will not be able to discriminate between fluke and frail falls. These indeed may share common risk as a robust person may be able to avoid the cat and a frail person may not, but the real answer may never be known.

The World Health Organization defines a fall as 'an event which results in a person coming to rest inadvertently on the ground or floor or other lower level' [16]. Currie [17] defines a fall for a non-hospitalised geriatric population as 'an event which results in a person coming to rest unintentionally on the ground or lower level, not as a result of a major intrinsic event (such as a stroke) or overwhelming hazard'. This latter definition would be compatible with a frail fall and likely cover some fluke falls considering that the hypothetical cat may not be classified as an overwhelming hazard, although some might.

In a systematic review of definitions and methods used to measure falls in randomised controlled trials [18], the wording used to describe falls represented an external perspective: 'involuntary', 'unintentional', 'unexpected', 'inadvertent', 'unplanned' or 'sudden'. Some definitions included the concept of a 'near' fall when someone may have tripped, slipped or stumbled but not fallen.

Having decided upon what type of fall is to be studied, it is often challenging to make sense of research reports on falls. The next sections will attempt to explain some of the typical ways that falls data are reported and analysed.

3.3 Statistical Methods Depend on the Type of Data Collected

Data are of two types: measured and counted. Many important health indicators or health outcomes are measured: blood pressure, weight, grip strength and walking capacity, to name a few relevant for the older population. When data are measured, the expectation is that, if a large number of people are measured, the distribution will be close to a normal distribution with few people at the extremes and the majority in the middle. With this distribution, the average value, along with a measure of how spread out the data are (standard deviation or SD), provide a good description of the distribution. When the data have this normal distribution, the mean and SD can be used to find out quite a lot about the sample. In particular, 68 % of the sample will fall within 1 SD on either side of the mean (±1 SD), 95 % will fall within 2 SD and 99 % within 3; effectively the range of values will lie within (±4 SD).

This type of data can be compared between groups or over time using parametric statistics such as a *t*-test or linear regression. The choice of statistical test will depend of course also on the 'exposure' or the variables under study that are hypothesised to explain variability in the measured data. A special feature of measured data is that the measurement scale is continuous indicating that the quantity being measured can take any value, depending on the precision of the measuring device. For example, weight can be measured in milligrams, grams or kilograms. In Great Britain, Australia and Ireland, weight is commonly measured in stone which is a unit weighing 14 lb based on an ancient and not very precise unit of weight, a rock weighing 14 lb, hence the name.

3.4 Falls Are Not Measured, They Are Counted: Hence, Falls Count

The other type of data arises from counting events that happen to people or counting the number of people that can be classified into different 'bins', such as by sex, age group, living arrangement or any other type of 'bin' that is relevant to the situation under study.

Falls are counted, they are not measured and, hence, it would not be appropriate to calculate an average number of falls in a group. This is because the mean will not represent the data well. The mean represents data that are normally distributed. With falls, it would not be true that few people have few or many falls and most have a middle number of falls. The vast majority will actually have 0 falls, the next largest group would have 1 fall and a small proportion would have 2 and very few 3 or more. For example, in an Australian [19] study of 704 community-dwelling people aged 65 years and older who reported on fall frequency in the previous 12 months, 66 % did not fall and 20 % fell once and 14 % fell twice or more. With this type of distribution, an average number of falls per person does not make sense as, amongst the 704 people, 246 falls occurred yielding an average of 0.34 per person. The calculated average does not apply to anyone, nor would the SD be a useful parameter to describe the distribution because it is based on an average deviation around a mean; if the mean is meaningless, so is the SD.

VIP

Falls cannot be measured they can only be counted. A person cannot have one-third of a fall indicating that falls are discrete quantities with fixed values such as 0, 1, 2 or 3, and the mean is meaningless.

Above, we counted the number of falls per person but this is only one kind of fall metric. Fall metrics are usually of four types: (1) falls, implying that people could fall more than once; (2) fallers meaning that once someone has fallen even one time, they are considered a faller; (3) rate of falls defined over a specified time period; and (4) time to fall, implying the time from some known starting point to the first fall episode. The statistical issues around using these different fall metrics will be illustrated as we work through different examples.

To choose the best way to analyse data collected on falls, it is necessary to consider what the investigator or observer wants to know. In other words: What is the research question [20]? Another important determinant of the choice of statistical methods is whether the investigator wishes to estimate a parameter, usually about the magnitude of risk across different groups, or simply wishes to find out if any observed differences could have occurred by chance. Thus, analyses are of two types, parameter estimation methods and hypothesis-testing methods. I leave you with the quote from Lord Kelvin to help the reader choose which method might provide more useful information:

> "When you can measure what you are speaking about and express it in numbers, you know something about it. When you cannot express it in numbers, your knowledge is of a meagre and unsatisfactory kind." Therefore, "To measure is to know" and "If you cannot measure it, you cannot improve it."

As falls are counted, it is most usual to use a statistical method that estimates the magnitude of risk, either in relative or absolute terms, associated with a factor or an intervention. The choice of statistical method depends on whether the outcome is binary (faller: yes/no), a rate (falls per person-time in view), ordinal (number of falls per person), or time to fall (first). Different models are used for each of these different fall metric outcomes and different parameters are estimated. However, they all relate to the risk for one group relative to the risk in a reference group. Parameters are expressed as point estimates and confidence intervals (CI) indicating the degree of confidence one can have about the finding in different samples. A 95 % CI that excludes 1.0 means that the factor or intervention either increases the risk (putative factor) or decreases it (protective); if the CI includes the null value of 1.0, there is no evidence that the factor acts one way of the other. The CI is interpreted in the context of repeated samples such that if the study was repeated over and over, say,

100 times, 95 % of the estimates from these samples would lie within the 95 % CI and only very rarely (total 5 %) would an estimate be below or above the boundaries.

The different statistical ways of dealing with falls data will be discussed in the context of particular questions that can be asked about falls.

3.5 What Kinds of Questions Can Be Asked About Falls?

3.5.1 *How Many People Fall?*

This is a question that will provide local knowledge. The assumption is that the population is stable and that more than one fall would be rare. It would be of value to know the number of people falling in different places, at different times of the day or days of the week, information that would be useful for considering environmental interventions.

Consider the time of day that people fall. This is of interest for ensuring appropriate services are in place at peak fall times, if the setting, for example, is an institution. If we divide the day up into 3 h periods, any 1 day has eight of these periods. If there is no effect of time of day on falls, then the expected proportion of falls would be the same for each time period (12.5 %: 100 %/8). To answer the questions as to whether there are more falls at certain times of the day, the observed number of falls is compared to the expected number and a chi-square test would be used to test the hypothesis that the observed distribution by time of day differs from the expected number. The only issue to be careful of here is in the number of degrees of freedom (df) which, in this situation, is 7 (categories-1). It is tempting to look at the data and see a lot of falls at one time point and then decide to test whether there are more falls then than other times and consider only 1 df. A degree of freedom in a table, with counts distributed into cells defined by rows (r) and columns (c), is the number of independent pieces of information as defined by (r-1)(c-1). With eight time periods there are 7 df. In a study of falls in a rehabilitation centre [21], the distribution across time periods differed significantly from uniform (12.5 %) and the chi-square test with 7 df was 34.2 ($p<0.05$). The two time periods that stood out with a higher than expected proportion of falls were 9 to noon (19.9 %) and noon to 3 pm (23.3 %) [21]. This is not surprising given that this is when people are up and about.

3.5.2 *Are Falls Getting More Common or Rarer?*

Answering this question can be quite challenging because the population of interest may change over time as people move in and out of the cohort. This can happen if people are hospitalised, institutionalised, die or move away; of course new people can move into the population as well. Thus, the size of the population at each time point

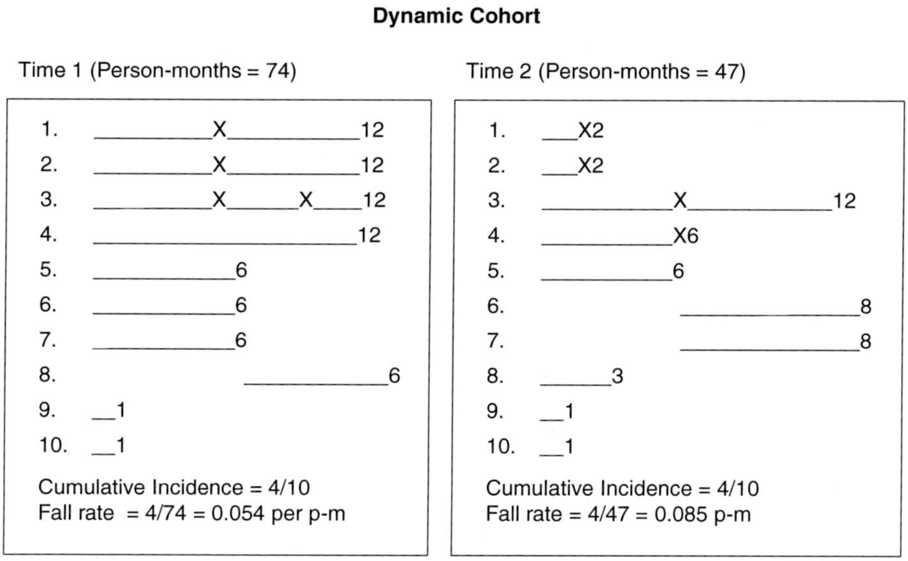

Fig. 3.1 Shows the fall experience of fictitious residents in an assisted living residence over a 1-year period for two time periods, Time 1 and Time 2

of interest needs to be known and how long each person has been ‘in view’ to have had a fall. The analysis needs to consider that each person has a unique ‘footprint’ on the data. Some people may be ‘in view’ for the whole time and others for less time of varying durations. If one of the reasons for short time in view are variables under study or because someone had a fall and was hospitalised, then ignoring the time in view will result in incorrect inferences about what has happened over time.

Consider the situation in Fig. 3.1.

In Time 1, ten people were included and four were in view for 12 months, three for 6 months and then exited because of illness, one was in view for 6 months but entered the cohort late and two were in view for only 1 month as they changed residences. Four falls were observed amongst three people in view for the entire 12-month period (one person fell twice). The cumulative incidence rate of falls is 4/10. The total number of person-months in view is 74 and so the incidence rate (IR) of falls is 4/74 or 0.054, commonly expressed per 100 person-months, so 5.4 per 100 p-m.

At Time 2, four falls were also observed but they were serious and resulted in hospitalisation without return to the residence. So although the cumulative incidence rate of falls is still 4/10, the IR is 4/47 yielding a rate of 8.5 per 100 p-m, a rate close to double that of Time 1. Without considering person-time in view, the rates of falls look that same at these two time points when in fact the rate was higher in Time 2 owing to an increase in fall severity. One should not be surprised that the IR is higher because the person-time-in-view is much less at Time 2.

A classic method of fall prevention is implement a programme targeting falls and study the effects before and after the programme has been put in place. The correct analysis of data arising from such a study is to consider the person-time-in-view for both time periods.

VIP
Are falls getting rarer or more common? To answer this question, the person-time in view needs to be considered and the parameter of interest is the incidence rate ratio (IRR).

3.5.3 What Are the Risk Factors for Falls?

There is a very substantial literature on risk factors for falls. The most important consideration when looking at this literature is that for a factor to be declared a 'risk factor', very specific methodological criteria need to have been met. Risk factors are identified using observational studies – either cohort or case-control studies – and these types of studies can have a number of biases that can affect the findings. To aid in the reporting on these kinds of studies, to clarify that all sources of bias have been addressed, recommendations summarised under the title 'Strengthening the Reporting of Observational Studies in Epidemiology (STROBE)' have been developed. These recommendations are also useful for readers of this literature as they provide explanation of methods and biases that are beyond the scope of this chapter [22].

Two key points are worth underlining for this chapter. First, for a factor to be declared a 'risk factor', the population 'at risk' needs to be defined, appropriately sampled and followed in its entirety over a defined period of time. Risk factors apply to populations, although specific subgroups may have a greater or lesser risk. Thus, risk factor studies are population based and with as complete follow-up as possible; when there are losses, reasons are not related to the presence or absence of the risk factor understudy (termed independent censoring assumptions). Without complete follow-up, the study can only conclude about that subgroup who 'survived' the study.

Second, 'risk factors' are important to identify because if they are causally associated with the outcome, here falls, interventions targeting the risk factors would likely reduce this risk. In order for a factor to be considered a 'cause', a number of pieces of evidence need to accumulate. These were first suggested by Sir Bradford Hill [23] and are summarised in Table 3.1.

Causes can be further classified as necessary and/or sufficient [25]. A cause is deemed necessary if this factor always precedes the effect, or, in other words, if without this factor the outcome will not occur. A cause is sufficient if, inevitably, the outcome will occur with this factor present [26]. Outside of infectious disease, and falls are no exception, there are very few examples of necessary and sufficient causes; rather we recognise component causes which collectively act to cause an effect [27].

VIP

All research on risk factors for falls aims to link a factor to the occurrence of falls, and the hypothesis is that the factor is causally associated. To infer causality, the factor must be shown to precede the fall and not be a consequence of falls; factors that are strongly associated are more likely causal as are factors that show a dose-response relationship.

Table 3.1 Bradford Hill's criteria for causality as applied to falls

Strength of the association	Relative risks >2.0 are less likely to be explained by unmeasured confounding variables
Dose-response gradient	Risk of falls increases with increasing levels of the risk factor. This was shown in the paper by Mayo et al. on the relationship between response time and falls [24]
Temporality	The development of the risk factor precedes the occurrence of the event; for example, fear of falling is often implicated as a risk factor for falls, but it is imperative that the fear of falling preceded the fall and was not a consequence of the fall
Consistency	An association has been observed by different persons in different places, at different times and under different circumstances
Biological plausibility	There is a reasonable biologic mechanism whereby the risk factor could cause the disease (of course, this is dependent on the knowledge of the day)
Coherence of the evidence	There is no conflict with what is generally known about falls from an epidemiologic and clinical perspective
Specificity	The association is specific to falls
Analogy	When there is an analogous situation with other similar risk factors, the balance of the evidence would not need to be so strong (e.g. if one medication has an association with falls, then similar drugs would be suspect
Experiment	Direct or indirect manipulation of the risk factor changes the rate of falls in the population

The component causes of falls are usually studied by creating a statistical model that includes several factors, with the aim of identifying independent factors for falls. Table 3.2 from the paper by Cesari et al. [28] presents a study of over 5500 people who were assessed at the time of entry into a home-care programme and followed for 90 days from assessment. In this paper, the authors identify that age, sex, cognition and limitations in activities of daily living were not causal factors but rather confounders, factors associated with both causal factors understudy and the outcome of 'faller' (binary variable). The model used was logistic regression which is described in Box 3.1 (a summary guide of statistical models). Amongst the potential causal factors, those independently associated with an increased risk of being classified as a 'faller', were foot problems, gait problems, wandering, depression and presence of environmental hazards. As evidence, odds ratios (OR) and 95 % CIs were presented. All these findings were further explored in their paper.

Table 3.2 Adjusted model for risk of falling in the study population from Cesari et al. [28]

	Adjusted model	
Characteristic	OR	95 % CI
Age (years)	1.01	1.00–1.02
Gender (female)	1.01	0.90–1.14
Activities of daily living impairment	1.06	1.04–1.09
Foot problems	1.19	1.04–1.37
Gait problems	2.13	1.81–2.51
Fear of falling	0.97	0.83–1.13
Visual impairment	0.98	0.87–1.11
Wandering	2.38	1.81–3.12
Depression	1.53	1.36–1.73
Urinary incontinence	1.06	0.93–1.20
Parkinsonism	0.93	0.74–1.17
Environmental hazards	1.51	1.34–1.69

Source: Reproduced with permission from Cesari et al. [28]
OR odds ratio, *CI* confidence interval

When such a model is presented, the interpretation of each factor is the effect of that factor 'adjusted for all other factors'. Statistically, this is done by assigning people the average value for other factors and then estimating the risk of each factor. Sometimes, such a complex model can be difficult to interpret, particularly if related variables are included. For example, in this paper from Cesari et al., both foot problems and gait problems were included, each 'adjusted' for each other. As these variables are related (most foot problems will produce a gait problem, but not all gait problems are caused by foot problems), both are competing to explain the same risk. Here the OR for foot problems is interpreted as that risk over and above the risk for gait problem. The implication is that interventions for both gait and foot problems are needed. To appreciate the extent to which these risk factors act synergistically, the authors presented Fig. 3.2, for the risk factors gait problems and wandering.

To interpret this figure, it is important to note that people with no wandering problems and no gait problems are the reference group as indicated by an OR of 1. The group with only wandering problems, but no gait problems, have an increased risk (OR: 1.34), but this increase is not statistically different as the 95 % CI includes the null value of 1, so their risk is likely similar to the group with neither problem. However, having gait problems does infer higher risk (OR: 2.25; 95 % CI: 1.99–2.54), but there is an unexpectedly higher risk when both risk factors are present (OR: 6.16; 95 % CI: 4.50–8.43). With two factors, the risk would be expected to be close to the sum or the multiplication of the two risks: 1.34 + 2.25 (3.59) or 1.34*2.25 (3.02); the observation that the risk associated with having both of these putative factors is >6 indicates that they act synergistically and that having both infers extra risk. This effect of the two factors combined is determined by fitting an interaction term in the regression model: Outcome (falls) = Gait problems + Wandering + Gait*Wandering.

VIP
Two factors may interact such that when both are present, the risk is much greater than would be expected by summing or multiplying the separate risks. Each one increases twofold, but both increase eightfold; this is interaction.

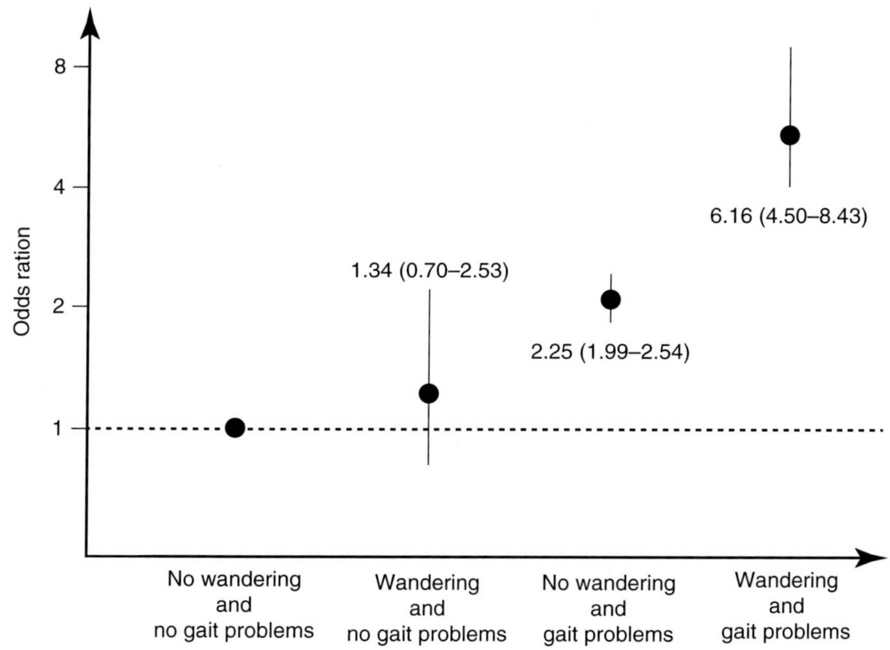

Fig. 3.2 Risk factors acting synergistically from Cesari et al. (Reproduced with permission from Cesari et al. [28]

Sometimes the association between risk factors and falls is presented in such a way that fallers and non-fallers are compared on levels of the risk factors. Instead of the model being as above [outcome (falls) =risk factor level], the model has been reversed [risk factor level = falls]. Table 3.1 in the Cesari paper did just this and found that the mean impairment on activities of daily living was higher for people who became fallers (4.81 ± 0.05) than those who remained fall-free (2.15 ± 0.03). This difference in means was tested using a *t*-test. This approach is used likely because of the perception that it is easier to compare two groups using simple t-tests or chi-square tests.

VIP
Beware when a paper compares fallers and non-fallers on level of risk. As the falls occurred in the future and the risk factor was measured in the past, this approach asks the question: Can the future predict the past? Always think of the causal model and hope that the statistical model matches the causal model.

The paper from Cesari et al. [28] illustrates the use of logistic regression because the outcome was binary. Another form of logistic regression can be applied when the outcome considers how often a person falls, 0, 1, 2, 3 times etc. Ordinal regression models are of two types, the proportional odds model or the cumulative odds model. In a study of risk factors for falls amongst 473 people with multiple sclerosis [29], the distribution of 0, 1 or ≥2 falls was 42 %, 13 % and 45 %. A number of health-related factors were associated with more falls, no matter how more falls is defined, using the proportional odds model: 1 vs. 0; ≥2 vs. 0 or 1.

A common feature of falls data is that, while the majority will not fall, the range of fall frequency can be very large with some people falling a very large number of times. Often, this wide range with few people is dealt with by creating a $\geq n$ category as in the Cesari paper. The people in this category can be quite heterogeneous invalidating the predictive model such as the Poisson model (see Box 3.1. Summary of Statistical Models Commonly Used for Estimating Impact of Factors or Interventions on Different Fall Metrics, in the Lessons Learned section) or ordinal model.

When risk factors are medications, a common way of considering risk is to measure the time to fall from the date of first prescription. Medications are one of the few risks that can be studied using this metric because there is an identifiable '0' time for all. The model for time to data is Cox proportional hazards [30]. Let us examine what these terms mean. Cox refers to Sir David Cox, a British statistician (July 15, 1924–). The hazard is the instantaneous risk of falling at time t_1, given the person has not fallen prior to time t_1. It is not a probability but an indicator of the risk of experiencing the fall; the higher the value of the hazard, the higher is the risk of falling. When two groups are compared, a ratio of the two hazards is estimated, the hazard ratio (HR). Proportional means that the risk of falling is higher in one group than the other by a consistent amount over time, that is, one group does not have a higher risk early on and then end up with a lower risk later on. This is a key assumption that needs to be tested if this model is to be used. If the hazard is not proportional, a solution is to stratify the time into chunks where the risks are proportional. Hazard ratios (HRs) are formed as a ratio of the two hazards (one for each group) and can be interpreted as a relative risk although relative risks reflect the cumulative risk over time at a defined end point. Hazard ratios evaluate the impact of an intervention throughout the whole study period.

The Cox model is one of several 'survival' models [31], all of which are concerned with time to fall. Survival is modelled as the conditional probability of 'surviving' – not falling – up to a particular time, conditional on the probability of being alive in a previous time period. The survival function is estimated using the Kaplan-Meier method and tested using the log-rank test. However, if there is a need to adjust for confounding variables, the Cox model needs to be used which models the 'hazard'.

An excellent example of using the Cox model to estimate risk of fall-related injury associated with opioid use was published by Buckeridge et al. [32]. This was a very large study because the sample was drawn from health administrative data on persons over the age of 65 years of age in the Province of Quebec, Canada. From these data, it was possible to identify the start and dates for prescriptions of an opioid, establishing a zero time. Amongst the 403,339 older adults studied, about 15 %

had been prescribed an opioid of different potencies, and 3.7 % had a fall-related injury in the ensuing year. In comparison to those not prescribed an opioid (although they could have been prescribed other types of drugs), the HR associated with a high-potency opioid was 1.43 (95 % CI: 1.05–1.95); the highest risk (OR: 2.30; 95 % CI: 2.23–2.36) was associated with a codeine combination drug. All HRs were adjusted for a number of variables thought to be associated with both getting an opioid and having a fall-related injury. As the sample was very large, even this very small event rate, 3.7 %, yielded a very large number of events making the estimates from the Cox model very precise.

All of the studies described above took the approach of identifying people with different levels of a risk factor and following them forward. This type of study is called a cohort study. With rare events, a large number of people have to be followed to have sufficient events for analysis. Another way of identifying risk factors for falls is to sample the other way, by fall status. People who fell are defined as cases, and controls, who match the cases on personal characteristics, are randomly chosen from the pool of people who did not fall. Risk factors are identified for the cases and controls from prior history or circumstances. This is termed a case-control study [33, 34] and, all things being equal, yields the same estimates of risk as the cohort study approach; all things equal are accurate information from past history, records or recall. Mayo et al. [35] carried out a case-control study of risk factors for falls in a rehabilitation hospital by establishing an admission-to-discharge cohort and identifying the first fall amongst the people in this cohort. Each person who fell for the first time since admission was defined as the case and one control, matched on age and sex and who had been admitted at the same time as the case (to control for time of exposure to falling in the hospital) was selected. As there were data for many days of hospitalisation, the data collection focused on three periods, admission, 7 days before the fall and 24 h before the fall. Cases and controls were compared on variables during those time periods. As there were over 1800 people admitted during the 2-year study period and only 356 cases, collecting data on only 356 controls is very efficient.

As the control selection is conditional on the characteristics of the case, a form of logistic regression for matched data was used, conditional logistic regression. Table 3.3 reproduces data from this study. Four risk factors were identified: one from variables present at admission (stroke), one from variables present in the week prior to the time the case fell and two from the 24-h period prior.

All of these studies report a parameter that is closely related to relative risk. However, high relative risks can occur with very rare exposures and as a result the absolute number of people at risk to fall can be very small. It is recommended that when reporting on relative risk, the absolute risk should also be reported; in the Buckeridge study [32], 3.7 % of people fell in the 1 year of follow-up. The highest HR was associated with codeine combination drugs, 2.27, making the absolute risk increase from 3.7 % to 8.4 %.

In evidence-based medicine, another parameter of interest is number needed to treat (NNT), which is defined as the number of people that need to be treated with an intervention to prevent one adverse health event [36]. In the context of the

Table 3.3 Factors associated with falls in a rehabilitation hospital from Mayo et al. [35]

Variable	Cases ($n=356$)	Control ($n=356$)	Adjusted[a] OR (95 % CI)
Stroke at admission			
Yes	124	50	3.99 (2.47–6.45)
No	232	306	1
Incontinence week prior to fall date of case			
Ever	137	56	2.80 (1.88–4.16)
Never	219	300	
Anticonvulsants 24 h prior to fall date of case			
Yes	36	19	2.98 (1.50–5.94)
No	320	337	
Topical eye preparations 24 h prior to fall date of case			
Yes	33	17	3.39 (1.62–7.10)
No	323	339	

Source: Reproduced with permission from Mayo et al. 35
[a]Adjusted for all other risk factors listed

Buckeridge study on falls [32], the use of a treatment for pain had a negative effect and hence the number needed to harm (NNH) is the parameter of interest. NNT or NNH is calculated as 1/risk difference which is 1/0.084–0.037 which yields 21. Thus, for every 21 people treated with codeine combination drugs, 1 will have a fall-related injury.

Another piece of the puzzle of how to understand the magnitude of the risk associated with a factor of interest. A key parameter is the population attributable risk (PAR) which is a function of relative risk and how common the risk factor is. PAR was estimated using the equation P(HR-1)/1+[P(HR-1)] [27] where P is the prevalence of exposure, which for codeine combinations is 9.3 %, and the HR is the approximation to the RR. Using this formula, 10 % of all fall-related injuries could be attributed to codeine combination drugs: $0.093(2.27-1)/1+[0.093(2.27-1)]$.

The consideration of risk has many features: the relative risk which can be expressed as RR, OR or HR, the absolute risk; the number who need to be exposed to the putative risk factor for one person to be harmed (NNH); and the proportion of the outcome in the population attributed to the risk factor (PAR). All of these parameters are helpful in considering risk and should be reported in papers of risk factors in order for the study to be informative to everyone concerned with these risks.

VIP

The importance of a risk factor is expressed both in relative and absolute risk. A high relative risk (RR) for a factor that is very rare would not be responsible for very many falls; a risk factor that is very common can be a very important contributor even if, relative to the absence of the factor, it is not very much higher.

3.5.4 Did Intervention Reduce Falls?

When it is important to know if people improve over time, it is easier to consider improvement on a measured variable. Consider improvement on walking capacity; values at Time 1 are compared to values at Time 2. It is quite obvious that the data are not independent, but paired, and thus, a paired *t*-test or other repeated measures analysis would be appropriate. The situation is the same when the data are counts, but how often would the research question relate to whether person falls less often over time? This question is not answerable because many events may have happened to the person pre- to post-intervention to change their fall risk so that, in the absence of a crystal ball to foresee how often someone would have fallen had they not had the intervention, no within person comparison can be made. This type of very important question can be answered, and there are several study designs and statistical methods that can be called upon as tools to help out.

VIP
Unless you have a crystal ball, you cannot know if the intervention prevented falls!

3.6 The Case of the Pre-/Post-implementation Study

Many institutional settings implement fall prevention programmes as part of quality improvement, and they wish to evaluate whether implementing the programme was successful in reducing falls. Such a study was conducted in the United Kingdom (UK) by Healey et al., published in 2014 [37], to deal with the serious issue of falls in hospitals. The FallSafe programme was implemented in 16 inpatient care settings in the South of England. They presented data (see Table 3.1 in their paper) that indeed things had changed for the better over time with respect to implementing safety procedures, and, hence, the authors wished to know if implementing this programme changed the rate of falls over time. Four 6-month time frames were of interest: baseline, introduction period, implementation period and sustainability. To answer this question, the authors counted the number of person-days in view (termed occupied bed days or OBD) for each month over these four time periods and counted the number of falls and calculated a rate of falls for each month. They did this for the 16 FallSafe units and for 16 other units where FallSafe had not been implemented (control settings). This type of design creates a time series and, when graphed, the rates can be quite variable from seasonal variation and other environmental factors. To smooth out the data so an overall trend can be seen, a common procedure is to calculate a 'moving' average which averages adjacent time periods with the months included moving. For example, months 1–4 are averaged and then 2–5, 3–6, 4–7, etc., until all the months have been covered. This smoothing showed

Table 3.4 Data comparing rates of falls per person-time in view across time for clinical settings with a fall prevention programme (FallSafe) and without (control) from Healey et al. [37]

	Pre-implementation		Post-implementation	
	Baseline	**Introduction**	**Implementation**	**Sustaining**
FallSafe	**Period 1**	**Period 2**	**Period 3**	**Period 4**
Bed days	33,583	35,822	33,495	32,942
N falls	366	430	329	234
Rate per 1000 bed days	10.90	12.00	9.82	7.10
	Period 1 and 2	**Period 3 and 4**		
Bed days	69,405	66,437		
N falls	796	563		
Rate per 1000 bed days	11.47	8.47		
RR (95 % CI)	Referent	0.75 (0.68–0.84)		
Control	**Period 1**	**Period 2**	**Period 3**	**Period 4**
Bed days	32,426	33,041	30,274	31,657
N falls	265	311	266	232
Rate per 1000 bed days	8.17	9.41	8.79	7.33
	Period 1 and 2	**Period 3 and 4**		
Bed days	65,467	61,931		
N falls	576	498		
Rate per 1000 bed days	8.80	8.04		
RR (95 % CI)	Referent	0.91 (0.81–1.03)		

Source: Reproduced with permission from Healey et al. [37]
RR rate ratio, adjusted

that, in the FallSafe settings, after 12 months following the introduction period, there was a downward trend in fall rates. No such trend was seen for the control settings.

To illustrate the challenge in comparing falls rates over time, data from this paper have been set out in Table 3.4. The first thing to note is that there were over 30,000 occupied bed days (OBD) in each period in the FallSafe and control settings. The number of falls counted in the several hundreds and the rate of falls was 10.90 per 1000 OBD at baseline in the FallSafe settings and 7.10 per 1000 OBD during the sustaining period. For the control settings, the rate of falls was less than the FallSafe setting but remained the same over time. To estimate the magnitude of change over time, a Poisson regression model was used dividing the four time periods into two, pre- and post-implementation. A Poisson model is used for rates when the denominator is person-time and is usually very large with respect to the numerator, which is an event such as a fall. The events must be independent, that is, one person falling will not affect another person falling. The Poisson model used here took the form of

Y (log of number of fallers/number of people or person-time) = Time (Post-implementation vs. Pre) + Setting (here FallsSafe vs. Control) + Time*Setting.

The regression parameter for time yields the incidence rate ratio and can be calculated directly from the data presented in the study. What cannot be calculated directly is the 95 % CI because each unit represents a cluster, such that the people in the cluster are more similar to each other than to people in other clusters. This is typical of hospital wards which tend to group similar patients together. The Poisson model was referred to as a mixed model meaning that the setting was considered as a 'random' variable but time as 'fixed' and so this model has a mix of random and fixed effects this model has a mix of random and fixed effects. This model adjusts the variance for clustering which is needed as otherwise the variance is too small owing to the similarity of patients within units.

Also tested was the interaction between time and setting denoted by the term, Time*Setting. The authors report that the interaction term was 'significant', meaning that the effect of setting depended on time, such that with time the fall rates in the settings grew apart as was expected owing to the implementation of the FallSafe programme.

This 'case' introduced bed days, rates, moving average, rate ratios, Poisson models, interaction and mixed effects models. This case also showed again the use of 95 % confidence intervals (CI).

3.7 The Case of the Simple Randomised Controlled Trial

The simple or classical RCT takes a group of people and randomly assigns them to two or more groups to evaluate a deliberate intervention, often an innovation in treatment [38]. The aim is to provide evidence to support a change in clinical practice. In 2014, Sherrington [39] reported on a trial of an intervention to enhance balance and mobility and prevent falls in a vulnerable senior population ($n=340$; mean age 80 years) who had recently been discharged following aged care, rehabilitation or orthopaedic care. Participants in the intervention group were shown an exercise programme by a physical therapist and were asked to exercise at home for 15–20 min up to six times weekly for 12 months. The control group received usual care and both groups were given a booklet on fall prevention. Members of both groups had fallen in the past, ~70 %, and randomization was successful in balancing the groups on proportion of fallers. A difference between groups at the end of the study on the proportion of people falling would be evidence of effectiveness, assuming a short fall in the intervention groups, and the interpretation is that the intervention 'prevented' falls as without the intervention the rate of falls would be that of the control group.

Table 3.5 Falls outcomes from Sherrington et al. [39]

	Control ($n=169$)	Intervention ($n=171$)	Difference between groups
Falls per participant, n (%)			
0	99(59)	73(43)	1.38 (1.11–1.73), $p=0.004$[a]
1	45 (27)	58 (34)	
2	12 (7)	16 (9)	
3	4 (2)	13 (8)	
≥4	9 (5)	11 (6)	
All falls (primary outcome)	123	177	1.43 (1.07–19.93), $p=0.017$[b]
Fall location			
Indoors	79	128	1.62 (1.13–2.33), $p=0.009$[b]
Outdoors	44	49	1.10 (0.71–1.69), $p=0.670$

Source: © 2014 Sherrington et al. [39] Open source. http://journals.plos.org/plosone/article?id=10.1371/journal.pone.0104412

[a]Relative risk, 95 % confidence interval and p-value from modified regression model for proportion of participants who had one or more falls in the 12-month follow-up period in the intervention group compared to the control group

[b]Incidence rate ratio, 95 % confidence interval and p-value from negative binomial regression model comparing the number of falls in the 12-month follow-up period in the intervention group compared to the control group

Of the 169 people in the intervention group, 67 % had one or more falls compared with 41 % in the control group, which was the opposite of what was desired. Table 3.5 is taken from this paper and illustrates a number of statistical methods. First, for the comparison of the proportion of people with one or more falls, Poisson regression was used with the numerator the number of falls and the natural logarithm of the group-specific population as the denominator.

3.8 The Case of the Complex Clustered Randomised Trial

A landmark study on falls prevention was conducted by Tinetti and colleagues and reported on in the New England Journal of Medicine in 1994[40]. A key feature of this study is that the subjects ($n=301$; mean age ~78 years) had one or more risk factors for falling including risky medications, health conditions and/or functional limitations, but not all had a history of falls (only about 40 % had fallen in the previous year). Two groups were formed by assigning their physicians randomly to two groups so half of the sample recieved the intervention which was multifactorial targeting personal risk profile and the other half to recieve usual care. The outcome was whether the person fell or not over the 1-year follow-up period. The results which were accumulated over the 1-year follow-up period showed that 35 % of the people in the intervention group fell as compared to 47 % in the usual care group. This was associated with an adjusted rate ratio (ratio of the two rates after adjusting for age, sex, number of targeted risk factors and falls in the previous year) of 0.69 (95 % CI 0.52, 0.90).

This study would today be classified as a clustered randomised trial although in that era, considering the clustering effect in the analysis would have been rare [41]. Pivotal work on the design and analysis of cluster randomised trials has been published by A. Donner, a well-known Canadian statistician [42–44]. A modern (2008) clustered randomised trial was conducted by Cummings et al. in Australia involving 3999 patients in 24 hospital wards (12 acute and 12 rehabilitation), elderly care wards randomised to a multifactorial intervention or usual care [45]. The intervention was based on recommendations from the literature and consisted of nursing and physical therapy involving prescription and training of appropriate walking aids and eye wear, modification to bedside environment, a drug review, exercises to enhance balance and function, practice of safe mobility, education and custom-designed alarms for ambulant patients with dementia or cognitive impairment. As the people in each ward share certain characteristics with each other but not with people from other wards, this inter-cluster correlation needs to be taken into account in estimating the variability, even if in reality the inter-cluster correlation is quite small. In this study, the analysis was of falls using negative binomial regression and generalised estimating equations (GEE), a form of regression that adjusts for clustering using ward as the clustering variable and group as the variable under study. There was no effect of intervention on falls, despite meta-analyses supporting an effect. The authors concluded that usual methods to reduce falls in senior wards were ineffective, and a more innovate whole system approach is needed targeting cognitive impairment, ward and bed redesign, use of hip protectors and heightened vigilance.

VIP

When units are randomised such as hospital wards or doctors but the intervention is delivered to the patients, the 'clustering' needs to be considered in the analysis. The patients in one unit are more similar to each other than they are to patients from other units, and this will affect the variance and make the effect look more significant than it should be.

3.9 The Case of the Observational or Non-randomised Trial

Van der Velde et al. [46] carried out a very innovative, real-life situation study to reduce falls amongst elderly fallers by withdrawing (if possible) 'fall risk-increasing drugs' or FRIDs for short. What is unique about this study is that it comprised a clinical sample of seniors ($n = 139$; mean age ~78 years) who had fallen one or more times in the past year. In addition, many of these people were taking FRIDs, 126 of the 139 (91 %) according to Table 3.2 of this paper. The clinical investigators were able to withdraw one or more FRIDs in 75 out the 126 patients taking FRIDs (remember 13 were not takers). In 67 patients, FRIDs were discontinued and in 8 the dose was reduced. For the other 64, including 13 non-FRIDs, withdrawal was either not possible or was attempted and failed.

So there are now two groups, one comprising 75 persons from whom withdrawal was carried out and 64 where FRIDs was not an issue ($n=13$) or not withdrawn ($n=51$). Now, these two groups did not differ on age or functional status, but they did differ on total drugs, total FRIDs and comorbidity with the withdrawal group, not surprising, having more of these putative factors.

Over 75 % of the total sample had fallen more than once in the past year, and ~25 % had one or more falls per month. As a result of this high fall occurrence rate, the impact of withdrawal of FRIDs was assessed over the subsequent 2 months using time to first fall from withdrawal attempt (same for both groups) as the outcome.

Most often, when the outcome is a negative health event, like a fall, the hypothesis is that the intervention will reduce the risk and the HR will be less than 1.0. In this study, the HR for withdrawing FRIDs is 0.48 with a 95 % confidence interval ranging from 0.23 to 0.99 when fully adjusted for all covariates. This essentially means that in any point in time, people who had FRIDs withdrawn were half as likely to fall as those remaining on FRIDs. However, the 95 % CI is wide and only barely excludes the null value of 1.0. The CI means that if a study such as this was repeated many times with different samples, the HRs from these studies would lie between 0.23 and 0.99, 19 times out of 20. So rarely would a sample be outside these bounds; however, in a proportion of samples, the effect of withdrawing FRIDs would not be very dramatic and could be close to null. In designing such a study, planning a sample size that would exclude a non-important HR would provide more confidence in the finding with respect to the effect that might be realised when the intervention implemented clinically. This study provides level II evidence for effectiveness of FRIDs withdrawal; level I evidence comes from RCTs.

Another novel feature of this study is that they also used a method of adjustment called propensity scoring [47], although they did not elaborate on this useful methodology. Propensity scoring calculates a conditional probability of exposure to a treatment, here FRIDs, given specific observed covariates, and combines in one score, the confounding effect of multiple variables without having to adjust for each variable separately. It would be wise to employ such a method in a small study such as this including many covariates in the model reduces to power to detect the main effect.

In reporting on HR or relative risks, it is important to place the effect in the context of the magnitude of the effect (absolute risk). An HR of 0.5 is not very impressive if the two risks are 0.02 (2 %) and 0.01 (1 %), respectively. In this study, the cumulative hazard of a fall was 0.18 for the FRIDs-withdrawal group and 0.37 for the group without FRIDs withdrawal, resulting in an absolute risk reduction of 19 % and a relative risk reduction of 49 %. This is helpful information to judge the clinical relevance of the intervention.

Using time-to-event as the outcome is optimal in this situation for reasons that might not apply to other types of studies. Here the sample consisted of people who commonly fell and hence would be likely to continue to do so even over a short time period, short enough for there not to be many health or life events changing the baseline fall risk.

3.10 The Case of the Stepped Wedge

A new methodology is making waves in the context of implementation science and that is the stepped-wedge design [48–50]. This design is optimal when the intervention to be tested has evidence for effectiveness and, hence, it would be unethical to have a completely untreated control group, and also when there are issues of resources and training such that not all participants can enter the intervention at the same time. The intervention is implemented sequentially to individuals or clusters over a number of time periods, and by the end of the study, all participants will have received the intervention. A critical feature is randomization of the order in which participants receive the intervention [51]. Figure 3.3 illustrates this design.

Hill et al. [52, 53] used this design to test the effectiveness of implementing a fall prevention patient education programme with the addition of staff training and feedback on rates of falls in eight rehabilitation units in Australia. In this design, the units are given the intervention in an order determined by randomization. The outcome was falls, analysed using negative binomial regression and taking into account that people are clustered in units. The variable indicating the effectiveness of the intervention was time since the start of the intervention and the unit of time was 5 periods of 10 weeks as the rehabilitation units were randomised two at a time. The hypothesis was that the more weeks of intervention, the lower would be the rate of falls. The incidence rate ratio (IRR) associated with step time was 0.95 and the CI

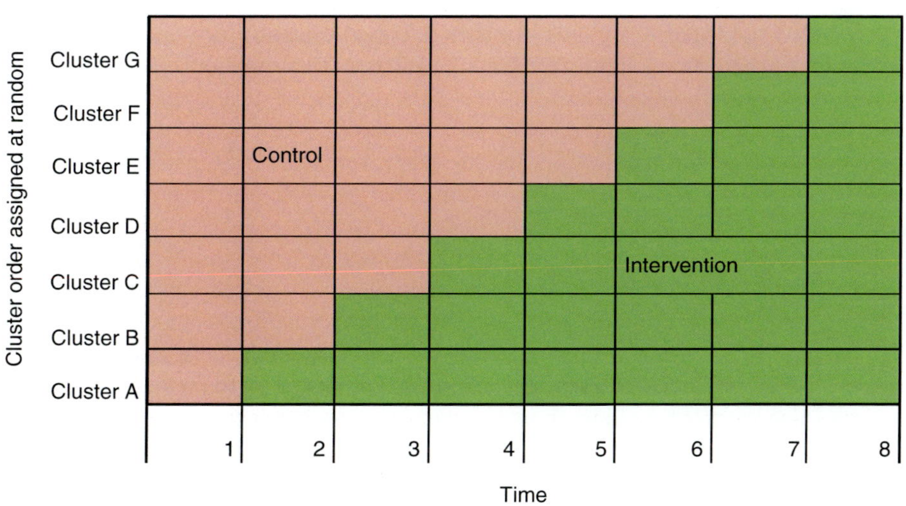

Fig. 3.3 Illustration of the stepped-wedge design

excluded the null value of 1.0 (0.92–0.99). Each unit of step time ($n = 5$) was associated with an estimated reduction of ~5 % such that over the 5 step-time periods, a total reduction of ~25 % would be expected (assuming linearity with time). This was born out by the raw data which showed a control period rate of falls of 13.78 % and an intervention period rate of falls of 7.80 %.

As there is much evidence for the effectiveness of fall prevention programmes, the future challenge will be in implementing this information so that existing knowledge can be translated in to routine clinical practice. The stepped-wedge design will be increasingly deployed in falls research.

VIP

There are a lot of effective interventions to reduce falls. It is time to implement these in our facilities, seniors' home and in the community. The stepped-wedge design is very good for studying the implementation of effective practices.

3.11 Lessons Learned

This chapter reviewed a lot of statistical material. Several important points were covered. *First*, falls are counted and not measured, and so statistics such as means and standard deviations and t-tests cannot be used to summarise or test hypotheses about falls. *Second*, it is important to know whether number of fallers or number of falls is being counted. If it is the number of falls, then the amount of person-time in view needs to be considered because a fall that causes an injury or death could shorten the time that the person could fall subsequently. A group that has more severe falls would spuriously look like they fall less frequently as the severity of the fall removed them from view. *Third*, numerous statistical methods can be used to analyse data on falls according to a level of a risk factor or an intervention. The choice of method will depend on what the research question is, and this will determine the outcome and its most optimal measurement scale (fall metric). The most useful methods for analysing falls are those that estimate parameters (remember Lord Kelvin) as they provide an estimated value for risk associated with different levels of a factor or intervention. Less useful are statistics that simply provide a yes/no answer as to whether the factor or intervention affects risk (hypothesis testing). Box 3.1 summarises the most common parameter estimation methods applied to analysing falls. *Fourth*, it is important to consider if people have an opportunity to fall and if this 'opportunity' changes over time. The best way to prevent a fall is to prevent someone from moving about on their own. As many seniors are sedentary, and this increases with ageing or with illness requiring a change in drug management, they may have less opportunity to fall as they do move around less. Few fall studies consider daily physical activity but technology is available to monitor this in real time. This is an opportunity to develop new avenues of fall research.

Box 3.1. Summary of Statistical Models Commonly Used for Estimating Impact of Factors or Interventions on Different Fall Metrics

Method	Parameter	Particulars
Logistic regression	Odds ratio (OR)	Outcome is binary; person is a faller or not; estimates the relative risk when the proportion of fallers is small (<20 %), termed the rare disease assumption
Ordinal regression	Odds ratio (OR)	Outcome is number of falls a person experienced in the study time which is an ordinal (and interval variable); as this number is usually not large (0 to <10 per person), this outcome could be modelled using a sliding cut-point to create different strata and the assumption is the OR is homogeneous across strata. Either the cumulative odds model (3 vs. 2; 2 vs. 1; 1 vs. 0) or proportional odds model (3 vs. 2, 1, 0; 2 vs. 1,0; 1 vs. 0) [54] can be used depending on fit to the data. A challenge with this model is that the distribution is often 'overdispersed', meaning that the variance exceeds the mean usually because people who fall 0 or 1 time is very large with respect to falling more often
Cox proportional hazards	Hazard ratio (HR)	Outcome is time to fall and the hazard function is determined by the instantaneous risk of falling at a particular time point, given that the person has not fallen prior to that time [30]
Poisson regression	Incidence rate ratio (IRR)	Outcome is a rate, number of falls per unit person-time; numerator is very small with respect to denominator. The assumption is that a) the recurrent events being counted are occurring independently of each other and randomly in time and b) the mean and variance are equal [26]
Negative binomial regression	Incidence rate ratio (IRR)	Outcome is number of falls; similar to Poisson model for overdispersed data (variance exceeds the mean) [55]

Falling to Conclusions

The reader may have noticed that the same statistical methods can be used to identify risk factors for falls or to test interventions. The choice of statistical method depends on the fall metric under study: fallers, rate of falls, number of falls or time to fall. These models produce a point estimate along with confidence bounds that indicate if repeated samples were observed, the estimates from these different samples would most often, 95 times out of 100, lie within these limits. The reader should look at the tables presented in the research papers to find these parameters, and remember, no matter if they are odds ratios (OR), incidence rate ratios (IRR), hazard ratios (HR), proportional odds ratios (POR) or cumulative odds ratios (COR), they all can be interpreted as reflecting relative risk. As falls are negative events, when the parameters from these values are greater than 1.0, they indicate that the factor is associated with a higher risk of falls; when <1.0, the factor or ideally the intervention is associated with a lower risk of falls. Therefore, to get the most out of a research paper on falls, look at the tables and look for the parameters discussed here.

References

1. Public Health Agency of Canada (PHAC) (2014) Falls in Canada: second report [Online]. Available: http://www.phac-aspc.gc.ca/seniors-aines/publications/public/injury-blessure/seniors_falls-chutes_aines/assets/pdf/seniors_falls-chutes_aines-eng.pdf. Accessed July 2015
2. Blake AJ, Morgan K, Bendall MJ, Dallosso H, Ebrahim SB, Arie TH et al (1988) Falls by elderly people at home: prevalence and associated factors. Age Ageing 17:365–372
3. Anonymous (1987) The prevention of falls in later life. A report of the Kellogg International Work Group on the Prevention of Falls by the Elderly. Dan Med Bull 34(Suppl 4):1–24
4. Ungar A, Rafanelli M, Iacomelli I, Brunetti MA, Ceccofiglio A, Tesi F et al (2013) Fall prevention in the elderly. Clin Cases Miner Bone Metab 10(2):91–95
5. Goodwin VA, Abbott RA, Whear R, Bethel A, Ukoumunne OC, Thompson-Coon J et al (2014) Multiple component interventions for preventing falls and fall-related injuries among older people: systematic review and meta-analysis. BMC Geriatr 14:15
6. Scott V, Wagar L, Elliott S (2010) Falls & related injuries among older Canadians: fall-related hospitalizations & intervention initiatives [Online]. Available: http://www.hiphealth.ca. Accessed July 2015
7. Svantesson U, Babagbemi B, Foster L, Alricsson M (2014) Influences on modern multifactorial falls prevention interventions and fear of falling in non-frail older adults: a literature review. J Clin Med Res 6(5):314–320
8. Martin JT, Wolf A, Moore JL, Rolenz E, DiNinno A, Reneker JC (2013) The effectiveness of physical therapist-administered group-based exercise on fall prevention: a systematic review of randomized controlled trials. J Geriatr Phys Ther 36(4):182–193
9. Canadian Institute for Health Information (CIHI) (2014) Preventing falls: from evidence to improvement in Canadian Health Care [Online]. Available: https://www.accreditation.ca/sites/default/files/falls-joint-report-2014-en.pdf. Accessed July 2015
10. Statistics Canada (2006) Portrait of seniors in Canada [Online]. Available: http://www.statcan.gc.ca/pub/89-519-x/89-519-x2006001-eng.pdf. Accessed July 2015
11. Merom D, Stanaway FF, Handelsman DJ, Waite LM, Seibel MJ, Blyth FM et al (2014) Swimming and other sporting activities and the rate of falls in older men: longitudinal findings from the Concord Health and Ageing in Men Project. Am J Epidemiol 180(8):830–837
12. Peeters GM, Verweij LM, van Schoor NM, Pijnappels M, Pluijm SM, Visser M et al (2010) Which types of activities are associated with risk of recurrent falling in older persons? J Gerontol Ser A Biol Sci Med Sci 65(7):743–750
13. Tuli T, Haechl O, Berger N, Laimer K, Jank S, Kloss F et al (2010) Facial trauma: how dangerous are skiing and snowboarding? J Oral Maxillofacial Surg 68(2):293–299
14. Barnett L, Green S, van Buerden E, Campbell E, Radvan D (2009) Older people playing ball: what is the risk of falling and injury? J Sci Med Sport 12(1):177–183
15. Bennett A, Gnjidic D, Gillett M, Carroll P, Matthews S, Johnell K et al (2014) Prevalence and impact of fall-risk-increasing drugs, polypharmacy, and drug-drug interactions in robust versus frail hospitalised falls patients: a prospective cohort study. Drugs Aging 31(3):225–232
16. World Health Organization (2008) WHO global report on falls prevention in older age [Online]. Available: http://www.who.int/ageing/publications/Falls_prevention7March.pdf. Accessed July 2015
17. Currie L (2008) In: Hughes RG (ed) Fall and injury prevention. Agency for Healthcare Research and Quality, Rockville
18. Hauer K, Lamb SE, Jorstad EC, Todd C, Becker C (2006) Systematic review of definitions and methods of measuring falls in randomised controlled fall prevention trials. Age Ageing 35(1):5–10
19. Lord SR, Ward JA, Williams P, Anstey KJ (1993) An epidemiological study of falls in older community-dwelling women: the Randwick falls and fractures study. Aust J Public Health 17(3):240–245

20. Mayo NE, Asano M, Barbic SP (2013) When is a research question not a research question? J Rehabil Med 45(6):513–518
21. Mayo NE, Korner-Bitensky N, Georges P, Becker R (1989) Preventing falls among patients in a rehabilitation hospital. Can J Rehabil 2:235–240
22. Vandenbroucke JP, von Elm E, Altman DG, Gotzsche PC, Mulrow CD, Pocock SJ et al (2007) Strengthening the reporting of observational studies in epidemiology (STROBE): explanation and elaboration. Ann Intern Med 147(8):W163–W194
23. Hill AB (1961) Principles of medical statistics. The Lancet, London
24. Mayo NE, Korner-Bitensky N, Kaizer F (1990) Relationship between response time and falls among stroke patients undergoing physical rehabilitation. Int J Rehabil Res 13(1):47–55
25. Mayo NE, Bronstein D, Scott SC, Finch LE, Miller S (2014) Necessary and sufficient causes of participation post-stroke: practical and philosophical perspectives. Qual Life Res 23(1):39–47
26. Porta M (2008) A dictionary of epidemiology. Oxford University Press, Oxford. New York, NY
27. Rothman KJ, Greenland S (1998) Modern epidemiology. Lippincott-Raven, Philadelphia
28. Cesari M, Landi F, Torre S, Onder G, Lattanzio F, Bernabei R (2002) Prevalence and risk factors for falls in an older community-dwelling population. J Gerontol A Biol Sci Med Sci 57(11):M722–M726
29. Matsuda PN, Shumway-Cook A, Bamer AM, Johnson SL, Amtmann D, Kraft GH (2011) Falls in multiple sclerosis. PM R 3(7):624–632
30. Cox DR, Oakes D (1984) Analysis of survival data. Chapman & Hall, New York
31. George B, Seals S, Aban I (2014) Survival analysis and regression models. J Nucl Cardiol 21(4):686–694
32. Buckeridge D, Huang A, Hanley J, Kelome A, Reidel K, Verma A et al (2010) Risk of injury associated with opioid use in older adults. J Am Geriatr Soc 58(9):1664–1670
33. Mayo NE, Goldberg MS (2009) When is a case-control study not a case-control study? J Rehabil Med 41(4):209–216
34. Mayo NE, Goldberg MS (2009) When is a case-control study a case-control study? J Rehabil Med 41(4):217–222
35. Mayo NE, Korner-Bitensky N, Becker R, Georges P (1989) Predicting falls among patients in a rehabilitation hospital. Am J Phys Med Rehabil 68(3):139–146
36. Laupacis A, Sackett DL, Roberts RS (1988) An assessment of clinically useful measures of the consequences of treatment. N Engl J Med 318(26):1728–1733
37. Healey F, Lowe D, Darowski A, Windsor J, Treml J, Byrne L et al (2014) Falls prevention in hospitals and mental health units: an extended evaluation of the FallSafe quality improvement project. Age Ageing 43(4):484–491
38. Mayo NE (2009) Randomized trials and other parallel comparisons of treatment. In: Bailar JC, Hoaglin DC (eds) Medical uses of statistics. Wiley & The New England Journal of Medicine, Hoboken, pp 51–89
39. Sherrington C, Lord SR, Vogler CM, Close JC, Howard K, Dean CM et al (2014) A post-hospital home exercise program improved mobility but increased falls in older people: a randomised controlled trial. PLoS One 9(9), e104412
40. Tinetti ME, Baker DI, McAvay G, Claus EB, Garrett P, Gottschalk M et al (1994) A multifactorial intervention to reduce the risk of falling among elderly people living in the community. N Engl J Med 331(13):821–827
41. Donner A, Brown KS, Brasher P (1990) A methodological review of non-therapeutic intervention trials employing cluster randomization, 1979–1989. Int J Epidemiol 19(4):795–800
42. Donner A, Klar N (2000) Design and analysis of cluster randomization trials in health research. Arnold Publishing Company, London
43. Donner A, Klar N (2004) Pitfalls of and controversies in cluster randomization trials. Am J Public Health 94(3):416–422
44. Donner A, Klar N (1996) Statistical considerations in the design and analysis of community intervention trials. J Clin Epidemiol 49(4):435–439

45. Cumming RG, Sherrington C, Lord SR, Simpson JM, Vogler C, Cameron ID et al (2008) Cluster randomised trial of a targeted multifactorial intervention to prevent falls among older people in hospital. BMJ 336(7647):758–760
46. van der Velde N, Stricker BH, Pols HA, van der Cammen TJ (2007) Risk of falls after withdrawal of fall-risk-increasing drugs: a prospective cohort study. Br J Clin Pharmacol 63(2):232–237
47. Rubin DB (1997) Estimating causal effects from large data sets using propensity scores. Ann Intern Med 127(8 Pt 2):757–763
48. Hemming K, Lilford R, Girling AJ (2015) Stepped-wedge cluster randomised controlled trials: a generic framework including parallel and multiple-level designs. Stat Med 34(2):181–196
49. Mdege ND, Man MS, Taylor nee Brown CA, Torgerson DJ (2011) Systematic review of stepped wedge cluster randomized trials shows that design is particularly used to evaluate interventions during routine implementation. J Clin Epidemiol 64(9):936–948
50. Brown CA, Lilford RJ (2006) The stepped wedge trial design: a systematic review. BMC Med Res Methodol 6:54
51. Mayo NE (2015) Dictionary of quality of life and health outcomes measurement: International Society for Quality of Life, Milwaukee, WI USA
52. Hill AM, McPhail SM, Waldron N, Etherton-Beer C, Ingram K, Flicker L et al (2015) Fall rates in hospital rehabilitation units after individualised patient and staff education programmes: a pragmatic, stepped-wedge, cluster-randomised controlled trial. Lancet 385(9987):2592–2599
53. Lamb SE (2015) The case for stepped-wedge studies: a trial of falls prevention. Lancet 385:2556–2557
54. Scott SC, Goldberg MS, Mayo NE (1997) Statistical assessment of ordinal outcomes in comparative studies. J Clin Epidemiol 50(1):45–55
55. Robertson MC, Campbell AJ, Herbison P (2005) Statistical analysis of efficacy in falls prevention trials. J Gerontol A Biol Sci Med Sci 60(4):530–534

Part II
Drugs and Falls: Why Are Older People at Risk?

Chapter 4
Polypharmacy

Susan K. Bowles

Abstract Polypharmacy is common among older adults, largely due to the need to treat the increasing number of diseases that present as a person ages. However, multiple medication use can lead to serious consequences such as adverse drug events and also contribute to geriatric syndromes. A number of strategies have been evaluated in an effort to improve polypharmacy. While such strategies consistently demonstrate significant reductions in inappropriate medication prescribing, their impact on clinical outcomes is equivocal. More research is needed to identify the most effective interventions to optimize medication use in the older population.

Abbreviations

ADE	Adverse drug event
ADL	Activity of daily living
CI	Confidence interval
LUTS	Lower urinary tract symptoms
MAI	Medication appropriateness index
MNA	Mini-nutritional assessment
NSAID	Nonsteroidal anti-inflammatory drug
OR	Odds ratio
OTC	Over the counter
PIM	Potentially inappropriate medication
RR	Relative risk
SIADH	Syndrome of inappropriate ADH secretion
SSRI	Selective serotonin reuptake inhibitor
STOPP	Screening tool of older person's prescriptions
US	United States

S.K. Bowles, PharmD, MSc (✉)
College of Pharmacy and Faculty of Medicine, Dalhousie University, Halifax, NS, Canada

Department of Pharmacy and Centre for Health Care of the Elderly, Nova Scotia Health Authority – Central Zone, Halifax, NS, Canada
e-mail: susan.bowles@cdha.nshealth.ca

© Springer International Publishing Switzerland 2016

A.R. Huang, L. Mallet (eds.), *Medication-related falls in older people*,
DOI 10.1007/978-3-319-32304-6_4

4.1 Introduction

The world's population is aging, with an estimated 12 % being 60 years of age or older in 2013 [1]. In North America, adults 65 years of age and older are estimated to make up 13 % of the US and 16 % of the Canadian population, respectively [2, 3]. Similar trends are observed in Europe [4]. Overall, the proportion of older individuals is projected to double in the next 40 years on a worldwide basis [1].

The aging process is associated with the onset of many chronic conditions, for which a wide variety of medications are used [2, 5]. Consequently, older individuals use more medications. It is estimated that those over 65 years of age account for 30–50 % of all prescribed medications and almost two-thirds of prescription drug costs across a number of international jurisdictions [6–9].

The use of multiple medications is referred to polypharmacy, although no standard definition has been agreed upon. The World Health Organization defines polypharmacy as "the administration of many drugs at the same time" or "the administration of an excessive number of drugs" [10]. Others have described polypharmacy as use of more medications than clinically indicated, unnecessary drugs, use of ineffective medication, and therapeutic duplication [11, 12]. Other definitions are based on the number of drugs, with a specific threshold (ranging from two to nine different agents), above which polypharmacy is deemed to be present [13, 14]. Despite the lack of consensus regarding its definition, recognition of polypharmacy as a geriatric syndrome is important. While the use of multiple drugs can be appropriate for the management of chronic disease in some situations, polypharmacy is associated with a number of iatrogenic consequences. These, in turn, result in emergency department visits, hospitalization, nursing home placement, and increased mortality [15–17].

4.2 Medication Use in Older Patients

The epidemiology of polypharmacy has been examined in various settings using numerous definitions. Regardless of this variability, however, several consistent findings emerge from the literature.

Firstly, the majority of people over 65 years of age take multiple drugs. US data indicate that 57 % of older women take five or more medications and 12 % take ten or more [18]. These data are similar to that observed in other jurisdictions. A large European study observed that half of older adults took six or more medications per day [19]. Review of Canadian publicly funded drug programs found that two-thirds of seniors had claims for at least five different drug classes and one-third had claims for ten or more [9].

Secondly, long-term care residents tend to use more drugs than their community counterparts. The US Nursing Home Survey found that almost 40 % were prescribed nine or more drugs [20]. Similarly, data from the European SHELTER study demonstrated that almost half of nursing home residents were prescribed between five and nine medications and almost one in five was prescribed ten or more agents [21]. Among Canadian residents of long-term care who were beneficiaries of provincial publicly funded drug programs, 60 % were found to have claims for ten or more drug classes [9]. Finally, use of ineffective medications, agents without a clinical indication and therapeutic duplication appears to be common. One study of older ambulatory patients found that 55 % were taking at least one medication lacking an indication, 30 % were taking agents deemed to be ineffective, and 16 % had a therapeutic duplication. In a group of ambulatory US veterans, 57 % were taking at least one medication that was not effective, not indicated, or a therapeutic duplication [22]. Within the hospital setting, one study found that one-third of patients were discharged with a prescription for at least one medication without a clear indication, of which 25 % were started during hospitalization [23]. In nursing homes, up to one-third of residents are prescribed at least one drug that is not clinically indicated [24–26].

Polypharmacy results from the use of prescription drugs, over-the-counter (OTC) medications, and supplements. The most frequently prescribed medications for older persons residing in the community include statins, antihypertensives, opioids, thyroid hormones, and antibiotics [9, 27]. Regular self-medication with OTC agents and/or supplements is also common with 46 % of prescription drug users reporting concurrent use with OTCs and 52 % concurrent use of supplements [7]. Analgesics (acetaminophen and NSAIDs), laxatives, antacids, and vitamins are the most frequently reported [7, 28]. Prescription drug classes differ somewhat for nursing home residents as use of antidepressants, benzodiazepines, and antibiotics is reported somewhat more frequently in this population [9, 27]. However, statins and antihypertensive agents are also among the top ten drug classes prescribed in the long-term care setting [9].

4.3 Contributing Factors

Many factors have been associated with polypharmacy. These include age, health status, number of health-care visits, and multiple prescribers [13, 29].

Of these, age is the most commonly identified [29]. As people age, they develop more chronic disease [2, 5, 6], so more guidelines apply, resulting in more drugs being prescribed. As many of these guidelines recommend multiple agents for treatment of a single condition, it is not surprising that adherence to guidelines results in the addition of numerous medications [30]. This can be even more pronounced in those with multiple comorbidities, who see different specialists for each individual condition, and who have medication prescribed based on guidelines for that single disease [30, 31]. Primary care providers are often hesitant to change or discontinue medications that other prescribers have initiated, especially if a drug is started during hospitalization or by a specialist, such that the number of drugs increases over time [32].

Importantly, however, older individuals with multiple comorbidities are usually excluded from, and therefore underrepresented in, the drug trials from which clinical guidelines are derived [33–36]. Consequently, the applicability of many clinical guidelines to older patients, particularly those who are frail and/or over 80 years of age, is questionable [37, 38]. Moreover, many guidelines generally do not address goals of care (symptom control versus longevity) and the lag time to benefit in the context of life expectancy [37, 39, 40]. Thus, there is a substantial gap between evidence for treatments for a particular disease and the reality of managing disease in frail, older patients with multiple comorbidities, where the risk of medication-related harms is high [38].

4.4 Consequences of Polypharmacy

Polypharmacy has many potential consequences. These include an increased likelihood of receiving an inappropriate medication, experiencing an adverse drug event, and multiple geriatric syndromes [13].

4.4.1 Exposure to Potentially Inappropriate Medications

The prevalence of inappropriate medication use varies across health-care settings, reported between 12 and 80 %, depending upon the patient population and the criteria used to define inappropriate use [41, 42]. Several different criteria, both explicit and implicit, have been used to measure the use of potentially inappropriate medication (PIM) use. Explicit criteria include Beers and STOPP. Beers Criteria, most recently updated in 2015, presents a list of medications, where risk of harm outweighs potential benefits [43]. These criteria also list drugs for which dose adjustment based on renal function is recommended and high-risk drug-drug interactions [43]. STOPP criteria, updated in 2014, includes medications with a high risk-benefit ratio in older persons, drugs that increase risk of falls, clinically important drug-drug and drug-disease interaction, as well as common therapeutic duplications [44]. Both STOPP and Beers criteria are grouped by organ system and provide an explanation of why a particular medication is considered inappropriate [43, 44]. The medication appropriateness index (MAI) is another measure, using implicit criteria, to identify inappropriate medication use. It consists of a ten questions regarding clinical indication, therapeutic duplication, medication effectiveness in an individual patient, dosing and duration, practicality of directions, drug-drug and drug-disease interactions, and cost considerations [45].

Regardless of the criteria used, the use of multiple medications increases the risk of receiving inappropriate medication. The number of both prescription and OTC medications increased the odds of inappropriate prescribing as defined by the MAI [46]. Likewise, polypharmacy has been shown to increase the risk of potentially inappropriate medications as defined by both Beers and STOPP criteria [19, 47–49].

As the number of drugs increase, the higher the prevalence of inappropriate medication use and the greater the risk of negative outcomes, such as adverse drug events [48, 50].

4.4.2 Adverse Drug Events

Adverse drug events (ADEs) are common in older adults, reported in up to 35 % of older outpatients and 40 % of hospitalized elderly, with 20 % experiencing an ADE following discharge [27, 51]. ADEs are a frequent, but often preventable, cause of emergency department visits and hospitalization [15, 17]. They can occur in the outpatient, inpatient, and long-term care settings.

Rather than being idiosyncratic in nature, ADEs in older adults tend to result from an exaggeration of the pharmacologic effect. This is thought to occur for a variety of reasons. Physiologic changes impact both the pharmacokinetics and pharmacodynamics of medications. The elimination of some drugs is impaired which can increase both peak and duration of effect, depending on the specific agent [52]. Increased sensitivity observed with some drugs may result from changes to neurotransmitters and receptors [52]. Frailty may also be an important factor as it can cause declining functional reserves and impaired homeostatic mechanisms, both of which can result in a more pronounced pharmacologic effect [52, 53]. While physiologic changes render older individuals more vulnerable to ADEs, the number of medications appears to be the most important risk factor. One survey-based study of approximately 3,100 Canadian seniors found that 27 % of them were taking five or more medications. Twelve percent experienced an ADE requiring medical attention in comparison to only 5 % who were taking two or fewer drugs [54]. In a study of 678 older veterans, the odds of having an ADE-related hospitalization was increased almost threefold (OR 2.85, 95 % CI 1.03–7.85) for those taking five to eight drugs and almost fourfold (OR 3.90, 95 % CI 1.43–10.61) with nine or more drugs [55]. The relationship between polypharmacy and ADEs has also been examined in the nursing home setting. Nursing home residents with nine or more medications were twice as likely (OR 2.33, 95 % CI 1.54–3.52) to experience an ADE in comparison to those taking fewer drugs [56]. Polypharmacy is also associated with an increased risk of ADEs secondary to drug interactions. Review of charts from 205 patients presenting to two emergency departments found an increasing risk of drug-drug/drug-disease interactions resulting in an ADE. The risk was 13 % with two drugs, 38 % with four drugs, and 82 % with seven or more drugs [57].

4.4.3 Geriatric Syndromes

The term "geriatric syndrome" has been used to describe commonly observed clinical conditions in frail older persons that cannot be diagnosed as a specific disease [58]. While the term "syndrome" generally refers to specific signs and symptoms that occur together leading to a specific diagnosis, a geriatric syndrome represents a health condition resulting from an accumulation of deficits across multiple systems that "render older persons vulnerable to situational changes" [58]. Multiple risk factors, including medication use, interact in a manner that leads to one or more of the geriatric syndromes. This results in increasing frailty, which in turn enhances the impact of risk factors and geriatric syndromes. Ultimately, the relationship between risk factors, geriatric syndromes, and frailty leads to increased disability [58].

Data suggests that polypharmacy is associated with a number of different geriatric syndromes. Different medications have the potential to impact multiple systems. The more medications a person uses, the more likely they will experience a drug-drug interaction, drug-disease interaction, or an ADE. Medication-related geriatric syndromes may represent a manifestation of the atypical presentation of one or more of these phenomena.

4.4.3.1 Functional Decline

Functional status refers to the ability of an individual to carry out their basic (ADLs) and instrumental activities of daily living (IADLs). Polypharmacy has been associated with functional decline in older individuals and therefore has a negative impact on the ability to remain independent. A study using data from 975 women participating in the Women's Health and Aging study found that use of five or more medications was associated with a decline in ability to carry out IADLs [59]. A prospective study of almost 300 older adults observed that both polypharmacy (six to nine drugs) and excessive polypharmacy (ten or more drugs) were both associated with a decline in IADLs [60]. Use of ten or more drugs also reduced physical function [60]. Other data from the Women's Health and Aging study showed that use of five or more medications was associated with incident disability in over 29,500 older women (RR 22.0, 95 % CI, 21.6–22.5) followed over a 3 year period [61]. In a cohort of almost 2,000 older community-dwelling adults with dementia, the use of five or more drugs was associated with greater functional decline than those using fewer medications [62].

4.4.3.2 Nutritional Status

It is well known that nutritional status can influence the pharmacological response of some medications. Conversely, and perhaps more importantly, drugs can impact nutritional status. There are a number of mechanisms by which different agents may affect nutritional status. Electrolyte abnormalities can occur as a result of a drug-related syndrome of inappropriate ADH secretion (SIADH), nausea, vomiting and/or diarrhea. Some medications may reduce the absorption (e.g., vitamin B12) of some nutrients or reduce their concentrations (e.g., folic acid) [63]. Others may decrease appetite, affect taste, or cause dry mouth, resulting in decreased food intake [63]. Indirect effects, such as drug-related tremor, could impact the ability of a person to eat independently [31]. Any or all of these drug effects have the potential to exacerbate preexisting muscle weakness, diminished energy levels, and cognitive impairment, thereby contributing to fall risk [31, 63].

Over 250 different medications have been identified as having an effect on the intake, absorption, metabolism, and excretion of nutrients [64]. Although the nutritional effects of individual drugs or drug classes are known, the overall impact of polypharmacy on nutritional status is poorly understood. A few studies have attempted to address this question. Among nursing home residents, an increasing number of drugs were found to be associated with a poorer nutritional status, as measured by the Mini-Nutritional Assessment (MNA), a validated tool incorporating both objective and subjective measures [65]. One community-based, prospective cohort study of 294 individuals 75 years of age or older observed that 50 % of those taking ten or more medications were either malnourished or at risk of malnourishment based on the MNA [60]. A survey of 1,000 community-dwelling persons 65 years of age and older found that polypharmacy (defined as five or more drugs) was associated with a reduced intake of B vitamins, fat-soluble vitamins, fiber, and minerals such as iron [66]. Conversely, an increased intake of cholesterol, sodium, and sugar was observed [66].

Polypharmacy has also been studied in the context of weight loss (ten or more pounds) in 885 community-dwelling persons 72 years of age and older. There was no relationship between weight loss in persons taking two or less medications (OR 1.48, 95 % CI 0.85–2.59) [67]. However, those taking three to four medications and those taking five or more drugs were found to be at increased risk of weight loss (OR 1.96. 95 % CI 1.08–3.54 and OR 2.78, 95 % CI 1.38–5.60, respectively) with a stronger association observed with the higher level of polypharmacy [67].

While these studies did not measure the clinical consequences of medication-related nutritional changes on overall health status, nor can they assume causality, they do provide implicit evidence of polypharmacy as a risk factor for poor nutrition and weight loss in older adults.

4.4.3.3 Lower Urinary Tract Symptoms and Urinary Incontinence

Lower urinary tract symptoms (LUTS) and urinary incontinence are common problems in older individuals, reported between 40 % and 50 % for men and women, respectively [68]. Notably, urinary incontinence, particularly the urge type, is associated with falls [69]. Many commonly used medications have the potential to exacerbate these symptoms depending on the pharmacologic action of the drug and type of incontinence. Several drug classes, such as calcium channel blockers, diuretics, SSRIs, and others, have been associated with increasing LUTS [70, 71]. One cross-sectional study of 390 patients 60 years of age and older attending an outpatient urinary incontinence clinic found that 60 % were taking at least one drug potentially contributing to their LUTS [72]. Not surprisingly, polypharmacy (five or more medications) was identified as a risk factor for taking a LUTS-worsening drug (OR 4.9, 95 % CI 3.1–7.9) [72].

However, the relationship between polypharmacy and LUTS is less clear as there are few studies examining this issue. A survey of 203 women, aged 70 years and older, found that polypharmacy was associated with an increased risk of LUTS [73]. Given that many drug classes are known to exacerbate LUTS and urinary incontinence, and impact of these conditions on frailty, patients should have a thorough medication review to identify and correct medication-related contributions to LUTS and urinary incontinence.

4.4.3.4 Cognitive Impairment

The potential for a number of different medications to negatively affect cognition is well known, but is not always recognized when it does occur. Exposure to agents with anticholinergic properties provides the greatest risk for cognitive impairment. The relationship between anticholinergic drug use and delirium is well known [51]. Generally, it has been thought that cognition should improve with discontinuation of these agents. More recently, however, data suggests that the cognitive impact of these agents may not be reversible and long-term use of anticholinergic agents may increase dementia risk, although this remains controversial [74].

Many other agents, other than those with anticholinergic properties, can also cause or contribute to cognitive impairment via a number of different mechanisms. These include antiparkinson drugs, SSRIs, anticonvulsants, H_2-receptor antagonists, corticosteroids, NSAIDs, and some antibiotics (e.g., quinolones) [75].

The relationship between polypharmacy and delirium was explored in a prospective study of 156 patients 65 years of age and older in a community hospital. The number of medications was significantly associated with delirium (OR 1.2, 95 % CI 1.01–1.49) [76]. Likewise, a study of 410 individuals 65 years of age or older admitted to an acute geriatrics service found a twofold increase in the odds of developing delirium in persons taking four or more drugs (OR 2.33, 95 % CI 1.23–4.41) [77].

Unlike delirium, the relationship between dementia and polypharmacy has not been well elucidated. A prospective, cohort study of 294 community-dwelling persons 75 years of age and older observed an increasing proportion of patients with cognitive impairment with an increase in the number of medications. Cognitive impairment was 22 % in those taking five or fewer medications, 33 % of those taking six to nine drugs, and 54 % when taking ten or more [60]. However, a similar relationship was not seen in a study of 572 individuals participating in the New Mexico Aging Process Study [78].

Despite a lack of clarity with regard to the relationship between polypharmacy and cognitive impairment, it is a risk factor for falls, so an understanding of those medications that precipitate or contribute to diminish cognitive abilities is an important strategy for reducing fall risk [79].

4.4.3.5 Falls

The risk of falling and sustaining a fall-related injury increases with age. The annual rate of falls is estimated as 0.7 falls per person among relatively healthy community-dwelling adults aged 65 years and older [80]. Rates for falls in the hospital and nursing home settings are higher than that in community, with an increased likelihood of injury in comparison [80]. Approximately 5 % of older adults residing in community will experience a fracture or require hospitalization following a fall versus 10–25 % of those in hospital or nursing home [80].

There is a clear relationship between medication use and falls, with the strongest association seen with psychotropic agents [81, 82]. Cardiovascular drugs, especially antihypertensives, also increase risk [82, 83]. Likewise, polypharmacy itself is an important risk factor for falls and fractures. In a large study of over 1,500 patients, 80 years of age and older, followed between 2009 and 2014 in a geriatric outpatient clinic, the risk of falls increased with the presence of polypharmacy (six to nine drugs) [84]. These data are supported by other smaller studies [85, 86]. Polypharmacy is also associated with injurious falls and fractures requiring hospitalization [87, 88]. Falls occur as a result of many interrelated factors; however, minimizing high-risk medications is an important and effective component of an overall fall risk reduction strategy [89]. Subsequent chapters in this book will explore these issues in detail.

4.5 Strategies to Reduce Polypharmacy

A number of strategies have been trialed in an attempt to minimize polypharmacy in ambulatory, hospital, and nursing home settings. A recent systematic review evaluated interventions to reduce polypharmacy. A total of 12 studies were included in the review, primarily involving multifaceted interventions delivered by prescribers and pharmacists, with one study evaluating a computerized decision support tool [90]. In general, these interventions decreased inappropriate medications, whether measured by implicit or explicit criteria [90]. A significant reduction in MAI scores was observed in pooled data from five studies [90]. Likewise, studies with Beers or STOPP criteria demonstrated reductions in the number of inappropriate medications [90].

Data regarding clinical outcomes, such as hospitalization, however, was equivocal [90]. Of the five studies included in the analysis, three observed reductions in hospital admissions between control and intervention groups [91–93] but two did not [94, 95]. No differences were observed in medication-related problems or quality of life. For all clinical outcomes, heterogeneity in measuring outcomes and expression of results precluded pooled analysis [90].

Overall, multidisciplinary interventions, involving pharmacists and physicians, can reduce prescribing of inappropriate medications, but whether or not they reduce hospitalizations or medication-specific outcomes such as ADEs remains to be elucidated.

References

1. United Nations Department of Economic and Social Affairs (2013) Population division. World population ageing. United Nations, New York
2. Federal Interagency Forum on Aging-related Statistics. Older Americans (2012) Key indicators of well-being. US Government Printing Office, Washington, DC

3. Statistics Canada. Population by sex and age group (2015). Available at: http://www.statcan.gc.ca/tables-tableaux/sum-som/l01/cst01/demo10a-eng.htm. Accessed 4 Jan 2016
4. European Commission (2015) The 2015 Ageing Report. Economic and budgetary projections of the 28 EU Member States (2013–2060);ISSN 1725-3217 Available at: http://europa.eu/epc/pdf/ageing_report_2015_en.pdf. Last accessed: April 15, 2016.
5. Canadian Institute for Health Information (2011) Analysis in brief – seniors and the health care System: what is the impact of multiple chronic conditions? Available at: https://secure.cihi.ca/free_products/air-chronic_disease_aib_en.pdf. Last accessed: April 15, 2016.
6. Department of Health (UK) (2001) Medicines and older people: implementing medicines-related aspects of the NSF for older persons Available at: http://www.wales.nhs.uk/sites3/documents/439/nsf%20for%20older%20people%20-%20medicines%20and%20older%20people.pdf. Last accessed: April 15, 2016.
7. Qato DM, Alexander GC, Conti RM, Johnson M, Schumm P, Lindau ST (2008) Use of prescription and over-the-counter medications and dietary supplements among older adults in the United States. JAMA 300(24):2867–2878
8. Martial L, Mantel-Teewisse AK, Jansen PAF (2013) Background paper 7.3 priority medicines for elderly Available at: http://www.who.int/medicines/areas/priority_medicines/Ch7_3Elderly.pdf. Accessed: April 15, 2016.
9. Canadian Institute for Health Information (2015) Drug use among seniors on public drug programs in Canada, 2012. Available at: https://secure.cihi.ca/free_products/Drug_Use_in_Seniors_on_Public_Drug_Programs_2012_EN_web.pdf. Accessed 8 Sept 2015
10. WHO Centre for Health Development (2004) Aging and health technical report volume 5. A glossary of terms for community health care and services for older persons. Available at: http://www.who.int/kobe_centre/ageing/ahp_vol5_glossary.pdf. Accessed 23 Nov 2015
11. Brager R, Sloand E (2005) The spectrum of polypharmacy. Nurse Pract 30(6):44–50
12. Bushardt RL, Massey EB, Simpson TW, Ariail JC, Simpson KN (2008) Polypharmacy: misleading, but manageable. Clin Interv Aging 3(2):383–389
13. Hajjar ER, Cafiero AC, Hanlon JT (2007) Polypharmacy in elderly patients. Am J Geriatr Pharmacother 5(4):345–351
14. Frazier SC (2005) Health outcomes and polypharmacy in elderly individuals: an integrated literature review. J Gerontol Nurs 31(9):4–11
15. Hohl CM, Dankoff J, Colacone A, Afilalo M (2001) Polypharmacy, adverse drug-related events, and potential adverse drug interactions in elderly patients presenting to an emergency department. Ann Emerg Med 38(6):666–671
16. Salvi F, Marchetti A, D'Angelo F, Boemi M, Lattanzio F, Cherubini A (2012) Adverse drug events as a cause of hospitalization in older adults. Drug Saf 35(Suppl 1):29–45
17. Canadian Institute for Health Information – Analysis in Brief (2013). Adverse drug reaction-related hospitalizations among seniors, 2006 to 2011. Available at: https://secure.cihi.ca/free_products/Hospitalizations%20for%20ADR-ENweb.pdf. Accessed 3 Sept 2015
18. Kaufman DW, Kelly JP, Rosenberg L, Anderson TE, Mitchell AA (2002) Recent patterns of medication use in the ambulatory adult population of the United States: the Slone survey. JAMA 287(3):337–344
19. Fialova D, Topinkova E, Gambassi G, Finne-Soveri H, Jonsson PV, Carpenter I et al (2005) Potentially inappropriate medication use among elderly home care patients in Europe. JAMA 293(11):1348–1358
20. Dwyer LL, Han B, Woodwell DA, Rechtsteiner EA (2010) Polypharmacy in nursing home residents in the United States: results of the 2004 National Nursing Home Survey. Am J Geriatr Pharmacother 8(1):63–72
21. Onder G, Liperoti R, Fialova D, Topinkova E, Tosato M, Danese P et al (2012) Polypharmacy in nursing home in Europe: results from the SHELTER study. J Gerontol A Biol Sci Med Sci 67(6):698–704
22. Steinman MA, Landefeld CS, Rosenthal GE, Berthenthal D, Sen S, Kaboli PJ (2006) Polypharmacy and prescribing quality in older people. J Am Geriatr Soc 54(10):1516–1523

23. Hajjar ER, Hanlon JT, Sloane RJ, Lindblad CI, Pieper CF, Ruby CM et al (2005) Unnecessary drug use in frail older people at hospital discharge. J Am Geriatr Soc 53(9):1518–1523
24. Stuijt CC, Franssen EJ, Egberts AC, Hudson SA (2008) Appropriateness of prescribing among elderly patients in a Dutch residential home: observational study of outcomes after a pharmacist-led medication review. Drugs Aging 25(11):947–954
25. Brulhart MI, Wermeille JP (2011) Multidisciplinary medication review: evaluation of a pharmaceutical care model for nursing homes. Int J Clin Pharm 33(3):549–557
26. Silva C, Ramalho C, Luz I, Monteiro J, Fresco P (2015) Drug-related problems in institutionalized, polymedicated elderly patients: opportunities for pharmacist intervention. Int J Clin Pharm 37(2):327–334
27. Maher RL, Hanlon J, Hajjar ER (2014) Clinical consequences of polypharmacy in elderly. Expert Opin Drug Saf 13(1):57–65
28. Hanlon JT, Fillenbaum GG, Ruby CM, Gray S, Bohannon A (2001) Epidemiology of over-the-counter drug use in community dwelling elderly: United States perspective. Drugs Aging 18(2):123–131
29. Hovstadius B, Petersson G (2012) Factors leading to excessive polypharmacy. Clin Geriatr Med 28(2):159–172
30. Wehling M (2011) Guideline-driven polypharmacy in elderly, multimorbid patients is basically flawed: there are almost no guidelines for these patients. J Am Geriatr Soc 59(2):376–377
31. Garfinkel D, Ilhan B, Bahat G (2015) Routine deprescribing of chronic medications to combat polypharmacy. Ther Adv Drug Safety 6(6):212–233
32. Anthierens S, Tansens A, Petrovic M, Christiaens T (2010) Qualitative insights into general practitioners views on polypharmacy. BMC Fam Pract 11:65–2296
33. Cherubini A, Oristrell J, Pla X, Ruggiero C, Ferretti R, Diestre G et al (2011) The persistent exclusion of older patients from ongoing clinical trials regarding heart failure. Arch Intern Med 171(6):550–556
34. Dodd KS, Saczynski JS, Zhao Y, Goldberg RJ, Gurwitz JH (2011) Exclusion of older adults and women from recent trials of acute coronary syndromes. J Am Geriatr Soc 59(3):506–511
35. Konrat C, Boutron I, Trinquart L, Auleley GR, Ricordeau P, Ravaud P (2012) Underrepresentation of elderly people in randomised controlled trials. The example of trials of 4 widely prescribed drugs. PLoS One 7(3):e33559
36. Cruz-Jentoft AJ, Carpena-Ruiz M, Montero-Errasquin B, Sanchez-Castellano C, Sanchez-Garcia E (2013) Exclusion of older adults from ongoing clinical trials about type 2 diabetes mellitus. J Am Geriatr Soc 61(5):734–738
37. Mutasingwa DR, Aaro LE (2001) Injury registration in a developing country. A study based on patients' records from four hospitals in Dar es Salaam, Tanzania. Cent Afr J Med 47(8):203–209
38. Cox L, Kloseck M, Crilly R, McWilliam C, Diachun L (2011) Underrepresentation of individuals 80 years of age and older in chronic disease clinical practice guidelines. Can Fam Physician 57(7):e263–e269
39. Holmes HM, Hayley DC, Alexander GC, Sachs GA (2006) Reconsidering medication appropriateness for patients late in life. Arch Intern Med 166(6):605–609
40. Lee SJ, Leipzig RM, Walter LC (2013) Incorporating lag time to benefit into prevention decisions for older adults. JAMA 310(24):2609–2610
41. Hill-Taylor B, Sketris I, Hayden J, Byrne S, O'Sullivan D, Christie R (2013) Application of the STOPP/START criteria: a systematic review of the prevalence of potentially inappropriate prescribing in older adults, and evidence of clinical, humanistic and economic impact. J Clin Pharm Ther 38(5):360–372
42. Wallace J, Paauw DS (2015) Appropriate prescribing and important drug interactions in older adults. Med Clin N Am 99(2):295–310
43. By the American Geriatrics Society 2015 Beers Criteria Update Expert Panel (2015) American geriatrics society 2015 updated beers criteria for potentially inappropriate medication use in older adults. J Am Geriatr Soc 63(11):2227–2246

44. O'Mahony D, O'Sullivan D, Byrne S, O'Connor MN, Ryan C, Gallagher P (2015) STOPP/START criteria for potentially inappropriate prescribing in older people: version 2. Age Ageing 44(2):213–218
45. Samsa GP, Hanlon JT, Schmader KE, Weinberger M, Clipp EC, Uttech KM et al (1994) A summated score for the medication appropriateness index: development and assessment of clinimetric properties including content validity. J Clin Epidemiol 47(8):891–896
46. Hanlon JT, Artz MB, Pieper CF, Lindblad CI, Sloane RJ, Ruby CM et al (2004) Inappropriate medication use among frail elderly inpatients. Ann Pharmacother 38(1):9–14
47. Cannon KT, Choi MM, Zuniga MA (2006) Potentially inappropriate medication use in elderly patients receiving home health care: a retrospective data analysis. Am J Geriatr Pharmacother 4(2):134–143
48. Hudhra K, Garcia-Caballos M, Casado-Fernandez E, Jucja B, Shabani D, Bueno-Cavanillas A (2015) Polypharmacy and potentially inappropriate prescriptions identified by Beers and STOPP criteria in co-morbid older patients at hospital discharge. J Eval Clin Pract 22(2):189–93
49. Oliveira MG, Amorim WW, de Jesus SR, Heine JM, Coqueiro HL, Passos LC (2015) A comparison of the Beers and STOPP criteria for identifying the use of potentially inappropriate medications among elderly patients in primary care. J Eval Clin Pract 21(2):320–325
50. Walsh KA, O'Riordan D, Kearney PM, Timmons S, Byrne S (2016) Improving the appropriateness of prescribing in older patients: a systematic review and meta-analysis of pharmacists' interventions in secondary care. Age Ageing 45(2):201–9
51. Gray SL, Lai KV, Larson EB (1999) Drug-induced cognition disorders in the elderly: incidence, prevention and management. Drug Saf 21(2):101–122
52. Sera LC, McPherson ML (2012) Pharmacokinetics and pharmacodynamic changes associated with aging and implications for drug therapy. Clin Geriatr Med 28(2):273–286
53. Petrovic M, van der Cammen T, Onder G (2012) Adverse drug reactions in older people: detection and prevention. Drugs Aging 29(6):453–462
54. Reason B, Terner M, Moses McKeag A, Tipper B, Webster G (2012) The impact of polypharmacy on the health of Canadian seniors. Fam Pract 29(4):427–432
55. Marcum ZA, Amuan ME, Hanlon JT, Aspinall SL, Handler SM, Ruby CM et al (2012) Prevalence of unplanned hospitalizations caused by adverse drug reactions in older veterans. J Am Geriatr Soc 60(1):34–41
56. Nguyen JK, Fouts MM, Kotabe SE, Lo E (2006) Polypharmacy as a risk factor for adverse drug reactions in geriatric nursing home residents. Am J Geriatr Pharmacother 4(1):36–41
57. Goldberg RM, Mabee J, Chan L, Wong S (1996) Drug-drug and drug-disease interactions in the ED: analysis of a high-risk population. Am J Emerg Med 14(5):447–450
58. Inouye SK, Studenski S, Tinetti ME, Kuchel GA (2007) Geriatric syndromes: clinical, research, and policy implications of a core geriatric concept. J Am Geriatr Soc 55(5):780–791
59. Crentsil V, Ricks MO, Xue QL, Fried LP (2010) A pharmacoepidemiologic study of community-dwelling, disabled older women: factors associated with medication use. Am J Geriatr Pharmacother 8(3):215–224
60. Jyrkka J, Enlund H, Lavikainen P, Sulkava R, Hartikainen S (2011) Association of polypharmacy with nutritional status, functional ability and cognitive capacity over a three-year period in an elderly population. Pharmacoepidemiol Drug Saf 20(5):514–522
61. Rosso AL, Eaton CB, Wallace R, Gold R, Stefanick ML, Ockene JK et al (2013) Geriatric syndromes and incident disability in older women: results from the women's health initiative observational study. J Am Geriatr Soc 61(3):371–379
62. Lau DT, Mercaldo ND, Shega JW, Rademaker A, Weintraub S (2011) Functional decline associated with polypharmacy and potentially inappropriate medications in community-dwelling older adults with dementia. Am J Alzheimer's Dis Other Demen 26(8):606–615
63. Pickering G (2004) Frail elderly, nutritional status and drugs. Arch Gerontol Geriatr 38(2):174–180
64. Zadak Z, Hyspler R, Ticha A, Vlcek J (2013) Polypharmacy and malnutrition. Curr Opin Clin Nutr Metab Care 16(1):50–55

65. Griep MI, Mets TF, Collys K, Ponjaert-Kristoffersen I, Massart DL (2000) Risk of malnutrition in retirement homes elderly persons measured by the "mini-nutritional assessment". J Gerontol A Biol Sci Med Sci 55(2):M57–M63
66. Heuberger RA, Caudell K (2011) Polypharmacy and nutritional status in older adults: a cross-sectional study. Drugs Aging 28(4):315–323
67. Agostini JV, Han L, Tinetti ME (2004) The relationship between number of medications and weight loss or impaired balance in older adults. J Am Geriatr Soc 52(10):1719–1723
68. Sexton CC, Coyne KS, Thompson C, Bavendam T, Chen CI, Markland A (2011) Prevalence and effect on health-related quality of life of overactive bladder in older americans: results from the epidemiology of lower urinary tract symptoms study. J Am Geriatr Soc 59(8):1465–1470
69. Chiarelli PE, Mackenzie LA, Osmotherly PG (2009) Urinary incontinence is associated with an increase in falls: a systematic review. Aust J Physiother 55(2):89–95
70. Tsakiris P, Oelke M, Michel MC (2008) Drug-induced urinary incontinence. Drugs Aging 25(7):541–549
71. Hall SA, Chiu GR, Kaufman DW, Wittert GA, Link CL, McKinlay JB (2012) Commonly used antihypertensives and lower urinary tract symptoms: results from the Boston Area Community Health (BACH) Survey. BJU Int 109(11):1676–1684
72. Kashyap M, Tu le M, Tannenbaum C (2013) Prevalence of commonly prescribed medications potentially contributing to urinary symptoms in a cohort of older patients seeking care for incontinence. BMC Geriatr 13:57–2318
73. Nuotio M, Jylha M, Luukkaala T, Tammela TL (2005) Health problems associated with lower urinary tract symptoms in older women. A population-based survey. Scand J Prim Health Care 23(4):209–214
74. Gray SL, Anderson ML, Dublin S, Hanlon JT, Hubbard R, Walker R et al (2015) Cumulative use of strong anticholinergics and incident dementia: a prospective cohort study. J Intern Med 175(3):401–407
75. Moore AR, O'Keeffe ST (1999) Drug-induced cognitive impairment in the elderly. Drugs Aging 15(1):15–28
76. Martin NJ, Stones MJ, Young JE, Bedard M (2000) Development of delirium: a prospective cohort study in a community hospital. Int Psychogeriatr 12(1):117–127
77. Hein C, Forgues A, Piau A, Sommet A, Vellas B, Nourhashemi F (2014) Impact of polypharmacy on occurrence of delirium in elderly emergency patients. J Am Med Dir Assoc 15(11):850.e11–850.e15
78. Oyarzun-Gonzalez XA, Taylor KC, Myers SR, Muldoon SB, Baumgartner RN (2015) Cognitive decline and polypharmacy in an elderly population. J Am Geriatr Soc 63(2):397–399
79. Zhao YL, Kim H (2015) Older adult inpatient falls in acute care hospitals: intrinsic, extrinsic, and environmental factors. J Gerontol Nurs 41(7):29–43; quiz 44–5
80. Rubenstein LZ, Josephson KR (2002) The epidemiology of falls and syncope. Clin Geriatr Med 18(2):141–158
81. Souchet E, Lapeyre-Mestre M, Montastruc JL (2005) Drug related falls: a study in the French pharmacovigilance database. Pharmacoepidemiol Drug Saf 14(1):11–16
82. Woolcott JC, Richardson KJ, Wiens MO, Patel B, Marin J, Khan KM et al (2009) Meta-analysis of the impact of 9 medication classes on falls in elderly persons. Arch Intern Med 169(21):1952–1960
83. Butt DA, Mamdani M, Austin PC, Tu K, Gomes T, Glazier RH (2012) The risk of hip fracture after initiating antihypertensive drugs in the elderly. Arch Intern Med 172(22):1739–1744
84. Wang R, Chen L, Fan L, Gao D, Liang Z, He J et al (2015) Incidence and effects of polypharmacy on clinical outcome among patients aged 80+: a five-year follow-up study. PLoS One 10(11):e0142123
85. Fletcher PC, Berg K, Dalby DM, Hirdes JP (2009) Risk factors for falling among community-based seniors. J Patient Saf 5(2):61–66
86. Kojima T, Akishita M, Nakamura T, Nomura K, Ogawa S, Iijima K et al (2012) Polypharmacy as a risk for fall occurrence in geriatric outpatients. Geriatr Gerontol Int 12(3):425–430

87. Lai SW, Liao KF, Liao CC, Muo CH, Liu CS, Sung FC (2010) Polypharmacy correlates with increased risk for hip fracture in the elderly: a population-based study. Medicine (Baltimore) 89(5):295–299
88. Lu WH, Wen YW, Chen LK, Hsiao FY (2015) Effect of polypharmacy, potentially inappropriate medications and anticholinergic burden on clinical outcomes: a retrospective cohort study. CMAJ 187(4):E130–E137
89. Panel on Prevention of Falls in Older Persons, American Geriatrics Society and British Geriatrics Society (2011) Summary of the updated American geriatrics society/British geriatrics society clinical practice guideline for prevention of falls in older persons. J Am Geriatr Soc 59(1):148–157
90. Cooper JA, Cadogan CA, Patterson SM, Kerse N, Bradley MC, Ryan C et al (2015) Interventions to improve the appropriate use of polypharmacy in older people: a Cochrane systematic review. BMJ Open 5(12):e009235, 2015-009235
91. Crotty M, Rowett D, Spurling L, Giles LC, Phillips PA (2004) Does the addition of a pharmacist transition coordinator improve evidence-based medication management and health outcomes in older adults moving from the hospital to a long-term care facility? Results of a randomized, controlled trial. Am J Geriatr Pharmacother 2(4):257–264
92. Taylor CT, Byrd DC, Krueger K (2003) Improving primary care in rural Alabama with a pharmacy initiative. Am J Health Syst Pharm 60(11):1123–1129
93. Trygstad TK, Christensen DB, Wegner SE, Sullivan R, Garmise JM (2009) Analysis of the North Carolina long-term care polypharmacy initiative: a multiple-cohort approach using propensity-score matching for both evaluation and targeting. Clin Ther 31(9):2018–2037
94. Spinewine A, Swine C, Dhillon S, Lambert P, Nachega JB, Wilmotte L et al (2007) Effect of a collaborative approach on the quality of prescribing for geriatric inpatients: a randomized, controlled trial. J Am Geriatr Soc 55(5):658–665
95. Gallagher PF, O'Connor MN, O'Mahony D (2011) Prevention of potentially inappropriate prescribing for elderly patients: a randomized controlled trial using STOPP/START criteria. Clin Pharmacol Ther 89(6):845–854

Chapter 5
Pharmacology of Drugs in Aging

Louise Mallet

Abstract General principles for appropriate prescribing for the elderly are described in this chapter. Age-related changes in pharmacokinetics (absorption, distribution, metabolism, and distribution) with normal aging and in frail elderly patients are presented. Tools to identify potentially inappropriate medications in the elderly, including the American Geriatrics Society Beers Criteria and the STOPP/START criteria, are described. The prescription cascade, where a side effect of a medication is misinterpreted as a new medical condition leading to the introduction of another drug, is also described. The association between geriatric syndromes and medication use is presented as well as strategies to reduce fall risk-increasing medications. Assessment and review of medications in frail elderly patients should be done every 6 months.

Abbreviations

ADE	Adverse drug events
ADL	Activity of daily living
AGS	American Geriatrics Society
FRID	Fall risk-increasing drug
ISMP	Institute for Safe Medication Practices
MAI	Medication appropriateness index
PIM	Potentially inappropriate medication
START	Screening tool to alert doctors to right treatment
STOPP	Screening tool of older person's prescriptions

> When an elderly patient presents with a status change, unless proven otherwise, it should be assumed to be a medication related problem. Jerry Gurwitz, M.D

L. Mallet, BScPharm, PharmD, CGP, FESCP
Faculty of Pharmacy, University of Montréal, Montréal, QC, Canada

Department of Pharmacy, McGill University Health Center, Montréal, QC, Canada
e-mail: Louise.mallet@umontreal.ca

© Springer International Publishing Switzerland 2016

A.R. Huang, L. Mallet (eds.), *Medication-related falls in older people*,
DOI 10.1007/978-3-319-32304-6_5

5.1 Background

Over the past century, life expectancy has greatly increased. Older people make up the largest growing segment of the global population. Traditionally the age of 65 years has been associated with the term "elderly" as well as with the age of retirement and social benefits such as a pension [1, 2]. More recently, older people have been categorized into the subgroups "young-old" (65–74 years), "old" (75–84 years), and "old-old" (85 years and older) [3].

Defining older people goes beyond chronological age. It is important to understand normal aging for frail older adults. Rather than using just the number of their age, factors such as multiple comorbidities, functional and cognitive status, frailty, geriatric syndromes, remaining life expectancy, therapeutic goals, time to benefit, and use of multiple medications have been suggested to better describe older patients [4]. Prescribing for the elderly has become an art. This chapter will review the factors which impact on the effects of medications taken by older people with the objective of understanding the principles of appropriate prescribing.

5.1.1 Age-Related Changes in Pharmacokinetics

5.1.1.1 Absorption

Normal aging is associated with a number of physiological changes that affect the absorption of medications. These include an increase in gastric acidity, a reduction in gastrointestinal motility, a decrease in splanchnic blood flow, and a decrease in the surface area of the intestinal mucous membrane [5]. However, recent studies suggest that these age-related changes have not been detected in the fit older person. The effect of these changes on drug absorption in the frail elderly is not fully understood [5]. Further studies are needed to clarify these changes.

There are limited studies of the effect of aging on the absorption of slow release formulations, transdermal patches, or gels. In frail elderly patients, muscle mass is often decreased. Absorption of a medication administered via the intramuscular or subcutaneous routes may be affected [6]. Often, elderly patients have swallowing difficulties which leads to people crushing pills to help with their ingestion. Taking multiple medications at the same time can potentially lead to less evident problems. For example, calcium tablets can chelate with medications such as quinolone antibiotics and levothyroxine, leading to a decreased absorption and efficacy [6]. Congestive heart failure can result in decreased blood flow to the gastrointestinal tract leading to a decrease in the absorption of some drugs. Oral absorption of furosemide can be impaired due to slow gastric emptying and can contribute to furosemide resistance in decompensated heart failure [6].

5.1.1.2 Distribution

With aging, an increase in total body fat of 18–36 % is reported along with a drop in lean body mass. The half-life of lipophilic medications such as long-acting benzodiazepines, antipsychotics, and antidepressants increases, resulting in prolonged effects and adverse drug events in older patients [7]. Frail elderly patients with low body weight and low muscle mass are at higher risk of presenting with serious side effects from these medications, especially if they are prescribed the drug in the "normal" adult dose range.

Total body water decreases by 10–15 % which proportionally decreases the volume of distribution for water-soluble drugs. Dosage adjustments are needed for drugs such as digoxin, lithium, oral hypoglycemic agents, and diuretics [7] to avoid potential toxicity. Hot weather can lead to older people becoming dehydrated, further exacerbating the risk for toxicity. The doses of water-soluble medications should be adjusted or discontinued during prolonged heat waves.

A decline in serum albumin in the frail or malnourished elderly individual is common [5]. In this situation an increase in the concentration of unbound drug can occur with drugs that are highly protein bound (usually more than 90 % to albumin), such as phenytoin, warfarin, valproic acid, or nonsteroidal anti-inflammatory drugs. The unbound drug is the portion that exerts its pharmacologic actions: both therapeutic effects and side effects. A serum albumin concentration can be helpful in the analysis of medication in the frail or malnourished elderly [7].

5.1.1.3 Metabolism

With aging, there is diminution of up to 40 % in liver volume and a decrease in hepatic blood flow [8]. Medications with a significant first-pass extraction by the liver, such as metoprolol, morphine, and verapamil, will be affected [8]. Recent studies have described the effect of frailty on enzymes involved in the metabolism of some drugs. Phase I reactions (oxidation, reduction, or hydrolysis) are reduced with aging. Esterases are phase I enzymes involved with the oxidative metabolism of several drugs; a decrease in their activities has been observed. Prodrugs such as enalapril need to be activated via hepatic esterases [5] and lower levels of enalaprilat; the active metabolite of enalapril has been observed. Other drugs such as amitriptyline, citalopram, sertraline, and venlafaxine, which undergo phase I metabolism (oxidation and reduction), need to have dosage adjustments because of a decrease in hepatic esterase activity in frail elderly. Studies have described pharmacokinetic modifications in phase II metabolism in frail elderly for metoclopramide and paracetamol [9, 10]. Glucuronidation of paracetamol and clearance of metoclopramide by sulfation were considerably reduced in frail patients [9, 10].

5.1.1.4 Elimination

Serum creatinine concentration does not change significantly in normal aging. However, a "normal" serum creatinine concentration hides the actual decline in kidney mass, renal blood flow, glomerular filtration rate, and tubular secretion rate because of a concurrent decline in muscle mass resulting in a decrease in creatinine production [4, 5]. An estimation of the creatinine clearance using the Cockcroft and Gault equation will help guide clinicians to adjust dosage for renally excreted drugs [11].

A formula to estimate creatinine clearance in patients with low muscle mass and low serum creatinine level is lacking. For frail elderly people, estimation of creatinine clearance using the patient serum creatinine concentration will overestimate the true value. Clinically, these patients often present with toxic effects due to the accumulation of renally excreted medications for which the calculation of the estimated creatinine clearance value was inaccurate.

Clinical judgment is needed to interpret the results. For frail elderly patients with low muscle mass and low creatinine levels, a "normal" value for serum creatinine concentration should be substituted for the actual measured value when used in the formula to estimate creatinine clearance. For example, using the Cockcroft and Gault equation to estimate the creatinine clearance for a 90-year-old woman, weighing 38 kg, and a measured serum creatinine concentration of 45 μmol/L, an overestimated value of 44 mL/min is calculated. "Adjusting" the serum creatinine value by substituting a "normal" value of 70 μmol/L results in an estimated creatinine clearance of 28 mL/min which should then be applied to adjust dosage for renally excreted medications. Table 5.1 illustrates the age-related changes in pharmacokinetics with normal aging and in frail elderly patients.

5.1.2 Potentially Inappropriate Medications

Explicit criteria to help clinicians avoid inappropriate medications in the elderly were first published by Beers in 1991 and updated in 2003, 2012, and 2015 [12–15]. Table 5.2 lists drugs with strong anticholinergic properties that should be avoided. Potentially inappropriate medications using the Beers Criteria have been associated with poor health outcomes such as confusion, falls and mortality [16, 17]. STOPP (Screening tool of older person's prescriptions) and START (Screening Tool to Alert doctors to Right Treatment) criteria represent another consensus list of PIMs developed in Ireland in 2008 and updated in 2014 [18, 19]. These lists of PIMs can help guide clinicians in clinical practice and can also be incorporated into clinical decision support systems that can flag PIMs at the time of prescribing [20]. A recent Cochrane systematic review evaluated different interventions aimed at improving the appropriate use of polypharmacy in older people, 65 years of age or older, in different healthcare settings, receiving 4 or more regular medicines and with 1 or more long term-care condition [21]. The primary outcomes of this systematic review were the change in the prevalence of appropriate polypharmacy and hospital admissions. Secondary outcomes included medication-related problems, medication adherence and quality of life. A number of 12 studies were included. Appropriateness was measured using validated tools such as Medication Appropriateness Index (MAI), Beers' criteria, STOPP criteria, Screening Tool to Alert doctors to Right Treatment (START) criteria. A reduction in inappropriate prescribing was detected but results on medication-related problems are conflicting [21]. A later Chap. 15, "Identifying Explicit

Table 5.1 Age-related changes in pharmacokinetics with normal aging and frail elderly patients

	Age-related changes	Clinical impact	Frail elderly
Absorption	No significant changes	No clinical impact	↓↓
Distribution	↑ Body fat	↑ volume of distribution for liposoluble drugs Adjust dosage for fat soluble drugs such as antipsychotics, antidepressants, benzodiazepines	↑↑
	↓ Total water	↓ Volume of distribution of water-soluble drugs Adjust dosage for water-soluble drugs such as digoxin, lithium, diuretics	↓↓
	↓ Albumin	↑ Free fraction of drugs for drugs >90 % bound to albumin such as phenytoin, valproic acid, warfarin	↓↓
Metabolism	↓ Hepatic blood flow	↓ First-pass extraction by the liver such as metoprolol, morphine, and verapamil	↓↓
	↓ Phase I metabolism	↓ Metabolism of oxidation reaction	Unchanged
	Esterase enzymes	↓ Metabolism of drugs metabolized by esterase enzymes. Decrease conversion of prodrug enalapril to enalaprilat	↓↓
	↓ Phase II metabolism	No changes with normal aging	↓↓ Changes in glucuronidation of acetaminophen and clearance of metoclopramide by sulfation
Elimination	↓ Glomerular filtration rate	↓ Elimination of drugs excreted renally such as ciprofloxacin, digoxin, pregabalin	↓↓
	↓ Tubular secretion	↓ Elimination of drugs excreted via tubular secretion such as cimetidine, trimethoprim	↓↓
	Serum creatinine	With normal aging, no change in serum creatinine	↓↓ For low-weight patient, with no muscle mass, decrease in serum creatinine level
	Creatinine clearance	↓ With normal aging	↓↓

Table 5.2 Drugs with strong anticholinergic properties listed in AGS Updated Beers Criteria 2015 [15]

Antiarrhythmic	Disopyramide
Antiemetic	Prochlorperazine, promethazine
Antihistamines	Brompheniramine, carbinoxamine, chlorpheniramine, clemastine, cyproheptadine, dexbrompheniramine, dimenhydrinate, diphenhydramine, doxylamine, hydroxyzine, meclizine, triprolidine
Antidepressants	Amitriptyline, amoxapine, clomipramine, desipramine, doxepin (>6 mg), imipramine, nortriptyline, paroxetine, protriptyline, trimipramine
Antimuscarinics	Darifenacin, fesoterodine, flavoxate, oxybutynin, solifenacin, tolterodine, trospium
Antiparkinsonian	Benztropine, trihexyphenidyl
Antipsychotics	Chlorpromazine, clozapine, loxapine, olanzapine, perphenazine, thioridazine, trifluoperazine
Antispasmodics	Atropine (excludes ophthalmic) belladonna alkaloids, clidinium-chlordiazepoxide, dicyclomine, homatropine (excludes ophthalmic), hyoscyamine, propantheline, scopolamine (excludes ophthalmic)
Skeletal muscle relaxants	Cyclobenzaprine, orphenadrine

Criteria for the Prevention of Falls," is devoted to PIMs. The Chap. 4 on "Polypharmacy" also discusses details on strategies to reduce polypharmacy.

5.1.3 *Prescribing Cascade*

Prescribing cascades are commonly observed in elderly patients but rarely detected and reported in the literature. This concept was initially reported by Rochon in 1997 [22]. A prescription cascade begins when a side effect of a medication is misinterpreted as new medical condition, which triggers the prescription of another drug [22].

For example, an 88-year-old man is seen in the emergency room for a fall because of leg pains. He is taking a statin and his creatine kinase level is normal. Recently, pregabalin was prescribed for his "leg pains." Prescribing pregabalin for leg pains associated with statin use represents a cascade.

An 85-year-old woman recently admitted to a long-term care facility presented to the emergency room with a fall following the prescription of betahistine to treat her dizziness symptoms. She is taking three different antihypertensive agents resulting in significant orthostatic hypotension. Since her admission to the long-term care facility, her medication adherence has been assured; hence, the full effectiveness and side effects of her multiple antihypertensive medications can now act. This case illustrates the cascade of prescribing betahistine to treat the "dizziness" symptoms secondary to orthostatic hypotension. Prescribing cascades increase the risk of adverse drug events in the elderly.

Patients should be asked about the presence of new symptoms especially if a new drug has recently been started or there has been a dose increase of an existing

Table 5.3 Examples of prescribing cascades from clinical practice

Furosemide → urinary incontinence → oxybutynin
Amlodipine → peripheral edema → furosemide
Donepezil → urinary incontinence → oxybutynin
Risperidone → rigidity → levodopa + carbidopa
Ciprofloxacin → hallucinations → risperidone
Antihypertensive drugs → dizziness → betahistine
Atorvastatin → leg pains → quinine
Venlafaxine → hyponatremia → salt supplements
Digoxin → nausea/vomiting → metoclopramide
Low TSH level (hyperthyroidism) → tremors → primidone

drug [23]. To avoid a potential prescribing cascade, new medications should always be prescribed at the lowest possible dose. A complete medication review can help identify a potential prescribing cascade, by clarifying the time frame of medication changes (new additions or dose changes) and the appearance of signs or symptoms. Tapering or stopping the last prescribed medication can help manage prescription cascades. Documentation in the medical record is strongly encouraged to help avoid future occurrences. Table 5.3 lists other examples of prescribing cascades.

5.1.4 Geriatric Syndromes

Geriatric syndromes define clinical conditions that are typically found in older patients and do not fit into specific illness categories [24]. They are common, are multifactorial in etiology, lead to functional impairment, and are associated with significant morbidity and poor outcomes in the elderly [24]. Examples of geriatric syndromes include delirium, falls, dizziness, urinary incontinence, syncope, and anorexia [24]. Table 5.4 illustrates the association between geriatric syndromes and some medications.

Wierenga et al. investigated if geriatric syndromes were associated with adverse drug events (ADEs) in a cohort of patients aged 65 years and older admitted for acute medical problems. Delirium was evaluated using the Confusion Assessment Method. A fall occurring before admission was extracted from the medical records. Overall 25 % of patients presented with an ADE on admission. The prevalence of delirium at admission was 25.9 % and 12 % for a fall prior to admission with 5.4 % of patients with both a fall and delirium. Antidepressants, antipsychotics, and antiepileptics were associated with delirium. Diuretics, coumarins, immunosuppressants, and nonsteroidal anti-inflammatory drugs were frequently associated with an ADE. More than half of the patients who had a fall were using antidiabetics, antidepressants, antihypertensives, and antipsychotics [25]. A fall may be an important sign associated with an ADE.

Lattanzio evaluated the association between geriatric syndromes and ADEs in patients 65 years or older admitted to acute care hospitals. The presence of a history

Table 5.4 Geriatric syndromes and medications

Geriatric syndromes	Medications
Falls	>4 drugs, antipsychotics, antidepressants, benzodiazepines
Delirium	Medications with anticholinergic properties
Anorexia	Digoxin, metronidazole, enalapril, lithium
Urinary incontinence	Diuretics, cholinesterase inhibitors, sedative hypnotics
Dizziness	Antidepressants, antihypertensive drugs, antipsychotics
Immobility	Antipsychotics

of falls and a loss in at least one activity of daily living (ADL) increased the risk of ADE in these patients. The exposure to neuropsychiatric drugs was more prevalent in the cases [26]. A history of falls and dependency in at least one activity of daily living appears to be a sign of vulnerability to the development of ADEs in older individuals [27]. Physicians should be aware of this association before prescribing drugs that may cause negative outcomes in elderly patients.

Health-care professionals need to be proactive. Scheduled medication reviews and deprescribing strategies can help manage potential fall risk related to medications. Considering the presence of a geriatric syndrome as an atypical presentation of an ADE should be included in the differential diagnosis of a clinical scenario.

5.2 Optimizing Drug Prescribing in the Elderly

The Institute for Safe Medication Practices (ISMP) Canada recently published an analysis of medication incidents associated with falls and risky fall-related situations [28]. The top medication classes associated with falls were opioids, psychotropics (including antipsychotics, sedative hypnotics, antidepressants), cardiac medications (including diuretics), and hypoglycemic agents (including insulin).

In their analysis, the authors identified four main themes associated with falls or risky fall-related situations [28].

1. *Failure to anticipate inherent risks of medications*

   Failure of patient engagement was identified as a risk for falls. A number of reviews, systematic reviews, and meta-analysis have been published on the risk associated with medication-related falls in the elderly [8, 29–31]. Dizziness, drowsiness, syncope, bradycardia, and muscle weakness are frequently documented with a fall. These falls can be associated with a prescribing cascade, use of PIMs, or geriatric syndromes. Increased awareness in patients, families, and prescribers about medication-related problems and their atypical clinical presentation in the elderly will help.
2. *Inadequate proactive clinical assessment*

   The following factors were identified that led to clinical assessments being absent or overlooked: failure to recognize a fall risk symptom, not recognizing the prescription of dosing regimens associated with an increased risk of fall, and failure to identify drug interactions that increased fall risk. In cases where potential falls were avoided, pharmacists or nurses were involved.

3. *Communication gaps*

   Absence or failure of medication reconciliation at hospital admission or discharge led to drug prescribing errors. Patients using their own medications during their hospital stay and not informing hospital staff also resulted in falls.
4. *Failure of medication-use processes*

   Seventy-five percent of the medication incidents were associated with problems in dispensing and medication administration processes in hospital. Administration of incorrect medications or dosages, the use of dangerous abbreviations, and the use of preprinted order sets not "geriatric friendly" are some risk factors identified with risk for falls in hospital. In the community pharmacy setting, the problems identified are processing multiple patient prescriptions at the same time, errors related to verbal orders, and dispensing errors.

5.3 Strategies to Reduce Fall Risk-Increasing Drugs

Safely prescribing medications in elderly patients with multiple comorbidities is complex and takes time and cognitive discipline. According to the AGS practice guidelines, "Patients who have fallen should have their medications reviewed and altered or stopped as appropriate in light of their risk of future falls. Particular attention to medication reduction should be given to older patients taking four or more medications and to those taking psychotropic drugs" [32].

A medication review of an older patient's medication should be done every 6 months. Review should also be done at transitions of care, for example, discharge from hospital, transfer to long-term care, and admission to hospital. The following list of actions should be considered when evaluating a geriatric patient. These can be completed over a period of time. A pharmacist can be asked to perform a detailed medication history and identify drug-related problems and fall risk-increasing drugs.

1. Obtain a detailed medication history, including prescribed medications, over-the-counter medications, natural products, pro re nata (prn) medications, health food supplements, and alcohol.
2. Advise the patient to see their community pharmacist for a medication reconciliation and review. Home visits are helpful for patients unable to leave their home.
3. Identify FRIDs.
4. Match each medication use to an appropriate indication.
5. Determine the onset and duration of the patient's current complaints or presenting problems. Are they related to geriatric syndromes: falls, delirium, etc.?
6. Identify the temporal relationship between adverse drug reaction and medications: prescribing cascade, PIMs, anticholinergic load, recent additions, or deletions. Document any adverse drug reaction and the consequences of this adverse drug reaction.

7. Evaluate the modalities of drug administration. How are the medications being taken? Can adherence be improved? Pill boxes? Blister packs? Engaging a caregiver?
8. Obtain a current weight.
9. Estimate a creatinine clearance and verify if any medication needs dosage adjustments to compensate for renal impairment.
10. Identify red flags for drug-drug or drug-disease interactions.
11. Document the therapeutic objective for each category of medications; for example, the target blood pressure for a 90-year-old woman may be higher than 160/90 mmHg. Time to benefit, remaining life expectancy, and expectation from the patient need to be discussed and documented when beginning a new treatment.
12. Simplify the drug regimen if appropriate; consider deprescribing with a stepwise approach by reducing one medication at the time with adequate follow-up. This can be done at each visit. Document benefit or harm when medications are discontinued.
13. Identify one physician that will prescribe to limit the number of prescribers and avoid adverse drug events.
14. Arrange for a follow-up when treatment is modified.
15. Involve a family member or caregiver.
16. Involve when needed other health-care professionals such as a pharmacist, nurse, physiotherapist, occupational therapist, and nutritionist.
17. Organize or refer for a home visit assessment when necessary.
18. Reevaluate treatment plans regularly: at least every 6 months.

5.4 Conclusions

Medications are one of the modifiable fall risk factors. Family, caregivers, and health-care professionals should be aware and appreciate the fall risks associated with medications. We can all strive to decrease medication-related falls in older adults.

> It takes one minute to prescribe a medication but years to discontinue it. Louise Mallet, January 2016.

References

1. World Health Organization (2016) Definition of an older or elderly person. http://www.who.int/healthinfo/survey/ageingdefnolder/en/. Accessed 19 Jan 2016
2. Sanderson WC, Scherbov S (2015) The characteristics approach to the measurement of population aging. Popul Dev Rev 39:673–685
3. Guimond J (2003) Médicaments et qualité de vie. In: Mallet L, Grenier L, Guimond J, Barbeau G (eds) Manuel des soins pharmaceutiques. Les Presses de l'Université Laval, Québec, pp 19–35

4. Hilmer SN, McLachlan AJ, Le Couteur DG (2007) Clinical pharmacology in the geriatric patient. Fundam Clin Pharmacol 21:217–230
5. Hubbard RE, O'Mahony MS, Woodhouse KW (2013) Medication prescribing in frail older people. Eur J Clin Pharmacol 69:319–326
6. Delafuente JC (2008) Pharmacokinetic and pharmacodynamic alterations in the geriatric patient. Consult Pharmacists 23:324–334
7. McLachlan SN, Hilmer S, Le Couteur DG (2010) Dosing errors, age-related changes in pharmacokinetics. In: Koch S, Gloth F, Nay R (eds) Medication management in older adults: a concise guide for clinicians. Springer, New York, pp 125–135
8. Huang AR, Mallet L, Rochefort CM, Eguale T, Buckeridge DL, Tamblyn R (2012) Medication-related falls in the elderly. Drugs Aging 29:359–376
9. Wynne HA, Cope L, Herd B, James OFW, Rawlins MD, Woodhouse KW (1990) The association of age and frailty with paracetamol conjugation in man. Age Ageing 19:419–424
10. Wynne HA, Yelland C, Cope LH, Boddy A, Woodhouse KW, Bateman DN (1993) The association of age and frailty with the pharmacokinetics and pharmacodynamics of metoclopramide. Age Ageing 22:354–359
11. Cockcroft DW, Gault MH (1976) Prediction of creatinine clearance from serum creatinine. Nephron 16:31–41
12. Beers MH, Ouslander JG, Rollingher I, Reuben DB, Brooks J, Beck JC (1991) Explicit criteria for determining inappropriate medication use in nursing home residents. Arch Intern Med 151:1825–1832
13. Fick DM, Cooper JW, Wade WE, Waller JL, Maclean JR, Beers MH (2003) Updating the Beers criteria for potentially inappropriate medication use in older adults: results of a US consensus panel of experts. Arch Intern Med 163(22):2716–2724
14. American Geriatrics Society 2012 Beers Criteria Update Expert Panel (2012) American Geriatrics Society updated Beers Criteria for potentially inappropriate medication use in older adults. J Am Geriatr Soc 60:616–631
15. American Geriatrics Society 2015 Beers Criteria Update Expert Panel (2015) American Geriatrics Society 2015 updated Beers Criteria for potentially inappropriate medication use in older adults. J Am Geriatr Soc 63:2227–2246
16. Stockl KM, Le L, Zhang S, Harada AS (2010) Clinical and economic outcomes associated with potentially inappropriate prescribing in the elderly. Am J Manage Care 16:e1–e10
17. Fick DM, Mion LC, Beers MH, Waller J (2008) Health outcomes associated with potentially inappropriate medication use in older adults. Res Nurs Health 31:42–51
18. Gallagher P, Ryan C, Byrne S, Kennedy J, O'Mahony D (2008) Screening Tool of Older Person's Prescriptions (STOPP) and Screening Tool to Alert doctors to Right Treatment (START). Consensus validation. Int J Clin Pharmacol Ther 46:72–83
19. O'Mahony D, O'Sullivan D, Byrne S, O'Connor MN, Ryan C, Gallagher P (2015) STOPP/START criteria for potentially inappropriate prescribing in older people: version 2. Age Ageing 44:213–218
20. Arvisais K, Bergeron S, Bouffard C, Michaud AS, Bergeron J, Mallet L et al (2005) A pharmacist-physician intervention using a computerized alert system to high-risk medication use in elderly patients. Drugs Aging 32:663–670
21. Cooper JA, Cadogan CA, Patterson SM, Kerse N, Bradley MC, Ryan C et al (2015) Interventions to improve the appropriate use of polypharmacy in older people: a Cochrane systematic review. BMJ 5:1–12
22. Rochon P, Gurwitz JH (1997) Optimising drug treatment for elderly people: the prescribing cascade. BMJ 315:1096–1099
23. Kalisch LM, Caughey GE, Roughead EE, Gilbert AL (2011) The prescribing cascade. Aust Prescr 34:162–166
24. Inouye SK, Studenski S, Tinetti ME, Kuchel GA (2007) Geriatric syndromes: clinical, research, and policy implications of a core geriatric concept. J Am Geriatr Soc 55:780–791

25. Wieranga PC, Buurman BM, Parlevliet JL, van Munster BC, Smorenburg SM et al (2012) Association between acute geriatric syndromes and medication-related hospital admissions. Drugs Aging 29:691–699
26. Lattanzio F, Laino J, Pedone C, Abbatecola AM, Corica F, Pranno L et al (2012) Geriatric conditions and adverse drug reactions in elderly hospitalized patients. J Am Med Dir Assoc 13:96–99
27. Lattanzio F, Landi F, Bustacchini S, Abbatecola AM, Corica F, Pranno L et al (2012) Geriatric conditions and the risk of adverse drug reactions in older adults. Drug Saf 35(Suppl 1):55–61
28. IMPS Canada (2015) Medication incidents that increase the risk of falls: a multi-incident analysis. ISMP Can Saf Bull 25:1–5
29. Leipzig RM, Cumming RG, Tinetti ME (1999) Drugs and falls in older people: a systematic review and meta-analysis: I. Psychotropic drugs. J Am Geriatr Soc 47:30–39
30. Leipzig RM, Cumming RG, Tinetti ME (1999) Drugs and falls in older people: a systematic review and meta-analysis: II. Cardiac and analgesic drugs. J Am Geriatr Soc 47:40–50
31. Woolcott JC, Richardson KJ, Wiens MO et al (2009) Meta-analysis of the impact of 9 medication classes on falls in elderly persons. Arch Intern Med 169:1952–1960
32. American Geriatrics Society (2010) American Geriatrics Society/Britisy Geriatrics Society (AGS/BGS) clinical practice guideline: prevention of falls in older persons. J Am Geriatr Soc 59:29–37

Chapter 6
Age-Related Physical and Physiologic Changes and Comorbidities in Older People: Association with Falls

Gustavo Duque

Abstract Several age-related changes that increase fall risk will be described. Changes in vision can result in impaired accuracy and sense of dimension. Changes in the vestibular system increase the response time to positional changes in older persons. Age-related muscle loss known as sarcopenia can lead to muscle weakness. The aging brain has a slower reaction time due to changes in intracerebral blood flow, neurotransmitter levels, cognitive impairment, and reductions in the neuron population. The heart and blood vessels become stiffer and the heart fills with blood more slowly. Stiffer arteries are less able to expand and results in increases in blood pressure. Orthostatic hypotension can be the result of the blunted vasoconstriction of stiffer blood vessels coupled with decreases in cardiac output. Medical comorbidities such as diabetes mellitus, dementia, Parkinson's disease, cerebrovascular disease, congestive heart failure, and chronic kidney disease can contribute to increased fall risk. Some comorbidities can involve changes in muscle mass (secondary sarcopenia) and calciotropic hormones leading to weaker muscles and bones.

6.1 Introduction

Falls in older persons are multifactorial. A combination of intrinsic and extrinsic factors affects the capacity of older persons to respond to changes in their interaction with the environment, thus inducing falls and predisposing them to injuries and death. Indeed, some of those intrinsic factors are associated with age-related physical and physiologic changes, which cannot be modified but only managed. Additionally older people have concurrent comorbidities some of which impact on key body systems, which are required to maintain sensory and locomotor function, thereby increasing

G. Duque, MD, PhD, FRACP
Australian Institute for Musculoskeletal Science (AIMSS), Melbourne Medical School – Western Campus, The University of Melbourne and Western Health, 176 Furlong Road, St. Albans, Melbourne, VIC 3021, Australia
e-mail: gustavo.duque@unimelb.edu.au

© Springer International Publishing Switzerland 2016

A.R. Huang, L. Mallet (eds.), *Medication-related falls in older people*,
DOI 10.1007/978-3-319-32304-6_6

the risk of falling. Contrary to normal and age-related physical and physiologic changes, which are irreversible, the optimal medical management of comorbidities are pivotal and effective interventions that can decrease fall risk in older persons.

In this chapter, those age-related changes that increase fall risk will be reviewed. Interventions intended to manage those changes focusing on fall prevention will be also reviewed. In addition, the impact of comorbidities will be considered from an intervention perspective intended to decrease their role in fall risk.

6.2 Age-Related Physical and Physiologic Changes

6.2.1 Sensory Changes

Locomotion and balance are essential components for mobility and independence and also to prevent falls in older persons. Balance disorders are considered a major risk factor for falling. Maintenance of balance involves a complex interaction between vision, vestibular function, proprioception, and other sensory functions [5]. With aging, and even in the absence of disease, visual accuracy is impaired with reduced capacity of accommodation and sense of dimension [1]. In addition, age-related changes in the vestibular system, mostly associated with the decreased mobility of the cilia within the utricle of the semicircular canals of the inner ear, increase the response time to positional changes in older persons. There is also age-related hearing loss due to sclerosis of the tympanic membrane. In addition, the brain may be impaired in its integration of normal afferent signals on vision, balance, and hearing or may not be able to adapt to the age-related changes or disease states affecting these sensory systems. These factors may all increase fall risk.

6.2.2 Postural and Mobility Changes

Compared to younger adults, older adults tend to move their center of mass more (increased postural sway) when standing still. Postural changes can occur as a consequence of age-related loss of lower limb muscle mass with resultant weakness. In addition, gait velocity becomes slower with age, a change that has been associated with poor outcomes, including falls, in older adults.

6.2.3 Musculoskeletal Changes

Aging is closely associated with changes in the musculoskeletal system, which is usually considered physiologic until certain clinical thresholds are exceeded. The normal age-related muscle loss – also known as sarcopenia – becomes clinical relevant after having an impact on gait velocity and grip strength. Nevertheless, muscle loss even in the absence of clinical criteria for sarcopenia is considered a risk factor for falls in older persons. Finally, in terms of the cartilage, age-related changes in the joints are associated with pain and stiffness, which can affect mobility and predispose to falls.

6.2.4 Changes in the Brain and Nervous System

The aging brain shows a slower reaction time, which is due to multiple factors including decreased intracerebral blood flow, changes in neurotransmitter levels, cognitive impairment, and reductions in the neuron population. Together, these changes reduce the capacity to react to sudden environmental changes thus predisposing to falls.

6.2.5 Changes in Heart and Blood Vessels

Under normal physiologic conditions, the older heart functions well and can provide adequate blood supply to tissues and organs. With aging the heart and blood vessels become stiffer and the heart fills with blood more slowly. The stiffer arteries are less able to expand when blood is pumped through them during each cardiac contraction and results in increases in blood pressure [3]. Conversely the blunted vasoconstriction of stiffer blood vessels coupled with decreases in cardiac output can predispose older people to orthostatic hypotension and falls when there are changes in blood volume such as with dehydration [15].

6.2.6 Changes in Kidney Function and Urinary Tract

In theory, age-related changes in kidney and urinary tract function should not be associated with falls [6]. However, changes, such as a reduction in the maximum bladder capacity, shortening of the length of the urethra in postmenopausal women, and prostatic enlargement in men, could predispose to the symptoms of urinary frequency and nocturia [9]. A combination of impaired mobility, orthostatic hypotension, and urinary frequency and nocturia has been associated with falls in older persons, sometimes in the absence of disease.

6.3 Comorbidities and Falls in Older Persons

The comorbidities that predispose older persons to fall have been well described [11]. Identification of these comorbidities and determining the impact of each on the risk of falls is an essential component of any fall prevention program. We will review the comorbidities from a system-based perspective while taking into consideration that some diseases could affect more than one system at the same time thus requiring a comprehensive assessment and care plan in order to reduce their impact on fall risk.

6.3.1 Endocrine System

The presence of diabetes mellitus is considered a major risk factor for falls in older persons [7–8]. Diabetes is also a highly prevalent disease in older people. Poor glycemic control has a negative effect on the neurosensory systems (impaired vision, the development of peripheral neuropathy, impaired proprioception, impaired brain circulation, etc.), which predisposes to falls. Diabetes mellitus also predisposes patients to cerebrovascular and cardiovascular disease, which can affect cognition, mobility, and vascular responsiveness. Optimizing glucose control and identification of affected organs in diabetic patients should be a priority in any fall prevention program.

Hypothyroidism is another endocrine disease that frequently predisposes to falls. Hypothyroid patients have increased reaction times. Myxedema predisposes them to sarcopenia and weaker muscles. Low heart rate and poor cardiovascular response increase their risk of orthostatic hypotension and falls.

Finally, Addison's disease could also be associated with falls due to changes in serum electrolytes, which can be associated with low blood pressure, delirium, and orthostatic hypotension.

6.3.2 Central Nervous System

Three comorbidities in this system have been highly associated with fall risk in older persons: dementia, Parkinson's disease, and cerebrovascular disease. Patients suffering from cognitive impairment, even at the mild cognitive impairment stage, are known to be at higher risk of falls. Use of cholinesterase inhibitors has been associated with improvement in gait and balance in those patients, resulting in reduced fall risk [12].

Patients with Parkinson's disease are at high risk of falls due to multiple changes associated with the disease. Postural instability is a common feature. Changes in gait and posture together with tremor predispose them to falls. Finally, the additional presence of orthostatic hypotension in these patients increases fall risk. Please refer to Chapter 11 on "Drugs for Neurologic Conditions: Antiparkinson Medications, Cholinesterase Inhibitors and Memantine" for a more detailed review of this topic.

Cerebrovascular disease is associated with falls for two reasons: (1) sequelae from cerebrovascular accident events, such as changes in muscle tone or strength or dyscoordination of movement [4], could predispose to falls by directly affecting mobility and reaction time and (2) cerebrovascular disease predisposes to the development of vascular dementia, which is highly associated with fall risk [16].

6.3.3 Cardiovascular System

Congestive heart failure is associated with high fall risk due to three major reasons: functional impairment related to fatigue or shortness of breath from heart failure, secondary muscle sarcopenia, and the side effects from medications used to manage this condition.

The assessment of functional changes and sarcopenia has become a common practice at heart failure clinics that focus on older patients. There is consensus that these patients require a comprehensive approach, which includes a multidisciplinary team and exercise programs focused on cardiac patients. These programs have demonstrated to be effective in reducing the incidence of poor outcomes in heart failure patients, including falls. Medications for heart disease, which could increase fall risk, are reviewed in Chapter 12, "Antihypertensives and Cardiovascular Medications."

6.3.4 Kidney and Urinary Tract

Older patients suffering from chronic kidney disease are at higher risk of falls due to changes in muscle mass (secondary sarcopenia) and alterations in the serum levels of calciotropic hormones (vitamin D and parathyroid hormone [PTH]) usually associated with low renal function [13].

Assessment for sarcopenia and measurement of serum levels of vitamin D and PTH is recommended [18]. While sarcopenia could be corrected by participating in an appropriate exercise program, serum levels of vitamin D could be normalized by appropriate supplementation, which is usually followed by normalization of serum PTH. Together, these interventions have been shown to reduce falls in this particular population.

6.3.5 Sensory Systems

As previously mentioned, age-related visual and vestibular impairments predispose to falls by limiting the capacity to perceive and interact with stimuli from the environment. Additional comorbidities that affect vision (e.g., cataracts, macular degeneration, etc.), hearing (otosclerosis), or vestibular function (positional vertigo, Meniere's disease, etc.) would also increase fall risk.

6.3.6 Nutritional Deficits

Vitamin D deficiency, even in absence of kidney disease, has been associated with high fall risk. This state results in reduced muscle mass and function as well as changes in balance and gait velocity. Indeed, vitamin D supplementation has been shown to improve balance and muscle function thus reducing fall risk.

Vitamin B12 deficiency has been associated with falls through three different mechanisms [14]. First, low levels of vitamin B12 lead to peripheral neuropathy, which results in proprioceptive sensory impairment. Second, it is associated with high levels of homocysteine, which is associated with the accelerated development of peripheral vascular disease. Finally, low vitamin B12 is also associated with cognitive impairment. Alone or in combination, these abnormalities observed in vitamin B12-deficient patients predispose them to falling. Vitamin B12 supplementation can only partially correct peripheral neuropathy, can potentially normalize homocysteine levels, and has not shown any therapeutic effect on cognitive decline.

Iron deficiency is also associated with falls due to anemia [10], which is closely associated with sarcopenia. Although the mechanisms explaining this association remain unknown, it is proposed that anemia is secondary to sarcopenia and not the opposite. Nevertheless, a combination of exercise plus iron supplementation has demonstrated to decrease fall risk in these patients [17].

6.3.7 Musculoskeletal Diseases

Osteosarcopenia, defined as a combination of osteopenia/osteoporosis and sarcopenia, corresponds to a subset of frailer older individuals at higher risk of falls and fractures [19]. Recent evidence has confirmed a particular phenotype in osteosarcopenic subjects including higher fall risk, vitamin D deficiency, high PTH, and higher prevalence of disability [20]. In the context of fall prevention, osteosarcopenic individuals should be treated by a multidisciplinary team and a specific care plan including osteoporosis treatment (if required), exercise program, vitamin D supplementation, and nutritional supplements [21].

Additionally, osteoarthritis is an important and highly prevalent comorbidity that predisposes to falls in older persons by affecting their mobility and predisposing them to sarcopenia and frailty [2]. Optimal analgesia and nonpharmacological interventions (e.g., hydrotherapy) are the treatments of choice in these patients.

6.4 Conclusion

Due to the multifactorial nature of falls, a comprehensive assessment should be performed in any older person considered at high risk of falling. This comprehensive assessment should include the identification of those age-related physical and physiologic changes that, although normal, may predispose those people to falls. In addition, the impact of frequently multiple comorbidities on fall risk and the design of care plans targeting those comorbidities are essential components in any fall prevention programs for older persons.

References

1. Dagnelie G (2013) Age-related psychophysical changes and low vision. Invest Ophthalmol Vis Sci 54:ORSF88–ORSF93
2. Li Y, Wei X, Zhou J, Wei L (2013) The age-related changes in cartilage and osteoarthritis. Biomed Res Int 2013:916530
3. Kohn JC, Lampi MC, Reinhart-King CA (2015) Age-related vascular stiffening: causes and consequences. Front Genet 6:112
4. Scherbakov N, Sandek A, Doehner W (2015) Stroke-related sarcopenia: specific characteristics. J Am Med Dir Assoc 16:272–276
5. Sturnieks DL, St George R, Lord SR (2008) Balance disorders in the elderly. Neurophysiol Clin 38:467–478
6. Denic A, Glassock RJ, Rule AD (2016) Structural and functional changes with the aging kidney. Adv Chron Kidney Dis 23:19–28
7. Malabu UH, Vangaveti VN, Kennedy RL (2014) Disease burden evaluation of fall-related events in the elderly due to hypoglycemia and other diabetic complications: a clinical review. Clin Epidemiol 6:287–294
8. Vinik AI, Vinik EJ, Colberg SR, Morrison S (2015) Falls risk in older adults with type 2 diabetes. Clin Geriatr Med 31(1):89–99
9. Coyne KS, Wein A, Nicholson S, Kvasz M, Chen CI, Milsom I (2013) Comorbidities and personal burden of urgency urinary incontinence: a systematic review. Int J Clin Pract 67:1015–1033
10. Balducci L (2010) Anemia, fatigue and aging. Transfus Clin Biol 17:375–381
11. Vu T, Finch CF, Day L (2011) Patterns of comorbidity in community-dwelling older people hospitalised for fall-related injury: a cluster analysis. BMC Geriatr 11:45
12. Montero-Odasso M, Wells J, Borrie M (2009) Can cognitive enhancers reduce the risk of falls in people with dementia? An open-label study with controls. J Am Geriatr Soc 57:359–360
13. Cook WL, Tomlinson G, Donaldson M, Markowitz SN, Naglie G, Sobolev B, Jassal SV (2006) Falls and fall-related injuries in older dialysis patients. Clin J Am Soc Nephrol 1:1197–1204
14. Nelson JM (2001) Vitamin B12 deficiency in the elderly. A major contributor to falls. Adv Nurse Pract 9:39–41
15. Kuritzky L, Espay AJ, Gelblum J, Payne R, Dietrich E (2015) Diagnosing and treating neurogenic orthostatic hypotension in primary care. Postgrad Med 127(7):702–715
16. Amboni M, Barone P, Hausdorff JM (2013) Cognitive contributions to gait and falls: evidence and implications. Mov Disord 28(11):1520–1533
17. Phu S, Boersma D, Duque G (2015) Exercise and sarcopenia. J Clin Densitom 18:488–492
18. Johnson K, Suriyaarachchi P, Kakkat M, Boersma D, Gunawardene P, Demontiero O, Tannenbaum C, Duque G (2015) Yield and cost-effectiveness of laboratory testing to identify metabolic contributors to falls and fractures in older persons. Arch Osteoporos 10:226
19. Huo YR, Suriyaarachchi P, Gomez F, Curcio CL, Boersma D, Gunawardene P, Demontiero O, Duque G (2015) Comprehensive nutritional status in sarco-osteoporotic older fallers. J Nutr Health Aging 19:474–480
20. Huo YR, Suriyaarachchi P, Gomez F, Curcio CL, Boersma D, Muir SW, Montero-Odasso M, Gunawardene P, Demontiero O, Duque G (2015) Phenotype of osteosarcopenia in older individuals with a history of falling. J Am Med Dir Assoc 16:290–295
21. Sanders KM, Scott D, Ebeling PR (2014) Vitamin D deficiency and its role in muscle-bone interactions in the elderly. Curr Osteoporos Rep 12:74–81

Chapter 7
Adverse Events and Falls

Shirley C.C. Huang and Alan J. Forster

Abstract Falls are a leading cause of fatal and nonfatal unintentional injuries among older people. Adverse events are often due to errors that may be preventable and have been well documented in hospitalized patients, in home care, and in nursing homes. Elderly patients are more vulnerable to sustaining an injury after an in-hospital fall, and these falls in general can be prevented. Medications are important risk factors for falls, and medication errors which result in falls are potentially preventable. Adverse drug events (ADEs) are defined as injuries resulting from medical intervention related to a drug. Older patients are four times as likely to develop ADEs as younger patients, and about half of ADEs are preventable. Falls may not only indicate the presence of "something wrong" in an older person (owing to the often multifactorial etiology of falls and atypical presentation of illnesses in the elderly), it can also signal a failure in the healthcare system resulting in decreased patient safety. Therefore, some falls in the geriatric population may be preventable. This chapter will present the total impact of falls and the role of medication use that contribute to falls. Understanding these factors is a crucial first step toward successful prevention of falls.

Abbreviations

ADE	Adverse drug event
AE	Adverse event
CI	Confidence interval
DAD	Discharge abstract database
MHRS	Mental health reporting system
NACRS	National ambulatory care reporting system

S.C.C. Huang, MD, MSc, FRCPC (✉)
Division of Geriatric Medicine, The Ottawa Hospital,
Ottawa, ON, Canada
e-mail: shhuang@toh.ca

A.J. Forster, MD, MSc, FRCPC
Department of Medicine, Ottawa Hospital Research Institute, University of Ottawa,
Ottawa, ON, Canada

© Springer International Publishing Switzerland 2016
A.R. Huang, L. Mallet (eds.), *Medication-related falls in older people*,
DOI 10.1007/978-3-319-32304-6_7

PFF	Proximal femoral fracture
RAI-HC	Resident assessment instrument for home care
SD	Standard deviation
WHO	World Health Organization

7.1 Introduction

In "To err is human: building a safer health system" published by the Institute of Medicine, it was estimated that more people die as a result of medical errors in a given year than from motor vehicle accidents, breast cancer, or AIDS [1]. In addition, it pointed out that more people die of medication errors alone on a yearly basis than workplace injuries, highlighting it as an important source of error [1]. The report served to put the spotlight on the importance and impact of patient safety issues and made several recommendations that target various levels of the healthcare community with the goal of improving patient safety. Since the publication of this report, there has been growing research, quality improvement efforts, and financial commitment from governments and the healthcare community to improve the safety of healthcare [2]. As a result, we have a developing understanding of the nature of adverse events in various healthcare settings and patient populations and of the strategies that may decrease these events and improve patient safety.

As one of the top "Geriatric Syndromes," falls have been well described in the literature as a leading cause of fatal and nonfatal unintentional injuries among people aged 65 and over [3]. In "To err is human," "safety" is defined as freedom from accidental injury [1]. As such, falls are clearly a safety issue in this population. When falls occur in the healthcare setting, they may constitute a patient safety concern and may be the result of an adverse event (AE) (i.e., injuries caused by medical management or complication rather than by the underlying disease itself, and ones that result in either prolonged healthcare, disability at the time of discharge from care, or both [4]) (Fig. 7.1).

This chapter will first summarize the overall impact of falls in the elderly population and in society as a whole and then provide an overview of the current literature on adverse events in general, adverse events in the elderly patient, and how falls and medications can play a role in resulting in adverse events in seniors.

7.2 Falls: A Preventable Public Health Crisis

Up to 30 % of seniors experience one or more falls each year [5], and about 10–15 % of falls can lead to serious injuries such as hip fractures and head injuries [3]. Aside from physical injuries, falls can lead to loss of confidence, reduced mobility and independence [6], admission to hospital [7], increased risk of admission to a nursing home [8] and even death [3]. As a result of these observations, falls in seniors are becoming an international challenge.

Falls in the elderly are a growing problem from the perspectives of their prevalence and their cost to seniors and society. With respect to prevalence, due to

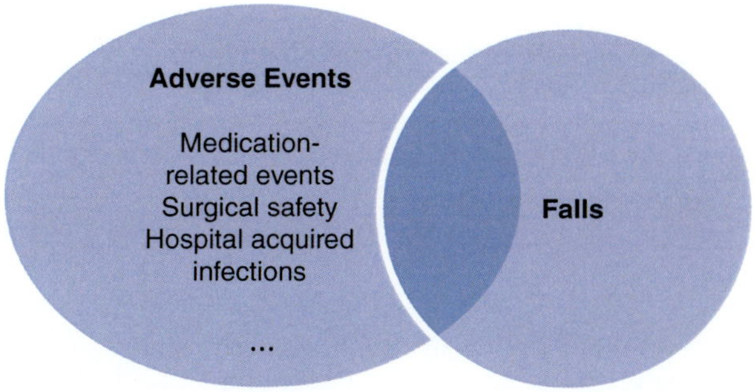

Fig. 7.1 When falls occur in the healthcare setting, they may constitute adverse events

advancements in medical sciences and improvements in social determinants of health, the numbers and proportions of older people are rising in most developed countries but also in many developing countries [3]. With increasing age, it has been shown that the relative rates of falls increased 5 % per year with cohort aging [9], and the higher rates of recurrent falling occur in the oldest-old (75 %) [10].

With respect to costs, not only do falls result in serious negative consequences in the health of many seniors, they also result in considerable economic burden. In Canada, falls account for 85 % of seniors' injury-related hospitalization, 95 % of all hip fractures, and $2 billion a year in direct healthcare costs [5]. In the United Kingdom (UK) in 1999, the rates of accident and emergency department attendance per 10,000 population for unintentional falls for those aged 60 and over and percentage admitted to hospital were 273.5 (12.6 %), and these numbers increase with increasing age [7]. The total cost of falls in the UK population aged 60 years and over was £981 million, and the highest overall cost component was attributed to inpatient admission, followed by long-term care [7]. In the United States (USA), about three-fourths of deaths due to falls occur in the 13 % of the population 65 years and over, and of those admitted to hospital after a fall, only about 50 % will be alive in 1 year [11]. The fall-related costs have been estimated at 1.5 % of the total healthcare expenditures in the USA, which corresponded to 0.2 % of the gross domestic product [12].

There have been many studies published looking into falls prevention strategies. Some studies have looked at the benefits of single interventions targeted toward specific fall risk factors (e.g., first-eye cataract surgery decreases falls in the visually impaired elderly) and others looked at multifaceted interventions that target multiple risk factors [13]. Many interventions have been found to reduce falls. For instance, individualized multifactorial interventions have been shown to decrease fall rates by 25–31 % [13]. Therefore, even though falls are significant problems for seniors and society in general, they are preventable to some degree, provided that appropriate evidence-based strategies are employed.

7.3 Adverse Events in the General Population

AEs may be unavoidable risks that can be associated with healthcare management, but often they are due to errors that may be preventable, which if better understood, can become foci of healthcare quality improvement efforts to improve patient safety (see Very Important Point). This section will provide a brief overview of what is known about AEs in the general population.

Very Important Point (VIP)
Common Adverse Events and Examples

1. Adverse drug event: For example, wrong dose of drug administered to patient resulting in morbidity
2. Surgical adverse event: For example, postoperative discovery of a surgical tool left inside the patient
3. Hospital-acquired infections: For example, patient developing urinary tract infection after insertion of a Foley catheter
4. Diagnostic error: For example, a diagnostic test performed on the wrong body part of the patient
5. System problem: For example, delays in elective surgery resulted in worsening symptoms in patient while waiting for surgery

Baker and colleagues published in 2004 *The Canadian Adverse Events Study*, where they sampled hospitals of various sizes across five provinces in Canada, in order to describe the incidence of AEs in hospitals in this country [14]. Using the random sample chart review protocol developed by the Harvard Medical Practice Study published in 1991, Baker and colleagues [14] found that the AE rate was 7.5 per 100 hospital admissions (95 % confidence interval [CI] 5.7–9.3). Of the AEs, 36.9 % (95 % CI 32.0–41.8 %) were felt to be preventable, 20.8 % (95 % CI 7.8–88.8 %) resulted in death, and of these 9 % were judged to have been preventable [14]. Therefore, the rate of preventable AEs across all hospitals studied was 2.8 per 100 admissions (95 % CI 2.0–3.6), and the rate of deaths from preventable AEs was 0.66 per 100 admissions (95 % CI 0.37–0.95) [14]. Not surprisingly, they also found that those who had an AE were significantly older than those who did not (64.9 vs. 62.0 years; $p = 0.016$) [14]. The rates of AE are somewhat comparable to those described in other countries, such as the reported 10.8 % in hospitals in the UK [15] and 10.6 % in Australia [16]. Vincent and colleagues [15] also found that patients who had an AE in UK hospitals were statistically significantly older than those who did not have an AE (median age 68.5 vs. 47.5, $p < 0.001$). Baker and colleagues [14] found that patients who had AEs had longer length of stay than those who did not suffer AEs, between 3.6 and 7.7 extra days depending on the type of hospital. The most frequently occurring AEs were associated with surgical procedures, followed by drug- or fluid-related event [14].

AEs that occurred in the ambulatory care setting have also been described. Woods and colleagues [17] looked at those AEs that occurred in the outpatient setting and resulted in hospitalization. They reported that about 11.9 % of AEs that occur in this setting led to hospitalizations, and 49.7 % of these were preventable [17]. Most of the AEs and the preventable AEs occurred in the physician's office and the emergency department [17]. The preventable AEs reported in this study include diagnostics (36.0 %), surgery (24.1 %), nonsurgical procedures (14.0 %), medication (13.1 %), and therapeutic events (12.3 %) [17].

Clearly, AEs in the general population are relatively common and potentially preventable in up to 50 % of the time. They occur in both inpatient and outpatient settings, may result in increased healthcare utilization, and are an international problem.

7.4 Adverse Events in the Elderly

Looking at AEs in the elderly population, a review of the literature showed that there is a relative paucity of research specifically designed to study the epidemiology of AEs in this group. Nonetheless, this section will summarize what is known about AEs in the elderly.

A systematic review published in 2013 by Long and colleagues attempted to look at studies that described AEs in older hospitalized medical patients [18]. They found that the AE rates in older people reported by large international adverse event studies that included patients of all ages were much lower (e.g., 5.29 % reported by Sari and colleagues [19]) than those reported by studies that were carried out to specifically document AEs in older patients (e.g., 58 % found by Lefevre and colleagues [20]). This variation is thought to be caused by the methodological differences between these study types and the fact that those that have a primary focus on the geriatric population tend to include AEs that are more common and relevant to the geriatric patient such as delirium and falls [18]. Regardless of whether the studies were designed specifically to investigate AEs in the older patient population, the signal is clear indicating that increasing age is associated with increased risk of developing an AE during hospitalization independently of disease severity and length of stay [18]. Aside from age, several other factors were found to be associated with statistically significant increased risk of AEs in the elderly, and they include functional impairment/nursing home residence, comorbidity and illness severity, being of Afro-American ethnicity and male, and having a prolonged length of stay in the emergency department [18]. In addition, over 50 % of AEs experienced by hospitalized geriatric patients are judged to be possibly preventable in the study of Lefevre and colleagues [20]. Two studies reviewed found that development of an AE is associated with increased length of stay up to twice as long as an admission without AE [18]. The types of adverse events reported can range from "geriatric syndromes" (e.g., falls and delirium), which are less likely to be detected in traditional adverse event studies, to more conventionally reported adverse events such as hospital-acquired infections and adverse drug events [18].

7.4.1 Adverse Events in the Home Care Setting

Two Canadian studies attempted to describe AEs among people of all ages who are recipients of formal or informal care at home [21, 22]. The data for these studies were gathered from available databases, including the Resident Assessment Instrument for Home Care (RAI-HC), Discharge Abstract Database (DAD), National Ambulatory Care Reporting System (NACRS), or Mental Health Reporting System (MHRS). In 2004–2005, the overall AE rate was 13.2 % [95 % CI 10.4–16.6 %] [21] and in 2008 and 2009, 12.72 % and 13.31 %, respectively [22]. The commonly documented AEs differed somewhat between these two studies, but the most common AEs in both studies were injurious falls and medication-related adverse events [21, 22]. Sears and colleagues [21] found that three factors in home care clients were significantly associated with the development of AEs: age over 65, living alone, and presence of communication difficulties due to cognitive causes. Under one-third of AEs were thought to have occurred as a result of care provided by home care workers or informal caregivers (family members or friends), but in 52.6 % (95 % CI 40.1–64.8 %) of AEs, self-care by clients was judged to have contributed to the AEs [21]. The latter point perhaps echoes the clients' decreased ability to care for themselves safely. 32.7 % of AEs were judged to be preventable, and interestingly, no significant differences were found in the preventability of AEs between those associated with care given by formal caregivers, informal caregivers, or by clients [21]. AEs in the home care setting are equally associated with deleterious consequences. Half of the AEs in the home care population studied resulted in moderate (recovery expected in 1 or more months to permanent impairment with ≤50 % disability) to serious impairment (permanent impairment with >50 % disability or death) [21].

7.4.2 Adverse Events in Long-Term Care

The studies available mostly focused on individual specific types of AEs, such as various categories of injuries, skin tears, or adverse drug events. For instance, Gurwitz and colleagues [23] attempted to describe the full range of AEs that affect the elderly in a long-term care facility. They carried out a retrospective review of resident incident reports from September 1990 to August 1991 in a 703-bed academic long-term care facility in the United States and found that 3,390 AEs were reported during this 1-year study period. The mean age of the residents in this facility was 88.5 years [23]. Out of these AEs, the most frequently reported AEs were falls (52.2 %), followed by non-fall-related injuries (41.9 %), and medication-related events (4.6 %) [23]. Van Gaal and colleagues [24] studied the concurrent incidence of pressure ulcers, urinary tract infections, and falls in 241 nursing home residents. These residents had a mean age of 78 years (SD = 10.3) [24]. The overall incidence rate of AEs was 0.09 AEs per patient week (95 % CI 0.08–0.1) [24].

Despite the relative paucity of studies targeting the elderly population, the available evidence already indicates that geriatric patients are particularly vulnerable to developing AEs in a variety of care settings. Similarly, AEs in this population are associated with increased morbidity and healthcare utilization, and some of them may be preventable. More studies specifically designed to study AEs relevant to the elderly population are needed.

7.5 Falls: A Potentially Preventable Adverse Event

The elderly population is more susceptible to falls and sustaining injuries in the event of a fall compared to the younger population due to a higher prevalence of medical comorbidities (e.g., Parkinson's disease and osteoporosis) and age-related physiological changes (e.g., changes in gait and balance). In the hospitalized elderly patients, this vulnerability is further amplified by the exacerbation of chronic health conditions or development of a new illness, increased contact with more healthcare professionals (and hence to increased possibility of human errors), and increased exposure to healthcare interventions (e.g., new tests, procedures, medications, etc.). This section will explore what is known about falls as AEs in the elderly population.

7.5.1 Rate of Falls as an AE in the Elderly

In English and Welsh hospitals, falls account for 32.3 % of all patient safety incidents; most of these were in acute care hospitals [25]. The mean standardized rates of falls per 1,000-bed days range from 2.1 in mental health units to 8.4 in community hospitals, and 82.6 % of falls occurred in people 65 years of age and over and 67.5 % in those over 75 years old [25]. Not surprisingly, when compared with occupied bed days by age, those over 85 years of age are the most vulnerable group for falls [25]. Most of the falls did not result in any injury, roughly one-third resulted in minor harm and 5 % resulted in moderate harm (e.g., requiring surgery or prolonged stay in hospital), severe harm (brain damage or permanent disability), or death [25]. In the USA, the fall rate has been reported as 3.56 falls/1,000 patient days in 1 study and about 1 in 10 resulted in moderate injury, less than 1 in 20 had major injuries (required surgery or neurology consult), and 2 in 1,000 injurious falls caused death [26]. The highest total fall and injurious fall rates occurred in medical units and lowest in surgery units [26]. However, the proportion of falls that occurred in patients 65 years and older was not reported in this study. In a German academic teaching hospital, the fall rate was reported as 10.0 per 1,000 hospital days, and the mean age of the patients was 80.3 [standard deviation (SD) = 8.7] [27].

7.5.2 Vulnerability to In-Hospital Fall-Related Injuries and Poor Outcomes

Elderly patients are more vulnerable to sustaining an injury after an in-hospital fall. Some studies have shown that there is a 19 % increased risk of fall-related injury for each added decade of age [28]. Fall-related injuries have been shown to have more severe consequences in in-hospital fallers than in community fallers. Murray and colleagues [29] collected data from hospital medical records and incident reports of all patients aged 75 and older who had falls resulting in a proximal femoral fracture (PFF) while hospitalized in one of nine public hospitals in a region of Australia. These subjects were matched (according to gender, age, and fracture date) with subjects who were admitted to hospital but had sustained their PFF after a fall in the community [29]. They found that the patients who sustained their PFF during a fall in hospital had a higher mean Charlson comorbidity index score owing to comorbidities acquired during their hospital stay [29]. They found that subjects with hospital-acquired PFF are more likely to die in the hospital ($p=0.03$), to be discharged to long-term nursing care facilities ($p=0.02$), and less likely to return to preadmission activity of daily living status ($p<0.001$) and ambulation ($p=0.004$) [29]. The median length of stay for this population was much longer, 46 days compared to 32 days for subject with PFF acquired in the community [29].

7.5.3 Falls in Home Care and Long-Term Care Settings

One study found that injurious falls accounted for 24.6 % of AEs in home care clients in Ontario, Canada, and 40 % of these resulted in fractures and 60 % resulted in lacerations or tissue injuries [21]. In the nursing home setting, Gurwitz and colleagues [23] found that the most common AEs in their study in nursing home residents were falls, but the majority of falls did not result in any injury. They found that under one-third resulted in minor injuries and 3 % resulted in a fracture [23]. Interestingly, the annual incidence of falls per 100 beds in this study varied according to resident care level and time of day. For instance, the rates were highest for semi-dependent (393 falls/100 beds) followed by dependent (269 falls/100 beds), and independent care residents (155 falls/100 beds) [23]. As for the association with time of day, the highest annual incidence rate of falls for semi-dependent residents occurred during the 6–8 am and the 6–8 pm time periods presumably when the highest density of care activities (e.g., assistance for transfers) were occurring [23]. In comparison, the highest incidence rate of falls for independent residents occurred during noon to 2 pm time period, likely when these residents are physically more active [23]. The former finding puts into question whether and how many of these falls during these times of potentially high care density would have been preventable. Unfortunately the study did not attempt to address this important question.

The annual incidence of fall-related injuries also varied according to resident care level and time of day and mirrors the trend seen for falls [23]. Some studies have reported a higher hip fracture incidence in home care clients than that reported for other community-dwelling populations (24.4 per 1,000 person-years of follow-up vs. 5.7 per 1,000 person-years) [30, 31]. The hip fracture incidence in these home care clients was similar to that reported for nursing home residents (23.0 per 1,000 person-years) [31]. These differences probably reflect the inherent variation in the health and functional status among these geriatric populations. It is not difficult to infer that those seniors who require home care or nursing home residence likely have functional impairment for various reasons affecting their ability to live independently, such as significant medical comorbidities, impaired mobility, cognitive impairment, and more advanced age, all of which are also characteristics that have been shown in the literature to increase one's risk for adverse events in care settings and falls.

7.5.4 Fall Prevention in Healthcare Setting

Several studies have shown that falls in the acute care setting can be prevented [32, 33]. For instance, von Renteln-Kruse and colleagues [27] looked at the effect of an inpatient fall prevention program on the incidence of falls and fall-related injuries. They showed that their prevention program was effective in reducing the rate of falls to 8.2 per 1,000 hospital days ($p<0.001$) from 10.0 per 1,000 hospital days, indicating that falls are preventable [27]. Unfortunately the fall prevention program did not significantly reduce the total number of injurious falls (26.9 % before and 27.6 % after introduction of prevention program) [27], perhaps indicating the inherent increased vulnerability of sustaining an injury after a fall in the hospitalized elderly. Another study found that a multi-intervention fall prevention program can decrease the number of falls by 30 % ($p=0.045$) and fall-related injuries by 28 % when compared to usual care in three subacute wards used for the rehabilitation and care of the elderly [34]. In care facilities, a Cochrane review found that multifactorial interventions can result in reduced rate of falls (rate ratio of 0.78, 95 % CI 0.59–1.04) and risk of falling (risk ratio of 0.89, 95 % CI 0.77–1.02) in this setting after looking at pooled data from seven trials (2,876 participants), but this evidence was not conclusive [33]. However, using pooled data from five studies (4,603 participants), vitamin D supplementation in care facilities has been shown to reduce the rate of falls (rate ratio of 0.63, 95 % CI 0.46–0.86) in elderly residents with vitamin D deficiency [33].

In summary, currently available literature has demonstrated that falls as AEs in the elderly population are common, potentially preventable, and result in more morbidity and higher healthcare utilization than falls that occur in the community. These findings further highlight the importance of falls in the healthcare setting as a significant patient safety issue for geriatric patients and the healthcare system.

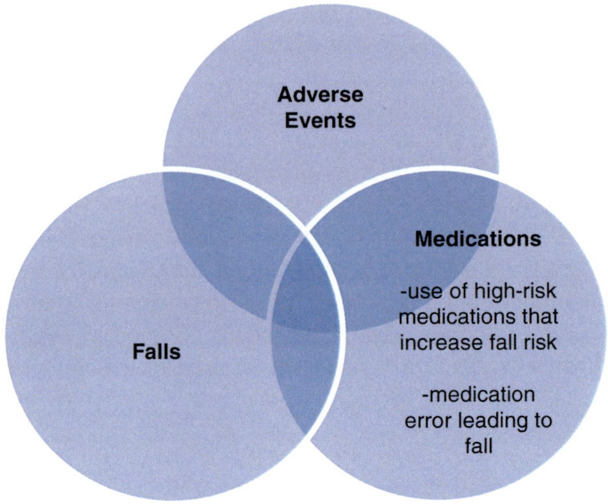

Fig. 7.2 Adverse events can independently involve falls and medication errors, but medication-related adverse event can also result in falls

7.6 Adverse Drug Events and Falls

The risk factors for falls are often multifactorial, and they can be generally categorized into intrinsic factors (e.g., age, neurocardiovascular conditions), which may be less modifiable, and extrinsic factors (e.g., use of high-risk medications such as benzodiazepines and antidepressants, environmental hazards), which may be modifiable [35, 36, 37]. Medications are particularly important as risk factors for falls not only because they are modifiable but also because medication-related falls may be caused by medication errors and thus potentially preventable. Indeed, medication-related AEs are one of the most common AEs in hospitalized patients [14]. As a result, it is not difficult to imagine that a complex interplay between medications and falls may exist (Fig. 7.2). This section will examine what is known about adverse drug events and their relationship to falls in elderly patients.

7.6.1 Epidemiology of Adverse Drug Events

Adverse drug events (ADEs) are defined as injuries resulting from medical intervention related to a drug [38]. Studies have shown that ADEs in care settings in the general population are common. In a prospective cohort study, Bates and colleagues found that in two tertiary care hospitals over a 6-month study period, ADE rates were 6.5 ADEs and 5.5 potential ADEs per 100 non-obstetrical admissions, and there were 7.3 preventable ADEs and potential ADEs combined per 100 admissions [38]. Up to 42 % of life-threatening and serious ADEs were deemed preventable [38]. Interestingly not all ADEs can be classified as an adverse event as defined by the WHO, as they may not have resulted in "prolonged healthcare, disability at the time of discharge from care or both" [4]. Bates and colleagues found that only 7.7 % of the ADEs met the WHO definition for AEs, and 37 % of these were preventable [38]. The most common drugs associated with ADEs in this study were analgesic drugs such as opioids (30 %) and antibiotics (24 %) [38]. With regard to preventable ADEs, 46 % were due to analgesics, sedatives, and antipsychotics combined, and the primary error occurred in the prescribing stage in nearly 50 % of events [38]. Classen and colleagues found that ADEs complicated 2.43 per 100 hospital admissions in their study population [39]. Not only do ADEs and preventable ADEs increase length of stay (by 2.2 days and 4.6 days, respectively) [40], they also increase risk of death by 1.88 fold (95 % CI 1.54–2.22) [39] and lead to excess healthcare costs ($5.6 million due to ADEs and $2.8 million due to preventable ADEs for a 700-bed teaching hospital in the USA) [40].

7.6.2 ADEs and the Falling Elderly Patient

Geriatric patients are four times as likely to develop ADEs as younger patients, and about 50 % of ADEs are preventable [41]. It is commonly recognized that the geriatric patient may not present typically when experiencing an ADE, but rather, the presence of an ADE may be heralded by the emergence of a "Geriatric Syndrome" such as falls or delirium [41]. Wierenga and colleagues studied geriatric patients newly admitted to a medicine ward during a study period of more than 3-years to a tertiary teaching hospital in Amsterdam and found that delirium was present at admission in 25.9 % of patients, a fall occurred prior to admission in 12 % of cases, and 5.4 % of patients had both. In their study, ADEs involving antidiabetics, antidepressants, antihypertensives, and antipsychotics were related to over 50 % of the falls [41]. Interestingly, in the multivariate logistic regression analysis, a preadmission fall and diuretic use were independently associated with an ADE-related hospital admission [41]. Unfortunately, they did not comment on the preventability of the ADE-associated falls. Chan and colleagues from Australia carried out a prospective, cross-sectional study in an acute care hospital looking at ADEs as potential causes of unplanned hospital admissions for seniors and whether they might have been preventable [42]. They found that up to 30.4 % of admissions may have been due to ADEs, and of these 53.4 % were judged to be definitely preventable [42]. The most common ADEs were falls and falls associated with postural hypotension (24 %), followed by heart failure (16.8 %), and delirium (14.4 %) [42].

7.6.3 ADEs and the Elderly in Ambulatory Care

Gurwitz and colleagues carried out a cohort study using all geriatric Medicare enrollees that attend a multispecialty group practice during a 1-year period [43]. They found that the overall rate of ADE was 50.1 per 1,000 person-years, and the rate of preventable ADE was 13.8 events per 1,000 person-years [43]. Over one-third were deemed to be serious, life threatening, or fatal, and more of these were deemed preventable compared to those ADEs that were less severe [43]. The most common errors associated with preventable ADEs occurred during prescribing (58.4 %) and monitoring (60.8 %), and the most common drugs implicated in preventable ADEs were cardiovascular drugs (24.5 %) and diuretics (22.1 %) [43]. Of all the ADEs reported in this study, falls with or without injury accounted for 1.5 %, and more of them were deemed preventable than non-preventable [43].

7.6.4 ADEs and the Elderly in Long-Term Care

Gurwitz and colleagues found that the annual incidence for adverse medication-related events in a single facility studied is 26 per 100 beds, and of these events, errors in dosing and administration were more prevalent than adverse drug reactions (72.2 % vs. 27.8 %), presumably indicating that most of these events might have been preventable [23]. Gurwitz and colleagues later published another study looking at all long-term care residents in Massachusetts, which included 18 nursing homes, and the incidence of adverse drug events in a cohort study [44]. The mean age of the study population was 84 ± 9 years. They found that the rate of adverse drug events was 1.89 per 100 resident-months, and the rate of preventable adverse drug events was 0.96 per 100 resident-months. The rate of potential adverse drug events was 0.65 per 100 resident-months [44]. Seventy-two percent of the fatal, life-threatening, or serious adverse drug events were deemed preventable, and the preventable adverse drug events were more likely to result in disability when compared to non-preventable adverse drug events (relative risk = 2.4, 95 % CI 1.2–4.7, $p<0.01$) [44]. Neuropsychiatric events (e.g., oversedation, delirium) were the most common types of both preventable and non-preventable adverse drug events, and falls occurred in 20 % of preventable adverse drug events but only 4 % of non-preventable events [44]. Once again, medication prescribing errors (68 %) and monitoring errors (70 %) were the most common causes of preventable events [44].

In summary, ADEs are relatively common, are preventable to some degree, and are associated with increased morbidity, mortality, and healthcare expenditure. Not only is the elderly population more likely to develop ADEs than other adults, ADEs can contribute to falls and thus to the negative consequences associated with falls in this population.

7.7 Conclusion

Regardless of the contributing etiologies or the locations where they occur, falls pose a significant challenge that is unique to the geriatric population, the people who care for them, and the healthcare system as a whole. The occurrence of falls may not only indicate the presence of "something wrong" in an older person (owing to the often multifactorial etiology of falls and atypical presentation of illnesses in the elderly), it can also signal a failure in the healthcare system resulting in decreased patient safety especially when looking at the various roles medications and other care interventions can play in increasing fall risk. Furthermore, falls in the geriatric population may be preventable. The task to reduce fall risk and fall-related injuries is no small feat, but it is certainly a worthwhile challenge for care providers and policy makers. Understanding the total impact of falls and the roles healthcare interventions such as medications can play in contributing to falls in the elderly is a crucial first step toward successful prevention of falls.

References

1. Kohn LT, Corrigan JM, Donaldson MS (eds) (2000) To err is human: building a safer health system. National Academy Press, Washington, DC
2. Forster AJ, Dervin G, Martin C et al (2012) Improving patient safety through the systematic evaluation of patient outcomes. Can J Surg 55:418–425
3. Peel NM (2011) Epidemiology of falls in older age. Can J Aging 30(1):7–19
4. World Health Organization (WHO) (2008) The conceptual framework for the international classification for patient safety. Version 1.0. World Health Organization (WHO), Geneva
5. Seniors' falls in Canada second report (2014) Public Health Agency of Canada. Available via Public Health Agency of Canada. http://www.phac-aspc.gc.ca/seniors-aines/publications/public/injury-blessure/seniors_falls-chutes_aines/assets/pdf/seniors_falls-chutes_aines-eng.pdf. Accessed 13 May 2015
6. Huang AR, Mallet L, Rochefort CM et al (2012) Medication-related falls in the elderly. Causative factors and preventive strategies. Drugs Aging 29(5):359–376
7. Scuffham P, Chaplin S, Legood R (2003) Incidence and costs of unintentional falls in older people in the United Kingdom. J Epidemiol Community Health 57:740–744
8. Tinetti ME, Williams CS (1997) Falls, injuries due to falls, and the risk of admission to a nursing home. N Engl J Med 337:1279–1284
9. Anstey KJ, Burns R, von Sanden C et al (2008) Psychological well-being is an independent predictor of falling in an 8-year follow-up of older adults. J Gerontol B Psychol Sci Soc Sci 63(4):249–257
10. Fleming J, Matthews FE, Brayne C, Cambridge City over-75s Cohort Study Collaboration (2008) Falls in advanced old age: recalled falls and prospective follow-up of over-90-year-olds in the Cambridge City over-75s Cohort study. BMC Geriatr 8(6):1–11
11. Rubenstein LZ (2006) Falls in older people: epidemiology, risk factors and strategies for prevention. Age Ageing 35–S2:ii37–ii41
12. Stevens JA, Corso PS, Finkelstein EA et al (2006) The costs of fatal and non-fatal falls among older adults. Inj Prev 12:290–295
13. Karlsson MK, Magnusson H, von Schewelov T et al (2013) Prevention of falls in the elderly – a review. Osteoporos Int 24:747–762
14. Baker GR, Norton PG, Flintoft V et al (2004) The Canadian Adverse Events Study: the incidence of adverse events among hospital patients in Canada. CMAJ 170:1678–1686
15. Vincent C, Neale G, Woloshynowych M (2001) Adverse events in British hospitals: preliminary retrospective record review. BMJ 322:517–519
16. Thomas EJ, Studdert DM, Runciman WB et al (2000) A comparison of iatrogenic injury studies in Australia and the USA. I: context, methods, casemix, population, patient and hospital characteristics. International J Qual Health Care 12:371–378

17. Woods DM, Thomas EJ, Holl JL et al (2007) Ambulatory care adverse events and preventable adverse events leading to a hospital admission. Qual Saf Health Care 16:127–131
18. Long SJ, Brown KF, Ames D et al (2013) What is known about adverse events in older medical hospital inpatients? A systematic review of the literature. Int J Qual Health Care 25:542–554
19. Sari AB, Cracknell A, Sheldon TA (2008) Incidence, preventability and consequences of adverse events in older people: results of a retrospective case-note review. Age Ageing 37:265–269
20. Lefevre F, Feinglass J, Potts S et al (1992) Iatrogenic complications in high-risk, elderly patients. Arch Intern Med 152:2074–2080
21. Sears N, Baker GR, Barnsley J et al (2013) The incidence of adverse events among home care patients. Int J Qual Health Care 25:16–28
22. Doran DM, Hirdes JP, Blais R et al (2013) Adverse events among Ontario home care clients associated with emergency room visit or hospitalization: a retrospective cohort study. BMC Health Serv Res 13(227):1–9
23. Gurwitz JH, Sanchez-Cross MT, Eckler MA et al (1994) The epidemiology of adverse and unexpected events in the long-term care setting. JAGS 42:33–38
24. Van Gaal BGI, Schoonhoven L, Mintjes-de Groot JAJ et al (2014) Concurrent incidence of adverse events in hospitals and nursing homes. J Nurs Scholarsh 46:187–198
25. Healey F, Scobie S, Oliver D et al (2008) Falls in English and Welsh hospitals: a national observational study based on retrospective analysis of 12 months of patient safety incident reports. Qual Saf Health Care 17:424–430
26. Bouldin ELD, Andresen EM, Dunton NE et al (2013) Falls among adult patients hospitalized in the United States: prevalence and trends. J Patient Saf 9:13–17
27. Von Renteln-Kruse W, Krause T, Geogr D (2007) Incidence of in-hospital falls in geriatric patients before and after the introduction of an interdisciplinary team-based fall-prevention intervention. JAGS 55:2068–2074
28. Cumbler E, Likosky D (2011) In-hospital falls: evaluation and response. Contin Lifelong Learn Neurol 17:1063–1076
29. Murray GR, Cameron ID, Cumming RG (2007) The consequences of falls in acute and sub-acute hospitals in Australia that cause proximal femoral fractures. JAGS 55:577–582
30. Stolee P, Poss J, Cook RJ et al (2009) Risk factors for hip fracture in older home care clients. J Gerontol A Biol Sci Med Sci 64:403–410
31. Sugarman JR, Connell FA, Hansen A et al (2002) Hip fracture incidence in nursing home residents and community-dwelling older people, Washington State, 1993–1995. JAGS 50:1638–1643
32. Stern C, Jayasekara R (2009) Interventions to reduce the incidence of falls in older adult patients in acute-care hospitals: a systematic review. Int J Evid Based Healthc 7:243–249
33. Cameron ID, Gillespie LD, Robertson CM et al (2012) Interventions for preventing falls in older people in care facilities and hospitals. Cochrane Database Syst Rev 12 DOI: 10.1002/14651858.CD005465.pub3
34. Haines TP, Bennell KL, Osborne RH et al (2004) Effectiveness of targeted falls prevention programme in subacute hospital setting: randomized controlled trial. BMJ 328:676
35. Clyburn TA, Heydemann JA (2011) Fall prevention in the elderly: analysis and comprehensive review of methods used in the hospital and in the home. J Am Acad Orthop Surg 19:402–409
36. Hartikainen S, Lönnroos E, Louhivuori K (2007) Medication as a risk factor for falls: critical systematic review. J Gerontol: Med Sci 62A:1172–1181
37. Kwan E, Straus SE (2014) Assessment and management of falls in older people. CMAJ 186:E610–E621
38. Bates DW, Cullen DJ, Laird N et al (1995) Incidence of adverse drug events and potential adverse drug events. JAMA 274:29–34
39. Classen DC, Pestotnik SL, Evans RS et al (1997) Adverse drug events in hospitalized patients. JAMA 277:301–306

40. Bates DW, Spell N, Cullen DJ et al (1997) The costs of adverse drug events in hospitalized patients. JAMA 277:307–311
41. Wierenga PC, Buurman BM, Parlevliet JL et al (2012) Association between acute geriatric syndromes and medication-related hospital admissions. Drugs Aging 29:691–699
42. Chan M, Nicklason F, Vial JH (2001) Adverse drug events as a cause of hospital admission in the elderly. Int Med J 31:199–205
43. Gurwitz JH, Field TS, Harrold LR et al (2003) Incidence and preventability of adverse drug events among older person in the ambulatory setting. JAMA 289:1107–1116
44. Gurwitz JH, Field TS, Avorn J et al (2000) Incidence and preventability of adverse drug events in nursing homes. Am J Med 109:87–94

Chapter 8
Risk Factors for Falls in the Elderly

E. Kwan, S. Straus, and J. Holroyd-Leduc

Abstract Falls can have significant impact on older adults including fractures and decreased quality of life. Individuals who are 65 years and older have a 30 % chance of falling per year, and this increases up to 37 % in those 80 years or older. In the community-dwelling older adult, various risk factors can contribute to falling. This chapter reviews the literature on risk factors for falling.

This chapter focuses on high-quality systematic reviews including adults aged 60 years and older. Reviews were assessed using A Measurement Tool to Assess Systematic Reviews (AMSTAR) and rated as high quality if they scored 7 or more out of 11. Thirteen systematic reviews were included. When assessing an older adult for falls, risk factors that encompasses extrinsic and intrinsic factors should be considered.

Abbreviations

ADL	Activities of daily living
AMSTAR	A measurement tool to assess systematic reviews
CI	Confidence interval
OR	Odds ratio
RR	Relative risk

8.1 Introduction

Falls cause serious injuries (e.g., fractures, brain contusions, subdural hematoma) and impact on quality of life for older adults [1, 2]. The definition of a risk factor for falling can be somewhat difficult to label. This can lead to problems in gathering

E. Kwan, MD, FRCPC (✉) • S. Straus, MD, MSc, FRCPC, HBSc
Section of Geriatrics, Department of Medicine, University of Calgary, Calgary, AB, Canada
e-mail: emily.kwan@ahs.ca

J Holroyd-Leduc, MD, FRCPC
Division of Geriatrics, Department of Medicine, University of Toronto, Toronto, ON, Canada

© Springer International Publishing Switzerland 2016
A.R. Huang, L. Mallet (eds.), *Medication-related falls in older people*,
DOI 10.1007/978-3-319-32304-6_8

data on risk factors [3]. There is no convention in defining fall risk factors. Take the case of a stroke that results in a gait abnormality, which then leads to a fall [3]. Should both stroke and gait abnormalities be considered risk factors for falls [3]? Overall, this can lead to contradictory results given there are so many ways to measure and look at fall risk factors [3].

One method to classify fall risk factors is to consider them as intrinsic or extrinsic. Intrinsic risk factors look at specific causes within an individual person, whereas extrinsic risk factors are those factors that are extrinsic to the individual [4]. Examples of intrinsic factors include age, gait and balance issues, and other neurological issues such as cognitive impairment. Extrinsic risk factors include medications and environmental hazards such as rugs and stairs [4, 5]. Extrinsic risk factors tend to be more modifiable. Another method for classifying fall risk factors includes the following categories: sociodemographic, balance/mobility, sensory/neuromuscular, psychological, medical, medications, and environmental factors [5].

More than 100 risk factors for falls have been identified in the literature. However, this chapter will focus on evidence-based risk factors that have been identified in high-quality systematic reviews (defined as ≥7 on A Measurement Tool to Assess Systematic Reviews (AMSTAR)) [6].

8.2 Search Strategy

A comprehensive search of the literature including MEDLINE, CINAHL, EMBASE, and COCHRANE was conducted from 2005 to March 2015. The following terms were used in the search: "falls," "accidental falls," "aged," "geriatric," "elderly," "senior," "old age," "risk factor," and "older adult." Additional articles were identified through review of reference lists of included articles and discussions with experts.

Only systematic reviews were considered for inclusion. The specific inclusion criteria were as follows: patients with average age of 60 years and greater, description of a risk factor associated with falls, and English language publications, published between 2005 and March 2015.

The systematic reviews on risk factors were assessed using the A Measurement Tool to Assess Systematic Reviews [6]. If multiple articles were identified on a topic, only those that were rated as high quality (defined as a score of 7 or more out of 11) were included.

8.3 Risk Factors of Falls

All risk factors mentioned in this chapter are also found in Table 8.1 and can be elicited in a comprehensive history with the patient.

Table 8.1 Risk factors for falls

Risk factors	Studies	Study quality	Number included (study design)	Results
Intrinsic risk factors				
Age	Ganz et al. [3]	8	19,178 (prospective studies)	Three studies reported LR (11 studies found):
				Risk was similar in two studies: for patients aged 65 through 74 years, the fall probability was 31–32 %; for those aged 70 through 74 years, 22–33 %; for those aged 75 through 79 years, 25–36 %; and for those 80 years or older, 34–37 %
				The third study found a statistically increased risk of falling at least once in the next 11 months among older patients (odds ratio per age category, 1.90; *P* 0.001): aged 65 through 69 years, the fall probability was 14 %; aged 70 through 74 years, 16 %; aged 75 through 79 years, 24 %; and aged 80 years and older, 34 %
				OR 1.00 (95 % CI, 1.00–1.01) and OR 0.86 (0.80–0.93) for multivariate analysis – in nursing home residents
				OR 1.04 (95 % CI, 1.01–1.06) (for a 5 year increase in age of hospital inpatient) and OR 1.06 (95 % CI, 1.00–1.13) in the multivariate analysis subgroup
	Deandrea et al. [7]	7	Varied sample size of 215–34,163 (prospective studies)	
Sex (female)	Deandrea et al. [7]	7	Varied sample size of 215–34,163 (prospective studies)	OR 1.00 (0.85–1.17) – nursing home residents
				OR 0.84 (0.64–1.11) overall, OR 0.72 (0.37–1.40) multivariate analysis – hospital inpatient
Previous falls	Ganz et al. [3]	8	19,178 (prospective studies)	4 studies reported LR (11 studies found in total): fall in the past year (LR range, 2.3–2.8)
	Deandrea et al. [7]	7	Varied sample size of 215–34,163 (prospective studies)	OR 3.06 (95 % CI, 2.12–4.41) (in nursing home residents)
				OR 2.85 (95 % CI, 1.14–7.15) and a multivariate subgroup
				OR 3.74 (95 % CI, 1.48–9.42) – hospital inpatients

(continued)

Table 8.1 (continued)

Risk factors	Studies	Study quality	Number included (study design)	Results
Balance impairment	Muir et al. [9]	8	60,602 (prospective studies)	Overall fall risk of OR of 1.98 (1.60, 2.46)
Gait and impairment of walking difficulty	Ganz et al. [7]	8	19,178 (prospective studies)	4 studies reported LR (15 studies found): clinically detected abnormality of gait or balance (LR range, 1.7–2.4)
Functional limitations, ADL disabilities	Ganz et al. [7]	8	19,178 (prospective studies)	2 studies reported LR (10 studies found):
				Inability to rise from a chair of knee height without using the chair arms was associated with an increased risk of 1 or more falls among men (LR 4.3; 95 % CI, 2.3–7.9)
				5 or more of 11 physical impairments (mostly activities of daily living) was associated with an increased risk of 1 or more falls (LR 1.9; 95 % CI, 1.4–2.6)
Functional limitations, ADL disabilities	Bloch et al. [10]	8	19,178 (RCT, observational studies (included cohort studies, case-control studies, and cross-sectional studies))	OR 2.26 (95 % CI, 2.09, 2.45) for disturbance in ADL and OR 2.10 (95 % CI, 1.68, 2.64) for IADL
	Deandrea et al. [7]	7	Varied sample size of 215–34,163 (prospective studies)	Moderate disability: OR 1.67 (95 % CI, 1.00–2.80) – nursing home residents
Medical condition	Deandrea et al. [7]	7	Varied sample size of 215–34,163 (prospective studies)	OR 2.08 (95 % CI, 1.88–2.31) – in nursing home residents
Parkinson's disease	Deandrea et al. [7]	7	Varied sample size of 215–34,163 (prospective studies)	OR 1.65 (95 % CI, 1.10–2.47) overall and 2.48 (95 % CI, 1.09–5.62) multivariate – nursing home residents

(continued)

Table 8.1 (continued)

Risk factors	Studies	Study quality	Number included (study design)	Results
Cognitive impairment	Ganz et al. [3]	8	19,178 (prospective studies)	2 studied reported LR (8 studies found):
				One study found that 5 or more errors on the Short Portable Mental Status Questionnaire was associated with 1 or more falls (LR 4.2; 95 % CI, 1.9–9.6)
				Other study reported that a history of dementia was associated with 1 or more falls (LR 17; 95 % CI, 1.9-149) and with 2 or more falls (LR 13; 95 % CI, 2.3–79)
				OR 1.20 (95 % CI, 0.52–2.79) – in nursing home residents
				OR 1.52 (1.18–1.94) overall, OR 1.65 (1.25–2.18) multivariate – in hospital inpatient
	Deandrea et al. [7]	7	Varied sample size of 215–34,163 (prospective studies)	
Stroke	Deandrea et al. [7]	7	Varied sample size of 215–34,163 (prospective studies)	OR 0.93 (0.81–1.07) – in nursing home residents; not significant
Incontinence	Deandrea et al. [7]	7	Varied sample size of 215–34,163 (prospective studies)	OR 1.28 (0.95–1.71) and OR 2.00 (1.27–3.14) for multivariate in nursing home residents
Extrinsic risk factors				
Depression	Kvelde et al. [11]	8	21,455 (in all 25 studies)	14 studies: (OR 1.46; 95 % CI, 1.27–1.67) of increased falls in higher level of depressive symptoms
	Deandrea et al. [7]	7	Varied sample size of 215–34,163 (prospective studies)	OR 1.21 (0.85–1.72) – in nursing home residents
Visual impairment	Ganz et al. [3]	8	19,178 (prospective cohort studies)	OR 1.6–2.0 range but no other results
	Deandrea et al. [7]	7	Varied sample size of 215–34,163 (prospective studies)	OR 1.29; 95 % CI, 0.89–1.85 – for nursing home residents; not significant

(continued)

Table 8.1 (continued)

Risk factors	Studies	Study quality	Number included (study design)	Results
Home hazards	Letts et al. [1]	7	25,145 (cross-sectional and cohort studies)	Home hazards (i.e., bathroom, environmental – indoor and outdoor, various list of hazards)
				OR 1.15, 95 % CI, 0.997–1.36
				High-quality studies only: OR 1.38 (95 % CI, 1.03–1.87)
				Use of mobility aids significantly increased fall risk in community (OR 2.07; 95 % CI,1.59–2.71)
				Institutional (OR 1.77; 95 % CI, 1.66–1.89)
	Deandrea et al. [7]	7	Varied sample size of 215–34,163 (prospective studies)	Use of walking aid: OR 2.08 (1.88–2.31) overall and OR 1.67 (1.00–2.80) for the multivariate subgroup – for nursing home residents
Being married	Bloch et al. [10]	8	19,178 (RCT, observational studies (included cohort studies, case-control studies, and cross-sectional studies))	OR 0.68 (95 % CI, 0.53–0.87) – protective against falling
Low education level	Bloch et al. [10]	8	19,178 (RCT, observational studies (included cohort studies, case-control studies, and cross-sectional studies))	OR 0.97 95 % CI, (0.83–1.13) – not significant
Married status	Bloch et al. [10]	8	19,178 (RCT, observational studies (included cohort studies, case-control studies, and cross-sectional studies))	OR 1.04 (95 % CI, 0.94–1.15) – not significant
Confined to bed	Bloch et al. [10]	8	19,178 (RCT, observational studies (included cohort studies, case-control studies, and cross-sectional studies))	OR 0.92 (95 % CI, 0.70–1.20) – not significant

(continued)

Table 8.1 (continued)

Risk factors	Studies	Study quality	Number included (study design)	Results
Orthostatic hypotension	Ganz et al. [3]	8	19,178 (prospective studies)	4 studies found no association when other risk factors were considered. One study found a weak association between an increased pulse rate of less than 6 per minute, measured 30 s after standing up predicts falls (LR 1.4; 95 % CI, 1.0–1.9)
	Angelousi et al. [12]	8	117,398 (28 prospective studies)	Insufficient data to assess the association of orthostatic hypotension with falls
Pain	Stubbs et al. [13]	9	9,581 (in the meta-analysis)	cixRecurrent falls with pain: OR 2.04 (95 % CI, 1.75–2.39)
				Comparison of fallers to non-fallers OR 2.18 (95 % CI, 1.26–1.64) with odds higher in single fallers than non-fallers
Wandering	Deandrea et al. [7]	7	Varied sample size of 215–34,163 (prospective studies)	OR 1.87 (95 % CI,1.68–2.09) – nursing home residents
Dizziness	Deandrea et al. [7]	7	Varied sample size of 215–34,163 (prospective studies)	OR 1.52 (95 % CI, 1.33–1.74) – nursing home residents

8.3.1 Age

Increasing age has been associated with falls. One review found two studies where those who are 65–74 years of age have a fall probability of 31–32 %, while those who are 80 years old or older have a fall probability of 34–37 % [3]. Among patients in acute care hospitals, for each 5 year increase in age, there was an increase in risk of falls (odds ratio (OR) 1.04 (95 % confidence interval (CI), 1.01–1.06)) [7]. However, among individuals living in nursing homes, there was no significant association between age and falls (OR 1.00 (95 % CI, 1.00–1.01)).

8.3.2 Sex

Sex does not appear to be a risk factor for falls. In both nursing home and acute care hospitals, there was no association between falls and sex (female versus male) with OR 1.00 (95 % CI, 0.85–1.17) for nursing home residents and OR 0.84 (95 % CI, 0.64–1.11) for hospitalized inpatients [7].

8.3.3 History of Falls

Previous falls have been shown to be associated with future falls. A fall in the last year can increase the risk of other falls in the next year [3]. Both nursing home residents and hospitalized inpatients with a history of falls were more likely to fall in the future (OR 3.06 (95 % CI, 2.12–4.41); OR 2.85 (95 % CI, 1.14–7.15), respectively) [7].

8.3.4 Functional Impairment

Functional impairment is associated with falls. Impairment is defined as any abnormality, partial or complete loss, or loss of the function of a body part, organ, or system. This impairment may be due directly or secondarily to pathology or injury and may be either temporary or permanent [8]. For example, balance impairment is associated with increased risk of falls (OR 1.98 (95 % CI, 1.60–2.46)) [7, 9]. The results are found in those with inability to rise from a chair of knee height [7].

Dependence in basic activities of daily living (defined as one or more basic ADL) or instrumental activities of daily living (defined as one or more instrumental ADL) is associated with falls (OR 2.26 (95 % CI, 2.09–2.45) for ADL; OR 2.10 (95 % CI, 1.68–2.64) for IADL) [10]. Overall, moderate disability is significantly associated with falls in nursing home residents (OR 1.67 (95 % CI, 1.00–2.80)) [7].

8.3.5 Medical Conditions

Having any medical condition can increase risk of falls in nursing home residents (OR 2.08 (95 % CI, 1.88–2.31)) [7]. However, the systematic review did not clarify what medical conditions were incorporated in this conclusion. Neither stroke (OR 0.93 (95 % CI, 0.81–1.07)) nor incontinence (unsure whether it is fecal and/or urinary; OR 1.28 (95 % CI, 0.95–1.71)) has not been found to be associated with falls in the nursing home population [7]. In contrast, Parkinson's disease has been found to be associated with falls among nursing home residents (OR 1.65 (95 % CI, 1.10–2.47)) [7].

8.3.6 Cognitive Impairment

Cognitive impairment was not found to increase risk of falls in nursing home residents (OR 1.20 (95 % CI, 0.52–2.79)), but was found to be associated with falls in hospitalized inpatients (OR 1.52 (95 % CI, 1.18–1.94)) [7].

8.3.7 Depression

Patients with a higher number of depressive symptoms (various measures used with different cutoffs for highest level of depressive symptomatology including Center for Epidemiologic Studies Depression Scale, Minimum Data Set for Home Care, Mental Health Inventory, Montgomery-Asberg Depression Rating Scale, Outcome and Assessment Information Set, Symptom Checklist, Cornell Scale, and Geriatric Depressions Scale) have increased fall risk (OR 1.46 (95 % CI, 1.27–1.67) or relative risk (RR) 1.5 (95 % CI, 1.19–1.84)) compared to those with fewer symptoms [11]. However, depression does not appear to be associated with falls in the nursing home population (OR 1.21 (95 % CI, 0.85–1.72)) [7].

8.3.8 Visual Impairment

There is a trend for a higher risk of falls in community-dwelling older adults with visual impairment compared to those without (OR range from 1.6 to 2.0) [3]. However, a recent article looking at nursing home residents found that visual impairment does not significantly increase the risk of falls (OR 1.29 (95 % CI, 0.89–1.85)) [7].

8.3.9 Home Hazards

Environmental hazards such as those found indoors (e.g., bathroom, stairs) are potential risk factors for falls (OR 1.15 (95 % CI, 0.997–1.36)) [1]. The use of gait aids by older people significantly increased fall risk in community-dwelling (OR 2.07 (95 % CI, 1.59–2.71)) and nursing home residents (OR 2.08 (95 % CI, 1.88–2.31)) [1, 7].

8.3.10 Orthostatic Hypotension

One review found no association when other risk factors were considered [3]. Another review that was solely looking at orthostatic hypotension found insufficient data to assess whether there is an association between orthostatic hypotension and falls [12].

8.3.11 Pain

Pain appears to be a risk factor for falls, both in recurrent (two or more falls over at least 12 months) fallers (OR 2.04 (95 % CI, 1.75–2.39)) and those who suffered only a single fall (OR 2.04 (95 % CI, 1.75–2.39)) [13].

8.3.12 Medications

Medications will be discussed more in-depth elsewhere in this book. However, various high-quality reviews have shown that several medications may increase risk of falls. One review found significantly more falls in women taking four or more medications (likelihood ratio (LR) 1.9 (95 % CI, 1.4–2.5)) but not in men, possibly due to a smaller sample of men in the studies [3]. High-risk medications include antidepressants (OR 1.68 (95 % CI, 1.47–1.91)), diuretics (OR 1.07 (95 % CI, 1.01–1.14)), narcotics (OR 0.96 (95 % CI, 0.78–1.18)), NSAIDs (OR 1.21 (95 % CI, 1.01–1.44)), neuroleptics and antipsychotics (OR 1.59 (95 % CI, 1.37–1.83)), benzodiazepines (OR 1.57 (95 % CI, 1.43–1.72)), and sedatives and hypnotics in general (OR 1.47 (95 % CI, 1.35–1.62)) [14, 15]. The risk of falling with antihypertensive medications is less clear. Some studies have found antihypertensive agents (OR 1.24 (95 % CI, 1.01–1.50)) and β-blockers specifically (OR 1.01 (95 % CI, 0.86–1.17)) to be risk factors [14–16]. However, in another high-quality systematic review, none of the antihypertensive medications evaluated showed an association with falling [17]. These conflicting results may have been related to differences in the study designs included, the antihypertensive medication included, the confounders adjusted, and drug dosages and duration of use [17].

Other medications that may contribute to falls include cholinesterase inhibitors and memantine [18].

8.4 Chapter Summary

Falls can cause many adverse health outcomes, and as such potentially modifiable risk factors should be considered and addressed to decrease an individual's risk of falling. In general, a complete history and physical examination are needed in order to consider all appropriate risk factors as discussed above. There may be other risk factors to consider, but the high-quality reviews included in this chapter did not look at them (e.g., poor foot care, footwear, hearing problems, ethnicity, income) [4]. Frailty overall may be a risk factor, but we found no data to specifically support this. Further confirmation of other risk factors associated with falls is still needed to be studied to provide strong quality evidence of these other risk factors.

The conclusions concerning medication-related falls found in the high-quality reviews that are reported in this chapter may not consistently support those reported in the other chapters in this book. These discrepancies illustrate the complexity and inhomogeneity of the syndrome of falls in older people and its study.

Acknowledgments The authors thank Andrew Tang and Luxey Sirisegaram who helped with the initial research.

References

1. Letts L, Moreland J, Richardson J et al (2010) The physical environment as a fall risk factor in older adults: systematic review and meta-analysis of cross-sectional and cohort studies. Aust Occup Ther J 57:51–64
2. Hartikainen S, Lönnroos E, Louhivuori K (2007) Medication as a risk factor for falls: critical systematic review. J Gerontol Ser A Biol Med Sci 62(10):1172–1181
3. Ganz D, Bao Y, Shekelle P, Rubenstein L (2007) Will my patient fall? JAMA 297:77–86
4. Huang AR, Mallet L, Rochefort CM, Eguale T, Buckeridge DL, Tamblyn R (2012) Medication-related falls in the elderly. Drugs Aging 29(5):359–376
5. Deandrea S, Lucenteforte E, Bravi F, Foschi R, La Vecchia C, Negri E (2010) Risk factors for falls in community-dwelling older people: a systematic review and meta-analysis. Epidemiology 21(5):658–668
6. Shea BJ, Grimshaw JM, Wells GA, Boers M, Andersson N, Hamel C et al (2007) Development of AMSTAR: a measurement tool to assess the methodological quality of systematic reviews. BMC Med Res Methodol 7(1):10
7. Deandrea S, Bravi F, Turati F, Lucenteforte E, La Vecchia C, Negri E (2013) Risk factors for falls in older people in nursing homes and hospitals. A systematic review and meta-analysis. Arch Gerontol Geriatr 56(3):407–415
8. Impairment (The Free Dictionary). http://www.thefreedictionary.com/impairment
9. Muir SW, Berg K, Chesworth B, Klar N, Speechley M (2010) Quantifying the magnitude of risk for balance impairment on falls in community-dwelling older adults: a systematic review and meta-analysis. J Clin Epidemiol 63:389–406
10. Bloch F, Thibaud M, Dugue B et al (2010) Episodes of falling among elderly people: a systematic review and meta-analysis of social and demographic pre-disposing characteristics. Clinics 65:895–903
11. Kvelde T, McVeigh C, Toson B, Greenaway M, Lord SR, Delbaere K, Close JC (2013) Depressive symptomatology as a risk factor for falls in older people: systematic review and meta-analysis. J Am Geriatr Soc 61(5):694–706
12. Angelousi A, Girerd N, Benetos A, Frimat L, Gautier S, Weryha G, Boivin JM (2014) Association between orthostatic hypotension and cardiovascular risk, cerebrovascular risk, cognitive decline and falls as well as overall mortality: a systematic review and meta-analysis. J Hypertens 32(8):1562–1571
13. Stubbs B, Schofield P, Binnekade T, Patchay S, Sepehry A, Eggermont L (2014) Pain is associated with recurrent falls in community-dwelling older adults: evidence from a systematic review and meta-analysis. Pain Med 15(7):1115–1128
14. Woolcott JC, Richardson KJ, Wiens MO et al (2009) Meta-analysis of the impact of 9 medication classes on falls in elderly persons. Arch Intern Med 169:1952–1960
15. Hegeman J, Van Den Bemt BJ, Duysens J, van Limbeek J (2009) NSAIDs and the risk of accidental falls in the elderly: a systematic review. Drug Saf 32:489–498
16. Sterke C, Verhangen A, van Beeck E et al (2008) The influence of drug use on fall incidents among nursing home residents: a systematic review. Int Psychogeriatr 20:890–910
17. Zang G (2013) Antihypertensive drugs and the risk of fall injuries: a systematic review and meta-analysis. J Int Med Res 41(5):1408–1417
18. Kim DH, Brown RT, Ding EL, Kiel DP, Berry SD (2011) Dementia medications and risk of falls, syncope, and related adverse events: meta-analysis of randomized controlled trials. J Am Geriatr Soc 59(6):1019–1031

Part III
Medications Associated with Falls in the Elderly

Chapter 9
Psychotropic Drugs

Andrea Iaboni and Benoit H. Mulsant

Abstract Available evidence suggests that antidepressants, antipsychotics, lithium, and antiepileptic drugs can increase the risks for falls and fractures in older adults. However, the relationship between falls and psychotropic medications is complex because the mental disorders treated with these psychotropic medications and their comorbidities are themselves significant and independent risk factors for falls. Thus, fall risk by itself is not a contraindication for the use of psychotropic medications in an older frail patient. Nevertheless, clinicians need to prescribe these medications judiciously and to follow principles of conservative prescribing to minimize the risk for falls. While some psychotropic medications may have a direct effect on balance, most falls and fractures are related to other side effects, in particular, orthostatic change in blood pressure, pro-arrhythmogenic effects, extrapyramidal symptoms (including Parkinsonism and akathisia), sedation, and cognitive impairment. Thus, careful selection of specific medications based on their differential side effect profile and monitoring of adverse effects is mandatory. Close monitoring is particularly important during the first few days or weeks after starting a new psychotropic medication or after a dose increase.

Abbreviations

AED	Antiepileptic drug
AGS	American Geriatrics Society
aRR	Adjusted relative risk
CI	Confidence interval

A. Iaboni, MD, DPhil, FRCPC (✉)
Department of Psychiatry, University of Toronto, Toronto, ON, Canada

Geriatric Rehabilitation Program, The Toronto Rehabilitation Institute,
University Health Network, Toronto, ON, Canada
e-mail: andrea.iaboni@uhn.ca

B.H. Mulsant, MD, FRCPC
Centre for Addiction and Mental Health, Toronto, ON, Canada

© Springer International Publishing Switzerland 2016

A.R. Huang, L. Mallet (eds.), *Medication-related falls in older people*,
DOI 10.1007/978-3-319-32304-6_9

DEXA	Dual-energy x-ray absorptiometry
EPS	Extrapyramidal signs and symptoms
OR	Odds ratio
PIM	Potentially inappropriate medications
SSRI	Selective serotonin reuptake inhibitors
TCA	Tricyclic antidepressants
TD	Tardive dyskinesia

9.1 Introduction

The relationship between falls and the use of psychotropic medication is complex: they are both highly prevalent in older adults and share a number of common risk factors (e.g., medical comorbidity, cognitive impairment). The underlying mental health problems for which psychotropic medications are prescribed can themselves be risks for falls. Thus, clinicians face a dilemma when they decide to prescribe psychotropic medications to older adults. This chapter reviews the magnitude and nature of the risk for falls associated with the use of psychotropic medication and discusses ways to moderate this risk.

The simplest way to prevent psychotropic-related falls is to avoid using psychotropics. Thus, a fundamental premise underlying this chapter is that for most mental health problems in later life, psychotropic medications should be used as a first-line intervention only when symptoms are severe, highly distressing, or dangerous. The evidence supporting the use of antidepressants for mild depression, sadness related to normal bereavement, or adjustment disorders is poor. Antipsychotics should not be used to treat sleep disturbances or mild behavioral symptoms associated with dementia. For many of these symptoms, non-pharmacologic interventions (brief individual psychotherapy, group programs, increased physical and social activity) are effective in promoting mental health in older adults, and they should be considered prior to initiating pharmacotherapy.

The rest of this chapter discusses the relationship between falls and antidepressants, antipsychotics, lithium, or antiepileptic drugs.

9.2 Antidepressants

Antidepressants are commonly prescribed in the elderly: about 19 % of older American females and 9 % of older American males are taking an antidepressant [73]. Thus, given this high prevalence of antidepressant use, even a small increase in the risk of falls would result in a large number of falls. It has been estimated that antidepressant use contributes to about 7 % of hip fractures in the United States [82].

There are a number of common on- and off-label uses for antidepressants, including the treatment of mood and anxiety disorders, pain disorders, sleep problems, and behavioral symptoms associated with dementia. Seniors facing these mental health problems tend to be older, be frailer, and have more cognitive and medical issues including a higher baseline history of falls [2, 7, 50, 95]. Thus, older adults who receive antidepressants overlap those who are most vulnerable to falls. That being said, the association between falls and antidepressants is stronger than the association between falls and antihypertensives or beta-blockers, two classes of drugs commonly prescribed to frail, medically complex elderly, that are perceived as having a high risk for falls [100].

In response to the evidence linking falls to antidepressants, the American Geriatrics Society (AGS) Beers criteria categorize (with high quality of evidence and strong recommendations) selective serotonin reuptake inhibitors (SSRIs) as potentially inappropriate medications (PIMs) for older adults with a history of falls or fractures [1]. Tricyclic antidepressants have long been considered PIMs for all older adults given their anticholinergic and cardiac side effects [1]. At present, other antidepressants have not been designated as PIMs due to lack of evidence of harm rather than evidence of safety in regard to falls.

9.2.1 Epidemiology of Antidepressant-Related Falls

Most of the evidence linking antidepressants to falls is observational in nature. They are thus subject to "confounding by indication," that is, confounding by the clinical condition for which the drug is prescribed. The strength of the association between antidepressants and falls is largely dependent on the population which is studied (community vs. nursing home), adjustment for confounders, the classes of antidepressants studied, and the study outcome measure (i.e., falls or fall-related injuries such as hip fractures) as has been comprehensively reviewed by Gebara et al. [30]. The odds ratio (OR) for a patient on antidepressants versus not on antidepressants experiencing a fall is 1.68 (95 % CI: 1.47–1.91) [110]. This is comparable to the fall risk associated with benzodiazepine and antipsychotic use.

Evidence related to class of antidepressant and risk for falls is mixed. Most studies have compared SSRIs and tricyclic antidepressants (TCAs), while a few studies have not been clear about which "antidepressants" they are examining. SSRIs have fewer fall-promoting side effects compared to older antidepressant drugs and would be expected to have less risk of falls. However, although some studies have found TCAs to be a higher risk [77], the fall risk associated with SSRIs and TCAs is comparable [24, 40]. A likely explanation for this finding is allocation bias: SSRIs are more likely than TCAs to be prescribed to those most likely to fall. A case-control study found that the risk associated with serotonin-norepinephrine reuptake inhibitors (SNRIs such as venlafaxine and duloxetine) is equivalent to that of TCA and SSRI [34]. Trazodone use in low doses in the context of long-term care has also been associated with falls [99]. There is little data about whether there are differences between individual SSRIs although one study found that they were all similar in risk [17]. In this study, mirtazapine was associated with a small increased risk of falls, although less so than SSRIs [17]. Little is known about the risk of bupropion. In one prospective study, bupropion combined with paroxetine was associated with a high rate of falls [44]; it is unclear if this was related specifically to bupropion or to its use in combination with paroxetine and the resulting drug-drug interaction.

The highest risk for falls and injuries is within the first few weeks after initiation of an antidepressant [3, 34, 40, 77, 99]. Several studies have also demonstrated that the risk for falls and injury have a relationship with medication dosage [8, 17, 99].

Several large epidemiological studies have also examined the outcome of injuries that are fall related, such as fragility fracture. In an uncontrolled longitudinal study, the attributable risk due to antidepressants was 4.7 % of hip fractures [3]. The risk of hip fracture does not appear to differ among different classes of antidepressants [57]. However, there is concern that chronic use of SSRIs and other serotonergic drugs may contribute to the risk of fractures through their direct effects on bone metabolism [22, 29, 83, 91].

9.2.2 Potential Mechanisms of Antidepressant-Related Falls and Fractures

Depression is an important risk factor for falls independent of antidepressant use [48, 109]. Like falls, depression is common in old age, with 15 % of community-dwelling seniors reporting clinically significant depressive symptoms [6, 69]. The relationship between depression and falls is complex and bidirectional (see Fig. 9.1). Some symptoms of depression may have a direct role in promoting falls, for example, insomnia [97] or poor nutrition [90]. Cognitive changes are also associated with depression in late life, in particular changes in attention, executive function, and processing speed [32, 63]. These cognitive domains are important in gait coordination and attention to the environment and thus may mediate some of the effect of depression on falls. Depression-associated gait disturbances, such as increased gait variability, are also associated with falls [36, 37, 60, 64]. "Vascular depression" is an increasingly recognized phenomenon that describes an accumulated burden of cerebrovascular disease associated with depression, cognitive impairment, frailty, and changes in balance and gait in late life [35].

Depression and falls may be mutually reinforcing phenomena. Depressive symptoms are particularly high in those who are recurrent fallers [95]. In a prospective study over an 8-year period, increase in depressive symptoms was associated with an increased rate of falls [2]. Activity restriction and decreased social participation can be a complication of recurrent falls [65]: the resulting social isolation is known to be a significant risk factor for depression in the elderly [107].

Multiple antidepressant-related side effects have been implicated in falls (Table 9.1). In a study of paroxetine, 38 % of subjects fell during the 21-week trial. Memory impairment at baseline and orthostatic changes in blood pressure during treatment were associated with falls [44]. Hyponatremia is a common and potentially serious adverse event complicating the use of SSRIs in the elderly [26], and it has been implicated in fractures in a small case-control study [87].

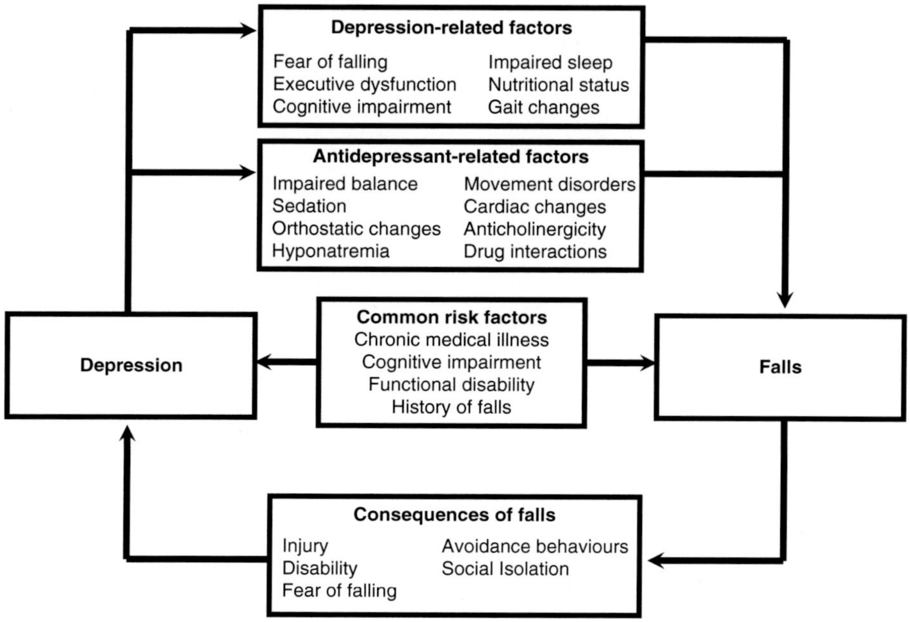

Fig. 9.1 The complex relationships between depression, antidepressant use, and falls (Reproduced with permission from [42])

Antidepressants may also directly impair postural control [115]. In healthy volunteer studies, only amitriptyline has shown an immediate effect on postural control after a single dose. However, increased postural sway was noted in depressed patients in the first week of treatment with sertraline when compared to nortriptyline or controls [49]. In a similar study, there was no change in balance over the course of 6 weeks of treatment with paroxetine or nortriptyline [61]. More studies are needed in this area to examine the effects of commonly used antidepressants in the period of highest risk for falls: the first few weeks of use.

A recent analysis compared different SSRI drugs for the side effect of "dizziness" in older adults [101]. Venlafaxine and duloxetine had a significantly greater risk of dizziness than placebo, while sertraline did not differ from placebo and other antidepressants trended towards being associated with a higher rate of dizziness than placebo.

Gagne et al. [28] compared incidence of fractures with antidepressants affinity for the serotonin transporter (5HTT) and their sedating potential. While the incidence of fractures increased with sedating potential for antidepressants with weaker 5HTT affinity, in the group with higher 5HTT affinity, low sedating potential was associated with fractures.

Many antidepressants have anticholinergic side effects that may impact on cognitive function and hence increase risk of falls (Table 9.1; [13]). Antidepressants may also have negative effects on cognition independent of their anticholinergic effects. This is particularly true in the treatment of "old-old"

Table 9.1 Fall-promoting side effects of commonly used psychotropic medications

	Orthostatic changes	Pro-arrhythmogenic effects[a]	Parkinsonism	Akathisia/agitation	Sedation	Anticholinergic potential	Drug-drug interaction
SSRI antidepressants							
Citalopram	–	+++	+/–	+/–	+	–	–
Escitalopram	–	+/–	+/–	+/–	+/–	–	–
Fluoxetine	–	–	+/–	+	–	+/–	+++
Paroxetine	–	–	+/–	+/–	++	++	++
Sertraline	–	–	+/–	+/–	+/–	–	+/–
Tricyclic antidepressants							
Amitriptyline	+++	+++	–	–	+++	+++	+++
Desipramine	+	++	–	–	+	++	++
Doxepin	++	+++	–	–	+++	+++	+
Nortriptyline	+	++	–	–	++	++	++
Other antidepressants							
Venlafaxine	+	+	+/–	+	+/–	–	++
Duloxetine	+/–	+/–	+/–	+	+/–	–	+
Bupropion	–	–	–	++	–	–	+
Mirtazapine	+/–	–	–	–	+++	+/–	+
Trazodone	+	+/–	–	–	+++	–	+
Second-generation antipsychotics							
Aripiprazole	+/–	+	+	++	–	–	+/–
Olanzapine	++	+	++	+	++	+++	+/–
Quetiapine	+++	++	+/–	+	+++	+/–	+/–
Risperidone	++	+	+++	++	+	+/–	+

[a]Increase in PR, QRS, or QTc intervals
– absent; +/– questionable; + mild; ++ moderate; +++ severe

patients, those with preexisting cognitive issues, and those who have not responded to treatment [18, 70, 79].

Older adults with depression often present with mild extrapyramidal signs and symptoms (EPS) [62]; and antidepressants have been reported to induce EPS in some patients [38], which may create a risk for falls. However, EPS induced by antidepressants are rare, and tricyclic antidepressants, SSRIs, and SNRIs have been used safely to treat depression in patients with Parkinson's disease [5, 12, 21, 94].

There is some evidence of a relationship between serotonergic antidepressant use and bone fractures, beyond what would be expected from the increased risk of falling, but this is somewhat controversial. This association has been observed in case-control studies [8, 57, 106] and prospective cohort studies [83, 114]. A recent meta-analysis found the relative risk of fractures related to SSRIs to be 1.72 (95 % CI: 1.51, 1.95) [111]. The effect of serotonin on bone metabolism may be the mechanism underlying this association between fractures and SSRI use. Serotonin transporters are present on bone cells, and central serotonin has a role in regulating bone mass through sympathetic outflow [86].

Depression is a significant confounder in studies of SSRIs and bone metabolism because depression itself has been associated with decreased bone mineral density and with fractures [96, 112]. Evidence for an association between SSRIs and bone loss is inconsistent [31]. Recent studies have shown some impact of antidepressant on bone formation. In one study, decreased bone formation (as measured by decreased P1NP-procollagen type N-terminal propeptide marker) was seen in patients on venlafaxine, particularly in those with the high-expressing 5HTTLPR genotype and the low-expressing HTR1B genotype (both involved in serotonin transport and binding) [29]. Another study found that the association between depression and fracture was mediated by the depressed patients' propensity to fall [108].

9.2.3 Prevention of Antidepressant-Related Falls

When making treatment decisions, clinicians need to weigh the risk of falls from untreated depression against the risk of falls associated with antidepressant medication. There are no prospective controlled data available to offer guidance. One uncontrolled study found that antidepressant treatment after 10 weeks improved depressive symptoms and gait parameters [75]. However, this study did not directly assess for gait changes during the higher-risk early treatment period and in treatment non-responders.

Basic principles in prescribing for older adults can be used to minimize risk ([88]; see Table 9.2). When an antidepressant can be selected to minimize fall-promoting side effects, SSRIs remain the first-line therapy ([68]; see Table 9.1). If an older antidepressant is required, the secondary amine nortriptyline is preferred: it has linear pharmacokinetics and a lower propensity to cause orthostasis, cardiac conduction defects, and anticholinergic effects than tertiary amines such as amitriptyline [13] even though both secondary and tertiary amines are considered to have "strong anticholinergic properties" according to the Beers criteria [1].

Table 9.2 Principles related to prescribing psychotropic medications to minimize risk of falls in older adults

Problems	Recommendations
Unnecessary prescription of psychotropic medications	Avoid using psychotropic mediations unless symptoms are severe, highly distressing, or dangerous
	Attempt dose decrease or discontinuation after period of symptomatic remission
Polypharmacy	Monitor and assess for effectiveness of current medications; discontinue those that have been shown to be ineffective
	Use augmenting strategies sparingly – replace an ineffective therapy rather than add new psychotropic medications
Falls in first days/weeks after starting medication	Address fall risk factors before starting new medications
	Start medications at low doses
	Only start one medication at a time
Inadequate monitoring	Obtain orthostatic vital signs
	Monitor for Parkinsonism (rigidity, tremor, shuffling gait, blunted affect, postural instability). Use lower doses or shift to lower potency agents if required
	Monitor levels, but treat the patient, not the level (i.e., if symptoms are controlled, "subtherapeutic" level may be adequate)
Sedation	Avoid sedating medications
	Start sedating medications in very small doses
	Provide education about risks of sedation, in particular risk for falls and effect on driving
Cognitive impairment	Select medications that are minimally anticholinergic
	Use lowest possible dose
	Get a baseline cognitive assessment before starting a new medication
	If evidence of cognitive decline, assess for toxicity – it could be due to the medication!
Adherence	Avoid prescribing medications that have a narrow therapeutic range or a short half-life in patients with poor adherence or risk factors for poor adherence (e.g., cognitive impairment)
	Use strategies to improve adherence (asking about adherence at every visit, screening for factors contributing to nonadherence, clear communication and instructions, simplified medication regimes)

Patients with depression are more likely to experience polypharmacy or received a potentially inappropriate medication [53, 74]. Polypharmacy (defined as greater than five medications) plus antidepressant use was found to be associated with a greater risk of falls (aRR: 1.28, 95 % CI: 1.06–1.54) and of multiple falls (aRR: 1.60, 95 % CI: 1.19–2.15) than either polypharmacy or antidepressant use alone [84]. Polypharmacy should be avoided, particularly the combination of two fall-promoting drugs at once. Special attention should be paid to pharmacokinetic and pharmacodynamic drug-drug interactions [67]. Many antidepressants are prone to drug-drug interactions (Table 9.1). In older persons, medications should be dosed lower and increased more slowly, especially during the first weeks of treatment. There is an increased risk of falls for at least 7 days following dose changes [116].

An overall assessment for fall risk is important when starting a new antidepressant. This would include an assessment of other fall-promoting medications, checking for drug interactions, observing gait and tone, and inquiring about fall history. In patients judged to be at high risk for falls, referral to fall prevention programs or home occupational therapy assessment can prove invaluable. In fact, such referrals to community supports or programs should be considered for all frail or isolated older adults with depression: their benefits to mood and level of activity may be as important an intervention as antidepressant therapy. In addition to assessing treatment response, cognitive impairment, orthostatic hypotension, extrapyramidal effects, and hyponatremia should also be monitored.

One may also be able to prevent fractures associated with falls. A simple intervention is to enquire about adherence to osteoporosis screening and treatment. Many patients with depression make poor use of preventative health interventions [66]. Current osteoporosis prevention guidelines recommend adequate calcium and vitamin D intake (often requiring supplementation), smoking cessation, decreasing caffeine intake, and regular weight-bearing exercise [16]. Screening recommendations are for dual-energy x-ray absorptiometry (DEXA) in those over 65 years of age and repeat DEXA scans every 2 years [16]. In younger patients (50–69 years) with osteoporosis risk factors, early screening is based on "risk factor profile." SSRI antidepressant use is now listed among other bone loss promoting medications in the current guidelines. In older adults with long-term SSRI use and who have other osteoporosis risk factors, early screening should be considered.

9.3 Antipsychotics

Most studies examining the relationship of antipsychotics and falls have focused on the frail dementia population or those living in long-term care homes. In these populations, antipsychotics are used largely (and controversially) for the management of behavioral symptoms of dementia [68]. Older adults with dementia have a number of intrinsic physiological changes that predispose them to falls such as changes in sensory, cardiovascular, neurological, and musculoskeletal function. They also have an increased sensitivity to the side effects of antipsychotics related to neurodegenerative changes such as decreased cholinergic reserve and increased dopaminergic receptor sensitivity [67, 104]. Behavioral symptoms are more likely to be present during the more advanced stages of dementia [59], which is another source of bias in observational studies of antipsychotics.

9.3.1 Epidemiology of Antipsychotic-Related Falls

Antipsychotics are associated with an increased risk of falls in the community [51] and in long-term care [72]: the increased odds in both cases are in the range of 40–60 %. Most studies have examined the relationship between antipsychotics and serious adverse events such as fractures in large epidemiological studies (reviewed in [80]). The strength of the association varies by study design and quality, approaches to minimizing bias, and study population (i.e., community-based or nursing home). In a meta-analysis of these studies, the OR of fracture was 1.68 (95 % CI: 1.43–1.99) in older adults using first-generation antipsychotics and 1.30 (95 % CI: 1.14–1.49) in those receiving second-generation antipsychotics [71].

In contrast, prospective studies have not found a relationship between antipsychotics and falls in the dementia population. For example, a secondary analysis of a prospective, controlled study examined the effect of risperidone on falls in patients with significant agitation and psychosis. In those who were the most agitated, 1 mg/day of risperidone decreased the rate of falls compared to placebo, whereas the rates of falls were similar with 2 mg/day of risperidone or placebo [45]. A recent meta-analysis of randomized placebo-controlled trials of antipsychotics for behavioral symptoms of dementia did not find an association between these medications and falls/injuries when compared to placebo (OR = 0.89; 95 % CI: 0.75–1.05) [98].

Second-generation antipsychotics produce fewer extrapyramidal symptoms [54, 85, 105], and they have a lower risk of falls and fractures than the first generation drugs [39, 43, 51]. When comparing specific second-generation agents, some studies have associated olanzapine and risperidone with higher risk [43, 56], while others have found quetiapine to be higher risk, particularly at higher doses [9, 41].

As with antidepressants, the risk of falls is highest during the first few weeks of treatment [81]. There is a dose relationship between antipsychotics and fractures [41].

9.3.2 Potential Mechanisms of Antipsychotic-Related Falls

Antipsychotics are associated with a host of fall-promoting side effects (Table 9.1). Parkinsonism is common: the rate is 30–50 % in older adults receiving first-generation ("conventional") antipsychotics [10] and 10–15 % in those receiving second-generation ("atypical") antipsychotics. There is a risk of prescribing cascades if the Parkinsonism is misdiagnosed as Parkinson's disease or if it is treated with an anticholinergic medication. Parkinsonism emerges within the first weeks of the initiation of an antipsychotic or after a dose increase. Parkinsonism is an established risk factor for falling: parkinsonian gait is prone to stumbling and freezing, postural instability, and rigidity; it decreases the ability to react to perturbations in balance and an impaired ability to transfer safely [103].

The prevalence of tardive dyskinesia (TD) in older adults who have been prescribed antipsychotics is 30–50 %. The annual incidence of TD is around 20 % for conventional agents and 5 % for atypical agents [11].

Akathisia associated with antipsychotic use presents as a paradoxical increase in psychomotor agitation, restlessness, anxiety, and distress. Although it appears to be as prevalent in older patients as in younger ones, it is more poorly recognized in older patients, particularly in those with dementia who are unable to articulate their distress. The rate of akathisia is about 20–40 % for conventional agents and 5 % for atypical agents [11]. However, among atypical antipsychotics, aripiprazole may be more likely to cause akathisia, particularly during the first weeks of treatment and with higher doses ([55]; Table 9.1).

Antipsychotics can also impact cognitive function, in particular in patients with dementia [67]. For example, in the Clinical Antipsychotic Trials of Intervention Effectiveness in Alzheimer's Disease (CATIE-AD) trial, the antipsychotic treatment group experienced cognitive changes comparable to 1 year's progression of dementia compared to the placebo group [89]. Older adults need to allocate attentional resources to walking to compensate for changes to motor and sensory functions. Thus, even small changes in cognitive function can have an impact on gait performance and fall risk [113].

Both conventional and atypical antipsychotics can also cause sedation and orthostatic changes in blood pressures, particularly during the first few weeks of treatment and after dose changes. Specific atypical antipsychotics differ in their propensity to cause these side effects (Table 9.1).

There is limited information about the effect of antipsychotics on bone health in older adults. Reduced bone mineral density in older adults receiving long-term treatment with antipsychotics may be mediated by antipsychotic-induced hyperprolactinemia, by lifestyle factors, or a combination of both [47]. In older adults, risperidone and paliperidone seem to be more likely to cause hyperprolactinemia than other atypical antipsychotics, but the possible significance of this differential effect on fractures has not been established [19, 46, 58].

9.3.3 Prevention of Antipsychotic-Related Falls

As with antidepressants, when using antipsychotics in older adults, the prevention of falls relies mostly on principles of conservative prescribing ([88]; see Table 9.2). First and foremost, clinicians should ensure that antipsychotics are clinically indicated. The use of antipsychotics for treating sleep disturbance or anxiety should be avoided because the risks (not just for falls) likely outweigh any potential benefits. When antipsychotic treatment is initiated in an older adult, close monitoring is required during the first few months of treatment and after each dose increase. Particular attention should be paid to EPS, sedation, orthostatic changes in blood pressures, and heart rate and the corrected QT interval (QTc) (Table 9.2). Even in patients receiving stable doses, regular monitoring for new abnormal movements is required to detect emergent TD.

In addition to regular monitoring, there is also good support for dose decreases or discontinuation of antipsychotic medications in patients with severe behavioral symptoms of dementia [4, 20]. Even in older patients with schizophrenia receiving long-term antipsychotic treatment, a recent study has shown that more than 80 % of patients who are stable clinically can tolerate a 25–40 % decrease in their antipsychotic dosage: the dose reduction was associated with improvement in their psychiatric symptoms and a reduction in EPS and hyperprolactinemia [33]. Since most antipsychotic side effects are dose dependent, even a small decrease in dose is a worthwhile clinical intervention. However, no studies to date have demonstrated that antipsychotic discontinuation has any impact, positive or negative, on rate of falls or injuries [76].

9.4 Other Psychotropic Medications

9.4.1 Lithium

Some limited evidence from one case-control study of psychiatric inpatients suggests that lithium may be associated with falls. However, this result needs to be interpreted with caution given the acuity of psychiatric illness and the degree of polypharmacy of these inpatients [52].

The main risk for falls associated with the use of lithium in older adults is due to the potential for lithium toxicity [23]. Pharmacokinetic changes related to aging, particularly changes in renal function, increase the risk of toxicity in older adults. Medical comorbidities and polypharmacy (most notably use of thiazide diuretics, angiotensin-converting enzyme inhibitors, and nonsteroidal anti-inflammatory drugs) increase the risk of lithium toxicity. Falls has been associated with lithium toxicity, and other symptoms suggestive of toxicity include ataxia, dizziness, confusion, and disorientation. Short of toxicity, older adults treated with lithium may experience some cognitive impairment related to the moderate anticholinergic potential of lithium [13].

Older patients need lower doses of lithium to achieve a therapeutic blood level. There is also a poor correlation between serum and brain levels of lithium in older adults [117]. Thus, beyond monitoring of blood levels, frequent monitoring of therapeutic response and signs of toxicity is important in older adults treated with lithium.

On the positive side, long-term lithium use has been associated with a decreased risk of bone fracture (adjusted OR, 0.63; 95 % CI, 0.43–0.9; [8]). This is consistent with animal experiments that suggest that lithium promotes bone formation [14].

9.4.2 Antiepileptic Drugs

More than 10 % of older adults residing in American long-term care homes are prescribed an antiepileptic drug (AED). About half of this use is for the treatment of seizure disorders [78]. AEDs are also commonly used in older adults for the treatment of bipolar disorder, pain disorders, and off-label for the behavioral symptoms of dementia.

Ataxia and impaired balance are commonly reported side effects of AEDs [27]. In general, carbamazepine, oxcarbamazepine, topiramate, phenytoin, and phenobarbital have the worst impact on balance, while lamotrigine, gabapentin, and levetiracetam are better tolerated. Many of these effects are dose dependent [93], and thus, lowest effective dosages should be used.

Few studies have examined the issue of AED-related falls. In one large prospective study, older women taking AEDs (largely phenytoin, carbamazepine, and phenobarbital) had significantly increased odds of falling (2.6; 95 % CI: 1.5–4.4) and of falling repeatedly [25]. Less is known about the antiepileptics used commonly as mood stabilizers such as divalproex, lamotrigine, and carbamazepine.

AED use is also linked to decreased bone mineral density and increased risk of fractures [92]. This is particularly true of the liver enzyme-inducing AEDs, likely through changes in vitamin D metabolism and sex hormone binding [15]. Steps should be taken to prevent loss of bone density in older adults prescribed AEDs, such as ensuring adequate vitamin D levels. Importantly, many AEDs are involved in clinically significant drug interactions because of their ability to induce or inhibit liver enzymes. Valproate-associated hyperammonemia is a rare but serious side effect of valproate therapy that can present in older adults with increased confusion, ataxia, and decreased level of consciousness [102].

9.5 Summary and Conclusions

Available evidence suggests that antidepressants, antipsychotics, lithium, and antiepileptic drugs can increase the risks for falls and fractures in older adults. However, the relationship between falls and psychotropic medications is complex because the mental disorders treated with these psychotropic medications and their comorbidities are themselves significant and independent risk factors for falls. Thus, fall risk by itself is not a contraindication for the use of psychotropic medications in an older frail patient. Nevertheless, clinicians need to prescribe these medications judiciously and to follow principles of conservative prescribing to minimize the risk for falls. While some psychotropic medications may have a direct effect on balance, most falls and fractures are related to other side effects, in particular, orthostatic change in blood pressure, pro-arrhythmogenic effects, extrapyramidal symptoms (including Parkinsonism and akathisia), sedation, and cognitive impairment. Thus, careful selection of specific medications based on their differential side effect profile and monitoring of adverse effects is mandatory. Close monitoring is particularly important during the first few days or weeks after initiation of a new psychotropic medication or after a dose increase.

References

1. American Geriatrics Society 2015 Beers Criteria Update Expert Panel (2015) American Geriatrics Society 2015 updated beers criteria for potentially inappropriate medication use in older adults. J Am Geriatr Soc 63:2227–2246
2. Anstey KJ, Burns R, von Sanden C, Luszcz MA (2008) Psychological well-being is an independent predictor of falling in an 8-year follow-up of older adults. J Gerontol B Psychol Sci Soc Sci 63:249–257
3. Bakken MS, Engeland A, Engesaeter LB, Ranhoff AH, Hunskaar S, Ruths S (2013) Increased risk of hip fracture among older people using antidepressant drugs: data from the Norwegian prescription database and the Norwegian hip fracture registry. Age Ageing 42:514–520
4. Ballard C, Hanney ML, Theodoulou M, Douglas S, McShane R, Kossakowski K, Gill R, Juszczak E, Yu LM, Jacoby R et al (2009) The dementia antipsychotic withdrawal trial (DART-AD): long-term follow-up of a randomised placebo-controlled trial. Lancet Neurol 8:151–157
5. Barone P, Scarzella L, Marconi R, Antonini A, Morgante L, Bracco F, Zappia M, Musch B, Depression/Parkinson Italian Study Group (2006) Pramipexole versus sertraline in the treatment of depression in Parkinson's disease: a national multicenter parallel-group randomized study. J Neurol 253:601–607
6. Beekman AT, Deeg DJ, van Tilburg T, Smit JH, Hooijer C, van Tilburg W (1995) Major and minor depression in later life: a study of prevalence and risk factors. J Affect Disord 36:65–75
7. Biderman A, Cwikel J, Fried AV, Galinsky D (2002) Depression and falls among community dwelling elderly people: a search for common risk factors. J Epidemiol Community Health 56:631–636
8. Bolton JM, Metge C, Lix L, Prior H, Sareen J, Leslie WD (2008) Fracture risk from psychotropic medications: a population-based analysis. J Clin Psychopharmacol 28:384–391
9. Bozat-Emre S, Doupe M, Kozyrskyj AL, Grymonpre R, Mahmud SM (2015) Atypical antipsychotic drug use and falls among nursing home residents in Winnipeg, Canada. Int J Geriatr Psychiatry 30:842–850
10. Caligiuri MP, Lacro JP, Jeste DV (1999) Incidence and predictors of drug-induced parkinsonism in older psychiatric patients treated with very low doses of neuroleptics. J Clin Psychopharmacol 19:322–328
11. Caligiuri MR, Jeste DV, Lacro JP (2000) Antipsychotic-induced movement disorders in the elderly: epidemiology and treatment recommendations. Drugs Aging 17:363–384
12. Chen P, Kales HC, Weintraub D, Blow FC, Jiang L, Mellow AM (2007) Antidepressant treatment of veterans with Parkinson's disease and depression: analysis of a national sample. J Geriatr Psychiatry Neurol 20:161–165
13. Chew ML, Mulsant BH, Pollock BG, Lehman ME, Greenspan A, Mahmoud RA, Kirshner MA, Sorisio DA, Bies RR, Gharabawi G (2008) Anticholinergic activity of 107 medications commonly used by older adults. J Am Geriatr Soc 56:1333–1341
14. Clement-Lacroix P, Ai M, Morvan F, Roman-Roman S, Vayssiere B, Belleville C, Estrera K, Warman ML, Baron R, Rawadi G (2005) Lrp5-independent activation of wnt signaling by lithium chloride increases bone formation and bone mass in mice. Proc Natl Acad Sci U S A 102:17406–17411
15. Cohen A, Lancman M, Mogul H, Marks S, Smith K (1997) Strategies to protect bone mass in the older patient with epilepsy. Geriatrics 52(8):70, 75–78, 81
16. Cosman F, de Beur SJ, LeBoff MS, Lewiecki EM, Tanner B, Randall S, Lindsay R, National Osteoporosis Foundation (2014) Clinician's guide to prevention and treatment of osteoporosis. Osteoporos Int 25:2359–2381
17. Coupland C, Dhiman P, Morriss R, Arthur A, Barton G, Hippisley-Cox J (2011) Antidepressant use and risk of adverse outcomes in older people: population based cohort study. BMJ 343:d4551

18. Culang ME, Sneed JR, Keilp JG, Rutherford BR, Pelton GH, Devanand DP, Roose SP (2009) Change in cognitive functioning following acute antidepressant treatment in late-life depression. Am J Geriatr Psychiatry 17:881–888
19. Deberdt WG, Dysken MW, Rappaport SA, Feldman PD, Young CA, Hay DP, Lehman DL, Dossenbach M, Degenhardt EK, Breier A (2005) Comparison of olanzapine and risperidone in the treatment of psychosis and associated behavioral disturbances in patients with dementia. Am J Geriatr Psychiatry 13:722–730
20. Declercq T, Petrovic M, Azermai M, Vander Stichele R, De Sutter AI, van Driel ML, Christiaens T (2013) Withdrawal versus continuation of chronic antipsychotic drugs for behavioural and psychological symptoms in older people with dementia. Cochrane Database Syst Rev (3):CD007726
21. Devos D, Dujardin K, Poirot I, Moreau C, Cottencin O, Thomas P, Destee A, Bordet R, Defebvre L (2008) Comparison of desipramine and citalopram treatments for depression in parkinson's disease: a double-blind, randomized, placebo-controlled study. Mov Disord 23:850–857
22. Diem SJ, Blackwell TL, Stone KL, Yaffe K, Cauley JA, Whooley MA, Ensrud KE, Study of Osteoporotic Fractures (2007) Depressive symptoms and rates of bone loss at the hip in older women. J Am Geriatr Soc 55:824–831
23. D'Souza R, Rajji TK, Mulsant BH, Pollock BG (2011) Use of lithium in the treatment of bipolar disorder in late-life. Curr Psychiatry Rep 13:488–492
24. Ensrud KE, Blackwell T, Mangione CM, Bowman PJ, Bauer DC, Schwartz A, Hanlon JT, Nevitt MC, Whooley MA (2003) Central nervous system active medications and risk for fractures in older women. Arch Intern Med 163:949–957
25. Ensrud KE, Blackwell TL, Mangione CM, Bowman PJ, Whooley MA, Bauer DC, Schwartz AV, Hanlon JT, Nevitt MC (2002) Central nervous system-active medications and risk for falls in older women. J Am Geriatr Soc 50:1629–1637
26. Fabian TJ, Amico JA, Kroboth PD, Mulsant BH, Corey SE, Begley AE, Bensasi SG, Weber E, Dew MA, Reynolds CF 3rd et al (2004) Paroxetine-induced hyponatremia in older adults: a 12-week prospective study. Arch Intern Med 164:327–332
27. Fife TD, Blum D, Fisher RS (2006) Measuring the effects of antiepileptic medications on balance in older people. Epilepsy Res 70:103–109
28. Gagne JJ, Patrick AR, Mogun H, Solomon DH (2011) Antidepressants and fracture risk in older adults: a comparative safety analysis. Clin Pharmacol Ther 89:880–887
29. Garfield LD, Muller DJ, Kennedy JL, Mulsant BH, Reynolds CF 3rd, Teitelbaum SL, Civitelli R, Dixon D, Todorov AA, Lenze EJ (2014) Genetic variation in the serotonin transporter and HTR1B receptor predicts reduced bone formation during serotonin reuptake inhibitor treatment in older adults. World J Biol Psychiatry 15:404–410
30. Gebara MA, Lipsey KL, Karp JF, Nash MC, Iaboni A, Lenze EJ (2015) Cause or effect? Selective serotonin reuptake inhibitors and falls in older adults: a systematic review. Am J Geriatr Psychiatry 23:1016–1028
31. Gebara MA, Shea ML, Lipsey KL, Teitelbaum SL, Civitelli R, Muller DJ, Reynolds CF 3rd, Mulsant BH, Lenze EJ (2014) Depression, antidepressants, and bone health in older adults: a systematic review. J Am Geriatr Soc 62:1434–1441
32. Gildengers AG, Butters MA, Chisholm D, Anderson SJ, Begley A, Holm M, Rogers JC, Reynolds CF 3rd, Mulsant BH (2012) Cognition in older adults with bipolar disorder versus major depressive disorder. Bipolar Disord 14:198–205
33. Graff-Guerrero A, Rajji TK, Mulsant BH, Nakajima S, Caravaggio F, Suzuki T, Uchida H, Gerretsen P, Mar W, Pollock BG et al (2015) Evaluation of antipsychotic dose reduction in late-life schizophrenia: a prospective dopamine D2/3 receptor occupancy study. JAMA Psychiatry 72:927–934
34. Gribbin J, Hubbard R, Gladman J, Smith C, Lewis S (2011) Serotonin-norepinephrine reuptake inhibitor antidepressants and the risk of falls in older people: case-control and case-series analysis of a large UK primary care database. Drugs Aging 28:895–902

35. Hajjar I, Yang F, Sorond F, Jones RN, Milberg W, Cupples LA, Lipsitz LA (2009) A novel aging phenotype of slow gait, impaired executive function, and depressive symptoms: relationship to blood pressure and other cardiovascular risks. J Gerontol A Biol Sci Med Sci 64:994–1001
36. Hausdorff JM, Rios DA, Edelberg HK (2001) Gait variability and fall risk in community-living older adults: a 1-year prospective study. Arch Phys Med Rehabil 82:1050–1056
37. Hausdorff JM, Peng CK, Goldberger AL, Stoll AL (2004) Gait unsteadiness and fall risk in two affective disorders: a preliminary study. BMC Psychiatry 4:39
38. Hawthorne JM, Caley CF (2015) Extrapyramidal reactions associated with serotonergic antidepressants. Ann Pharmacother 49:1136–1152
39. Hien le TT, Cumming RG, Cameron ID, Chen JS, Lord SR, March LM, Schwarz J, Le Couteur DG, Sambrook PN (2005) Atypical antipsychotic medications and risk of falls in residents of aged care facilities. J Am Geriatr Soc 53:1290–1295
40. Hubbard R, Farrington P, Smith C, Smeeth L, Tattersfield A (2003) Exposure to tricyclic and selective serotonin reuptake inhibitor antidepressants and the risk of hip fracture. Am J Epidemiol 158:77–84
41. Huybrechts KF, Schneeweiss S, Gerhard T, Olfson M, Avorn J, Levin R, Lucas JA, Crystal S (2012) Comparative safety of antipsychotic medications in nursing home residents. J Am Geriatr Soc 60:420–429
42. Iaboni A, Flint AJ (2013) The complex interplay of depression and falls in older adults: a clinical review. Am J Geriatr Psychiatry 21:484–492
43. Jalbert JJ, Eaton CB, Miller SC, Lapane KL (2010) Antipsychotic use and the risk of hip fracture among older adults afflicted with dementia. J Am Med Dir Assoc 11:120–127
44. Joo JH, Lenze EJ, Mulsant BH, Begley AE, Weber EM, Stack JA, Mazumdar S, Reynolds CF 3rd, Pollock BG (2002) Risk factors for falls during treatment of late-life depression. J Clin Psychiatry 63:936–941
45. Katz IR (2004) Optimizing atypical antipsychotic treatment strategies in the elderly. J Am Geriatr Soc 52:S272–S277
46. Kinon BJ, Stauffer VL, McGuire HC, Kaiser CJ, Dickson RA, Kennedy JS (2003) The effects of antipsychotic drug treatment on prolactin concentrations in elderly patients. J Am Med Dir Assoc 4:189–194
47. Kishimoto T, De Hert M, Carlson HE, Manu P, Correll CU (2012) Osteoporosis and fracture risk in people with schizophrenia. Curr Opin Psychiatry 25:415–429
48. Kvelde T, Lord SR, Close JC, Reppermund S, Kochan NA, Sachdev P, Brodaty H, Delbaere K (2015) Depressive symptoms increase fall risk in older people, independent of antidepressant use, and reduced executive and physical functioning. Arch Gerontol Geriatr 60:190–195
49. Laghrissi-Thode F, Pollock BG, Miller M, Altieri L, Kupfer DJ (1995) Comparative effects of sertraline and nortriptyline on body sway in older depressed patients. Am J Geriatr Psychiatry 3:217–228
50. Lakey SL, LaCroix AZ, Gray SL, Borson S, Williams CD, Calhoun D, Goveas JS, Smoller JW, Ockene JK, Masaki KH et al (2012) Antidepressant use, depressive symptoms, and incident frailty in women aged 65 and older from the women's health initiative observational study. J Am Geriatr Soc 60:854–861
51. Landi F, Onder G, Cesari M, Barillaro C, Russo A, Bernabei R, Silver Network Home Care Study Group (2005) Psychotropic medications and risk for falls among community-dwelling frail older people: an observational study. J Gerontol A Biol Sci Med Sci 60:622–626
52. Lavsa SM, Fabian TJ, Saul MI, Corman SL, Coley KC (2010) Influence of medications and diagnoses on fall risk in psychiatric inpatients. Am J Health Syst Pharm 67:1274–1280
53. Lee D, Martini N, Moyes S, Hayman K, Zolezzi M, Kerse N (2013) Potentially inappropriate medication use: the Beers' criteria used among older adults with depressive symptoms. J Prim Health Care 5:182–190
54. Lee PE, Gill SS, Freedman M, Bronskill SE, Hillmer MP, Rochon PA (2004) Atypical antipsychotic drugs in the treatment of behavioural and psychological symptoms of dementia: systematic review. BMJ 329:75

55. Lenze EJ, Mulsant BH, Blumberger DM, Karp JF, Newcomer JW, Anderson SJ, Dew MA, Butters MA, Stack JA, Begley AE et al (2015) Efficacy, safety, and tolerability of augmentation pharmacotherapy with aripiprazole for treatment-resistant depression in late life: a randomised, double-blind, placebo-controlled trial. Lancet 386:2404–12
56. Liperoti R, Onder G, Lapane KL, Mor V, Friedman JH, Bernabei R, Gambassi G (2007) Conventional or atypical antipsychotics and the risk of femur fracture among elderly patients: results of a case-control study. J Clin Psychiatry 68:929–934
57. Liu B, Anderson G, Mittmann N, To T, Axcell T, Shear N (1998) Use of selective serotonin-reuptake inhibitors of tricyclic antidepressants and risk of hip fractures in elderly people. Lancet 351:1303–1307
58. Madhusoodanan S, Zaveri D (2010) Paliperidone use in the elderly. Curr Drug Saf 5:149–152
59. Majic T, Pluta JP, Mell T, Treusch Y, Gutzmann H, Rapp MA (2012) Correlates of agitation and depression in nursing home residents with dementia. Int Psychogeriatr 24:1779–1789
60. Maki BE (1997) Gait changes in older adults: predictors of falls or indicators of fear. J Am Geriatr Soc 45:313–320
61. Mamo DC, Pollock BG, Mulsant B, Houck PR, Bensasi S, Miller MC, Redfern MS, Reynolds CF III (2002) Effects of nortriptyline and paroxetine on postural sway in depressed elderly patients. Am J Geriatr Psychiatry 10:199–205
62. Mamo DC, Sweet RA, Mulsant BH, Pollock BG, Miller MD, Stack JA, Begley AE, Reynolds CF 3rd (2000) Effect of nortriptyline and paroxetine on extrapyramidal signs and symptoms: a prospective double-blind study in depressed elderly patients. Am J Geriatr Psychiatry 8:226–231
63. McDermott LM, Ebmeier KP (2009) A meta-analysis of depression severity and cognitive function. J Affect Disord 119:1–8
64. Michalak J, Troje NF, Fischer J, Vollmar P, Heidenreich T, Schulte D (2009) Embodiment of sadness and depression – gait patterns associated with dysphoric mood. Psychosom Med 71:580–587
65. Miller RR, Ballew SH, Shardell MD, Hicks GE, Hawkes WG, Resnick B, Magaziner J (2009) Repeat falls and the recovery of social participation in the year post-hip fracture. Age Ageing 38:570–575
66. Mitchell AJ, Malone D, Doebbeling CC (2009) Quality of medical care for people with and without comorbid mental illness and substance misuse: systematic review of comparative studies. Br J Psychiatry 194:491–499
67. Mulsant BH, Pollock BG (2015) Psychopharmacology. In: Steffens DC, Blazer DG, Thakur ME (eds) Textbook of geriatric psychiatry, 5th edn. American Psychiatric Publishing, Arlington
68. Mulsant BH (2014) Challenges of the treatment of neuropsychiatric symptoms associated with dementia. Am J Geriatr Psychiatry 22:317–320
69. Mulsant BH, Ganguli M (1999) Epidemiology and diagnosis of depression in late life. J Clin Psychiatry 60(Suppl 20):9–15
70. Nagane A, Baba H, Nakano Y, Maeshima H, Hukatsu M, Ozawa K, Suzuki T, Arai H (2014) Comparative study of cognitive impairment between medicated and medication-free patients with remitted major depression: class-specific influence by tricyclic antidepressants and newer antidepressants. Psychiatry Res 218:101–105
71. Oderda LH, Young JR, Asche CV, Pepper GA (2012) Psychotropic-related hip fractures: meta-analysis of first-generation and second-generation antidepressant and antipsychotic drugs. Ann Pharmacother 46:917–928
72. Olazarán J, Valle D, Serra JA, Cano P, Muñiz R (2013) Psychotropic medications and falls in nursing homes: a cross-sectional study. J Am Med Dir Assoc 14:213–217
73. Olfson M, Marcus SC (2009) National patterns in antidepressant medication treatment. Arch Gen Psychiatry 66:848–856
74. Onder G, Liperoti R, Fialova D, Topinkova E, Tosato M, Danese P, Gallo PF, Carpenter I, Finne-Soveri H, Gindin J et al (2012) Polypharmacy in nursing home in Europe: results from the SHELTER study. J Gerontol A Biol Sci Med Sci 67:698–704

75. Paleacu D, Shutzman A, Giladi N, Herman T, Simon ES, Hausdorff JM (2007) Effects of pharmacological therapy on gait and cognitive function in depressed patients. Clin Neuropharmacol 30:63–71
76. Pan YJ, Wu CS, Gau SS, Chan HY, Banerjee S (2014) Antipsychotic discontinuation in patients with dementia: a systematic review and meta-analysis of published randomized controlled studies. Dement Geriatr Cogn Disord 37:125–140
77. Payne RA, Abel GA, Simpson CR, Maxwell SR (2013) Association between prescribing of cardiovascular and psychotropic medications and hospital admission for falls or fractures. Drugs Aging 30:247–254
78. Perucca E, Berlowitz D, Birnbaum A, Cloyd JC, Garrard J, Hanlon JT, Levy RH, Pugh MJ (2006) Pharmacological and clinical aspects of antiepileptic drug use in the elderly. Epilepsy Res 68(Suppl 1):S49–S63
79. Porsteinsson AP, Drye LT, Pollock BG, Devanand DP, Frangakis C, Ismail Z, Marano C, Meinert CL, Mintzer JE, Munro CA et al (2014) Effect of citalopram on agitation in Alzheimer disease: the CitAD randomized clinical trial. JAMA 311:682–691
80. Pratt N, Roughead EE, Salter A, Ryan P (2012) Choice of observational study design impacts on measurement of antipsychotic risks in the elderly: a systematic review. BMC Med Res Methodol 12:72
81. Pratt N, Roughead EE, Ramsay E, Salter A, Ryan P (2011) Risk of hospitalization for hip fracture and pneumonia associated with antipsychotic prescribing in the elderly: a self-controlled case-series analysis in an Australian health care claims database. Drug Saf 34:567–575
82. Prieto-Alhambra D, Petri H, Goldenberg JS, Khong TP, Klungel OH, Robinson NJ, de Vries F (2014) Excess risk of hip fractures attributable to the use of antidepressants in five European countries and the USA. Osteoporos Int 25:847–855
83. Richards JB, Papaioannou A, Adachi JD, Joseph L, Whitson HE, Prior JC, Goltzman D, Canadian Multicentre Osteoporosis Study Research Group (2007) Effect of selective serotonin reuptake inhibitors on the risk of fracture. Arch Intern Med 167:188–194
84. Richardson K, Bennett K, Kenny RA (2015) Polypharmacy including falls risk-increasing medications and subsequent falls in community-dwelling middle-aged and older adults. Age Ageing 44:90–96
85. Rochon PA, Stukel TA, Sykora K, Gill S, Garfinkel S, Anderson GM, Normand SL, Mamdani M, Lee PE, Li P et al (2005) Atypical antipsychotics and parkinsonism. Arch Intern Med 165:1882–1888
86. Rosen CJ (2009) Bone: serotonin, leptin and the central control of bone remodeling. Nat Rev Rheumatol 5:657–658
87. Sandhu HS, Gilles E, DeVita MV, Panagopoulos G, Michelis MF (2009) Hyponatremia associated with large-bone fracture in elderly patients. Int Urol Nephrol 41:733–737
88. Schiff GD, Galanter WL, Duhig J, Lodolce AE, Koronkowski MJ, Lambert BL (2011) Principles of conservative prescribing. Arch Intern Med 171:1433–1440
89. Schneider LS, Dagerman K, Insel PS (2006) Efficacy and adverse effects of atypical antipsychotics for dementia: meta-analysis of randomized, placebo-controlled trials. Am J Geriatr Psychiatry 14:191–210
90. Shahar D, Levi M, Kurtz I, Shany S, Zvili I, Mualleme E, Shahar A, Sarid O, Melzer I (2009) Nutritional status in relation to balance and falls in the elderly: a preliminary look at serum folate. Ann Nutr Metab 54:59–66
91. Shea MLO, Garfield LD, Teitelbaum S, Civitelli R, Mulsant BH, Reynolds III CF, Dixon D, Doré P, Lenze EJ (2013) Serotonin-norepinephrine reuptake inhibitor therapy in late-life depression is associated with increased marker of bone resorption. Osteoporos Int 24:1741–9
92. Shen C, Chen F, Zhang Y, Guo Y, Ding M (2014) Association between use of antiepileptic drugs and fracture risk: a systematic review and meta-analysis. Bone 64:246–253
93. Sirven JI, Fife TD, Wingerchuk DM, Drazkowski JF (2007) Second-generation antiepileptic drugs' impact on balance: a meta-analysis. Mayo Clin Proc 82:40–47

94. Skapinakis P, Bakola E, Salanti G, Lewis G, Kyritsis AP, Mavreas V (2010) Efficacy and acceptability of selective serotonin reuptake inhibitors for the treatment of depression in Parkinson's disease: a systematic review and meta-analysis of randomized controlled trials. BMC Neurol 10(1):1–11; doi:10.1186/1147-2377-10-49
95. Somadder M, Mondal S, Kersh R, Abdelhafiz AH (2007) Are recurrent fallers depressed? J Am Geriatr Soc 55:2097–2099
96. Spangler L, Scholes D, Brunner RL, Robbins J, Reed SD, Newton KM, Melville JL, Lacroix AZ (2008) Depressive symptoms, bone loss, and fractures in postmenopausal women. J Gen Intern Med 23:567–574
97. Stone KL, Ancoli-Israel S, Blackwell T, Ensrud KE, Cauley JA, Redline S, Hillier TA, Schneider J, Claman D, Cummings SR (2008) Actigraphy-measured sleep characteristics and risk of falls in older women. Arch Intern Med 168:1768–1775
98. Tan L, Tan L, Wang HF, Wang J, Tan CC, Tan MS, Meng XF, Wang C, Yu JT (2015) Efficacy and safety of atypical antipsychotic drug treatment for dementia: a systematic review and meta-analysis. Alzheimers Res Ther 7:20, 015-0102-9.
99. Thapa PB, Gideon P, Cost TW, Milam AB, Ray WA (1998) Antidepressants and the risk of falls among nursing home residents. N Engl J Med 339:875–882
100. Thorell K, Ranstad K, Midlov P, Borgquist L, Halling A (2014) Is use of fall risk-increasing drugs in an elderly population associated with an increased risk of hip fracture, after adjustment for multimorbidity level: a cohort study. BMC Geriatr 14:131; doi:10.1186/1471-2318-14-131
101. Thorlund K, Druyts E, Wu P, Balijepalli C, Keohane D, Mills E (2015) Comparative efficacy and safety of selective serotonin reuptake inhibitors and serotonin-norepinephrine reuptake inhibitors in older adults: a network meta-analysis. J Am Geriatr Soc 63:1002–1009
102. Tseng YL, Huang CR, Lin CH, Lu YT, Lu CH, Chen NC, Chang CC, Chang WN, Chuang YC (2014) Risk factors of hyperammonemia in patients with epilepsy under valproic acid therapy. Medicine (Baltimore) 93:e66
103. van der Marck MA, Klok MP, Okun MS, Giladi N, Munneke M, Bloem BR, Falls Task Force NPF (2014) Consensus-based clinical practice recommendations for the examination and management of falls in patients with Parkinson's disease. Parkinsonism Relat Disord 20:360–369
104. van Doorn C, Gruber-Baldini AL, Zimmerman S, Hebel JR, Port CL, Baumgarten M, Quinn CC, Taler G, May C, Magaziner J et al (2003) Dementia as a risk factor for falls and fall injuries among nursing home residents. J Am Geriatr Soc 51:1213–1218
105. van Iersel MB, Zuidema SU, Koopmans RT, Verhey FR, Olde Rikkert MG (2005) Antipsychotics for behavioural and psychological problems in elderly people with dementia: a systematic review of adverse events. Drugs Aging 22:845–858
106. Vestergaard P, Rejnmark L, Mosekilde L (2008) Selective serotonin reuptake inhibitors and other antidepressants and risk of fracture. Calcif Tissue Int 82:92–101
107. Vink D, Aartsen MJ, Schoevers RA (2008) Risk factors for anxiety and depression in the elderly: a review. J Affect Disord 106:29–44
108. Whooley MA, Kip KE, Cauley JA, Ensrud KE, Nevitt MC, Browner WS (1999) Depression, falls, and risk of fracture in older women. study of osteoporotic fractures research group. Arch Intern Med 159:484–490
109. Williams LJ, Pasco JA, Stuart AL, Jacka FN, Brennan SL, Dobbins AG, Honkanen R, Koivumaa-Honkanen H, Rauma PH, Berk M (2015) Psychiatric disorders, psychotropic medication use and falls among women: an observational study. BMC Psychiatry 15:75; doi:10.1186/s12888-015-0439-4
110. Woolcott JC, Richardson KJ, Wiens MO, Patel B, Marin J, Khan KM, Marra CA (2009) Meta-analysis of the impact of 9 medication classes on falls in elderly persons. Arch Intern Med 169:1952–1960
111. Wu Q, Bencaz AF, Hentz JG, Crowell MD (2012) Selective serotonin reuptake inhibitor treatment and risk of fractures: a meta-analysis of cohort and case-control studies. Osteoporos Int 23:365–375

112. Yirmiya R, Bab I (2009) Major depression is a risk factor for low bone mineral density: a meta-analysis. Biol Psychiatry 66:423–432
113. Yogev-Seligmann G, Hausdorff JM, Giladi N (2008) The role of executive function and attention in gait. Mov Disord 23:329–342
114. Ziere G, Dieleman JP, van der Cammen TJ, Hofman A, Pols HA, Stricker BH (2008) Selective serotonin reuptake inhibiting antidepressants are associated with an increased risk of nonvertebral fractures. J Clin Psychopharmacol 28:411–417
115. De Groot MH, Van Campen JPCM, Moek MA, Tulner LR, Beijnen JH, Lamoth CJC (2013) The effects of fallrisk-increasing drugs on postural control: A literature review. Drugs and Aging 30(11):901–920
116. Echt MA, Samelson EJ, Hannan MT, Dufour AB, Berry SD (2013) Psychotropic drug initiation or increased dosage and the acute risk of falls: a prospective cohort study of nursing home residents. BMC Geriatr 13:19
117. Forester BP, Streeter CC, Berlow YA, Tian H, Wardrop M, Finn CT, et al (2009) Brain lithium levels and effects on cognition and mood in geriatric bipolar disorder: a lithium-7 magnetic resonance spectroscopy study. Am J Geriatr Psychiatry 17(1):13–23

Chapter 10
Benzodiazepines

Annemie Somers and Mirko Petrovic

Abstract Benzodiazepines are used for a variety of indications. Age-related changes in the pharmacokinetics and pharmacodynamics of benzodiazepines place older people at increased risk for side effects. Decreased hepatic blood flow, albumin level, lean body mass, and an increased elimination half-life of active metabolites all play a role. These drugs can result in excessive sedation, cognitive impairment, delirium, agitation, and balance problems leading to falls and fractures. Consistent adverse effects related to benzodiazepine use have been reported in the community, in nursing homes, and in hospitals. Guidelines for rational use of benzodiazepines in older individuals should be followed. If needed, short-term treatment (i.e. less than 4 weeks for insomnia) might be considered using an intermediate-acting benzodiazepine. Patients should be clearly informed of the risk of falls when using these drugs. Long-term prescribing should be avoided. Benzodiazepine withdrawal strategies should be proposed to chronic users with proper psychological support and a drug tapering schedule adjusted to the patient's individual needs.

Abbreviations

BZD	Benzodiazepine
CI	Confidence interval
CNS	Central nervous system
FRID	Fall risk-increasing drug

A. Somers, PharmD, PhD (✉)
Department of Pharmacy, Ghent University Hospital, De Pintelaan 185, Ghent 9000, Belgium

Faculty of Pharmaceutical Sciences, Ghent University, Ghent, Belgium
e-mail: annemie.somers@uzgent.be

M. Petrovic, MD, PhD
Department of Geriatrics, Ghent University Hospital, Ghent, Belgium

Faculty of Medicine, Ghent University, Ghent, Belgium

© Springer International Publishing Switzerland 2016

A.R. Huang, L. Mallet (eds.), *Medication-related falls in older people*,
DOI 10.1007/978-3-319-32304-6_10

GABA	Gamma-aminobutyric acid
HR	Hazard ratio
OR	Odds ratio
Z-drug	Zolpidem, zopiclone, eszopiclone, zaleplon

10.1 Introduction

Benzodiazepines (BZDs) are the most frequently used drugs within the category of hypnosedatives. BZDs have sedative, hypnotic, anxiolytic, anticonvulsive, and muscle relaxing properties and are used in a variety of indications such as insomnia, anxiety, agitation, panic, seizures, and alcohol dependence. In this chapter, we will focus on the oral use of BZDs, used for insomnia and anxiety. BZDs are widely prescribed, but their long-term use is a reason for concern, because of dependency, side effects, and cost [1–3]. Older patients are especially at risk for impaired cognitive and movement function, with an increased risk of inappropriate sedation, falls, and fractures [4–6]. It is well known that the worldwide use of BZDs is high, both in the community and within the hospital. Different risk factors for BZD use have been explored, among which (socio)demographic, clinical, and patient personality traits. Older age and central nervous disorders seem to be consistent risk factors for BSD use. Numerous studies have highlighted the associated risk of falls in patients using BZDs [4, 7–17].

There is a general awareness that long-term BZD use is inappropriate in older patients, and discontinuation should be recommended. As a consequence, the long-term use of BZDs has been imbedded in different explicit criteria for potentially inappropriate drug use in older patients [18–22]. Different interventions to reduce BZD-related falls exist, with the aim to safely reduce and stop long-term BZD use. Although no unanimous recommendations concerning withdrawal exist, it seems possible to stop BZD use by using an approach tailored to the needs of the individual patient [23].

10.2 Benzodiazepines

Benzodiazepines are organic bases composed of a benzene ring fused to a seven member diazepine ring. Nearly all effects of the BZDs result from actions on the central nervous system (CNS). Molecular targets for BZD actions in the CNS are the gamma-aminobutyric acid (GABA) receptors (different subtypes) [24]. BZDs bind to the GABA receptor, modulate its activity, and thus facilitate GABA neurotransmission. GABA is the main inhibitory neurotransmitter of the CNS, and GABA activation results thus in reduced electrical activity of large neurons both in the brain and in the spinal cord. The reduced electrical activity in the cerebellum leads

Table 10.1 Benzodiazepines (for oral use) by elimination half-life (list compiled from the Martindale, Lexi-Comp, and Clinical Pharmacology databases)

Category	Benzodiazepine	Usual single adult dose (oral) (mg)	Oral peak (hours)	Half-life (hours)
Short acting	Oxazepam	10–30	2–4	5–15
	Triazolam	0.125–0.25	0.7–2	2–3
Intermediate acting	Alprazolam	0.25–0.5	1–2	6–27
	Bromazepam	2–6	1–2	8–20
	Lorazepam	0.5–3	2–4	10–20
	Temazepam	7.5–30	1–2	8–15
Long acting	Clobazam	10–20	0.5–4	36–42
	Clonazepam	0.25–0.5	1–2	18–50
	Clorazepate	7.5–15	1–2	Desmethyldiazepam: several days
	Chlordiazepoxide	5–25	0.5–4	5–30
				Desmethyldiazepam: several days
	Diazepam	2–10	0.5–1	20–50
	Flunitrazepam	0.5–2	1–2	16–35
	Flurazepam	15–30	0.5–1	N-desalkylflurazepam: 47–100

to anxiolytic and hypnosedative effects and to muscle relaxing actions for the neurons in the spinal cord and striatum [25].

There are marked differences in potency, duration of action, metabolite activity, and rate of elimination between the different BZDs, determined by the various side chains in the molecular structure [26]. The equivalent dose may vary as much as 20-fold, which should be kept in mind when substituting one BZD by another. Almost all of the BZDs are completely absorbed when taken orally; some of them reach the systemic circulation only in the form of active metabolites. The BZD and their metabolites have a high affinity for binding to plasma proteins. The extent of binding correlates with lipid solubility and varies from 70 % to 99 %. Most BZD have a large volume of distribution due to their high lipid solubility. The concentration in the cerebrospinal fluid is nearly equal to the concentration of free drug in plasma. BZDs are metabolized primarily in the liver; most of these compounds can be classified as low clearance drugs [27]. Benzodiazepines are commonly classified into three main categories based upon the elimination half-life, i.e., short-acting agents (<12 h), intermediate-acting agents (12–24 h), and long-acting agents (>24 h) (Table 10.1).

Short-acting benzodiazepines generally have few active metabolites, do not accumulate with repeated doses, and demonstrate clearance that is largely unaffected by age and liver disease. Examples include triazolam and oxazepam. Intermediate-acting benzodiazepines include the widely used drugs lorazepam and temazepam. Long-acting benzodiazepines generally have pharmacologically active metabolites, accumulate in tissues after multiple doses, and demonstrate impaired clearance in older patients and those with liver disease. Examples include diazepam and chlordiazepoxide.

10.3 Benzodiazepines: Effects and Adverse Effects

Most BZDs are used for the purpose of their hypnosedative and anxiolytic effects. Some BZDs are also used as anticonvulsive agents or muscular relaxants. BZDs can also cause amnesic effects. In the short term, BZDs may be used safely in certain clinical conditions, but in long-term use, the effect on sleep quality does not improve, and the effect on anxiety is only symptomatic [25]. In a recent study in ten Belgian nursing homes, it was found that sleep quality in chronic BZD users significantly decreased over 1 year and was significantly worse than in nonusers at the end of this period. Depressive symptoms seemed an important factor in the deterioration of sleep quality. This study suggests that using BZDs chronically does not maintain or improve sleep quality [28].

Well-known side effects of long-term BZD use includes drug tolerance, rebound insomnia, hangover, dependence, and paradoxical stimulation. Tolerance, dependence, and withdrawal effects may turn into major clinical problems such as delirium-like symptoms. Older patients are especially susceptible to the CNS adverse reactions of BZDs such as excess sedation, lethargy, memory problems, and impaired coordination, as well as impaired learning and psychomotor performance. As a consequence, the risk of falls induced by BZDs is higher with older age [6].

10.4 Susceptibility of Older Patients to Benzodiazepines

Changes in BZD pharmacokinetics have been observed in older people. A prolongation of the half-life of the oxidized drugs has been reported in this age group, but the clearance or half-life of the glucuronidated drugs is less affected. As a result, the BZDs metabolized by oxidation, such as flurazepam and diazepam, should not prescribed in older patients, since higher plasma concentrations for a given drug dosage and consequently enhanced clinical effects are to be expected [29]. Other important and frequently seen age-related changes that may influence BZD metabolism include decreased liver blood flow, plasma albumin, and lean body mass. Reduced hepatic blood flow can modify the plasma concentration-time profile and increase peak concentrations. Decrements in plasma albumin levels will affect protein-binding capacity. Distribution volume may increase as a consequence of decreased lean body mass and increased proportion of fat. This results in an increased elimination half-life, prolonged effects on the days after administration, and accumulation of active metabolites.

Modifications of pharmacodynamics may also occur, as a consequence of increased sensitivity of the drug receptors. Older patients are more sensitive to the influence of BZDs on cognitive function, especially at higher dosages.

When looking at the clinical effects of BZD use in older patients, a high risk of adverse effects has been reported. These include excessive sedation, cognitive impairment, delirium, night wandering, and agitation, as well as impaired balance, ataxia, falls, and fractures [30, 31].

In a meta-analysis of 24 randomized trials (2417 patients) that evaluated the impact of pharmacotherapy in adults older than 60 years with insomnia, there was an improvement of sleep quality, total sleep time, and frequency of nighttime awakening [6]. However, the magnitude of these benefits was relatively small compared with the two- to fivefold increase in adverse cognitive or psychomotor events. This suggests that additional caution is necessary when deciding whether pharmacotherapy is indicated for an older patient with insomnia.

10.5 Benzodiazepine-Related Falls

BZDs have, among other drug classes, been reported to increase the risk of falls. Leipzig and Woodcott reviewed fall risk-increasing drugs (FRIDs), mainly psychotropic and cardiovascular drugs [32, 33]. Numerous studies have reported the increased risk of falls in older patients taking BZDs, in various settings (community, nursing homes, and hospitals) and in different study designs.

In the B-vitamins for the prevention of osteoporotic fractures (B-PROOF) study, concerning 2407 community-dwelling older patients, BZD use was associated with an increased fall risk (HR 1.32, [95 % CI 1.02, 1.71]) [16]. Ensrud et al. reported on falls in BZD using community-dwelling older women with one fall (OR = 1.51 [95 % CI 1.09, 1.63]) or frequent falls (OR = 1.51 [95 % CI 1.14, 2.01]) [17]. In a prospective cohort study of 1412 patients admitted to 11 acute care hospitals in Australia, falls were recorded prospectively (in hospital) and retrospectively (in the 90 days prior to admission). However, incidence rates of falls inhospital and prior to admission for users and nonusers of BZDs were not statistically different; only use of diazepam at admission was positively associated with a history of falls [7].

In a review, studies exploring postural instability and consequent falls and hip fractures associated with use of hypnotics in older people were compared. Large-scale surveys consistently reported increases in the frequency of falls and hip fractures when hypnotics are used in older people (twofold risk) [13].

A retrospective cohort study in the Netherlands was performed with 404 patients who visited the day clinic of the department of geriatric medicine and found that psychotropic medication, including short-acting benzodiazepines, strongly increased the frequency of falls (hypnotics and anxiolytics, OR 1.81 [95 % CI 1.05–3.11]; short-acting benzodiazepines or Z-drug, OR 1.94 [95 % CI 1.10–3.42]) [9].

In a cross-sectional study within three health centers in the North-East of France, 7643 community-dwelling volunteers aged 65 and older were included. The results showed that age, female gender, and the use of clobazam or prazepam were related to the recurrence of falls [10]. Benzodiazepine use was significantly associated with the occurrence of injurious falls, increasing with age, in a nested case-control study using data from a community-based cohort collected during 10 years (the personnes âgées QUID- PAQUID or 'older people as subject matter' cohort) [12]. In this study, the incidence of injurious falls in subjects aged 80 or more years exposed to BZDs was 2.8 per 100 person-years. More than 9 % of these falls were fatal. According to the results of this study and to recent population estimates, BZD use could be held responsible for almost 20,000 injurious falls in subjects aged 80-years or older every year in France and for nearly 1800 deaths.

10.6 Risk Factors for Benzodiazepine Use

Since BZDs are associated with possible adverse drug reactions in long-term use, it is valuable to detect patients at risk. For hospitalized patients, the influence of age, length of stay, and comorbidities has been found in various studies [34–36]. One study also found a higher BZD use in patients who were not coming from home and who were suffering from CNS disorders [36]. This study also showed that 88 % of the hypnosedative users had not been informed by the treating physician about the risk of dependence and had not been advised to reduce BZD use.

Petrovic et al. also studied the socio-epidemiological status and personality traits in older hospitalized patients and showed that long-term older BZD users are typically widowed females with dysthymic disorder, anxiety, predisposition to alcohol dependence, and borderline disorder [37]. Therefore, it is important to recognize the nature of the older population at risk for BZD use and to consider a broader-ranging therapeutic management of the predisposing personality traits.

In a very large, prospective database cohort study in Quebec, Canada, involving more than 253,000 patients, the risk of injury associated with the new use of individual benzodiazepines and their dosage regimens was studied with 5 years of follow-up [4]. It was found that 27.6 % of these patients were dispensed at least one prescription for a benzodiazepine, and 17.7 % of these users were treated for at least one injury during follow-up, of which fractures were the most common. The risk of injury varied by benzodiazepine, independent of half-life, as did the risk associated with increasing dosage for individual products. Higher doses of oxazepam, flurazepam, and chlordiazepoxide were associated with the greatest risk of injury.

10.7 Approach and Interventions

Since older patients are particular vulnerable to the adverse effects of BZDs, a number of approaches can be taken in order to prevent long-term use. Risk factors such as CNS disorders which predispose patients to start BZD should be estimated. Firstly, guidelines for the rational use of BZDs in older patients should be followed, including the use of non-pharmacological measures. Secondly, short-term treatment duration with an intermediate-acting BZD should be accompanied, when possible, with information to patients about the CNS-related adverse effects and the risk of falls, and thirdly, BZD use should be properly recorded, as well as falls, in order to limit long-term use. This documentation will facilitate recommendations to reduce and stop BZDs when performing medication review, e.g., by application of explicit criteria for potentially inappropriate prescribing [18–22]. Healthcare providers can also act upon reminders, alerts, and guidelines by using computer-assisted prescribing systems.

Finally, the use of withdrawal protocols for BZDs should be encouraged and individualized to improve success rates, taking into account withdrawal symptoms. The treatment of BZD withdrawal includes suitable psychological support together with a gradual dosage tapering. In most of the cases, sleep symptoms progressively improve after withdrawal. Petrovic et al. showed that a short-term BZD withdrawal program for older patients is possible in the hospital setting [23]. In this randomized study, two-thirds of chronic BZD users could successfully be withdrawn using a single step of dose reduction, over 1 week. In the hospital setting, withdrawal symptoms can be more easily recognized and managed. However, general practitioners should be involved in the decision to stop the BZD treatment, in addition to the follow-up after discharge from the hospital.

In general, a multifaceted approach is needed in order to reduce long-term BZD use in older patients, since patients underestimate the risk for adverse effects like falls and overestimate the effect on the quality of sleep. Moreover, BZDs are relatively cheap medications, but a reduction in dose or stopping these drugs often requires psychological support and follow-up which is time-consuming and costly. Multidisciplinary cooperation between healthcare providers is necessary to stop long-term BZD use but also to ensure that patients do not restart these drugs. National quality programs should include awareness campaigns to avoid long-term use of BZD in all citizens, with special focus on older patients. Hospitals and nursing home facilities should implement quality criteria consisting of the detection of patients at risk, as well as preventive measures to limit new BZD users.

10.8 Conclusion

Benzodiazepines are one of the fall risk-increasing drug classes, and the long-term use of BZD in older patients should be discouraged. The sedation due to BZD use in older patients is a main risk factor for falls and other adverse effects. There is a general awareness that BZD use is inappropriate in many patients, and therefore, discontinuation should be recommended and actively encouraged. Different strategies for reduced long-term use of BZD should be combined, both for community-dwelling and for institutionalized older patients, including risk assessment and withdrawal protocols, tailored to the needs of the individual patient.

References

1. Buscemi N, Vandermeer B, Friesen C, Bialy L, Tubman M, Ospina M et al (2007) The efficacy and safety of drug treatments for chronic insomnia in adults: a meta-analysis of RCTs. J Gen Intern Med 22(9):1335–1350
2. Holbrook AM, Crowther R, Lotter A, Cheng C, King D (2000) Meta-analysis of benzodiazepine use in the treatment of insomnia. CMAJ 162(2):225–233
3. Panneman MJ, Goettsch WG, Kramarz P, Herings RM (2003) The costs of benzodiazepine-associated hospital-treated fall injuries in the EU: a pharmo study. Drugs Aging 20(11):833–839
4. Tamblyn R, Abrahamowicz M, Du BR, McLeod P, Bartlett G (2005) A 5-year prospective assessment of the risk associated with individual benzodiazepines and doses in new elderly users. J Am Geriatr Soc 53(2):233–241
5. Petrovic M, Mariman A, Warie H, Afschrift M, Pevernagie D (2003) Is there a rationale for prescription of benzodiazepines in the elderly? Review of the literature. Acta Clin Belg 58(1):27–36
6. Glass J, Lanctot KL, Herrmann N, Sproule BA, Busto UE (2005) Sedative hypnotics in older people with insomnia: meta-analysis of risks and benefits. BMJ 331(7526):1169
7. Ballokova A, Peel NM, Fialova D, Scott IA, Gray LC, Hubbard RE (2014) Use of benzodiazepines and association with falls in older people admitted to hospital: a prospective cohort study. Drugs Aging 31(4):299–310
8. Softic A, Beganlic A, Pranjic N, Sulejmanovic S (2013) The influence of the use of benzodiazepines in the frequency falls in the elderly. Med Arch 67(4):256–259
9. van Strien AM, Koek HL, van Marum RJ, Emmelot-Vonk MH (2013) Psychotropic medications, including short acting benzodiazepines, strongly increase the frequency of falls in elderly. Maturitas 74(4):357–362
10. Rossat A, Fantino B, Bongue B, Colvez A, Nitenberg C, Annweiler C et al (2011) Association between benzodiazepines and recurrent falls: a cross-sectional elderly population-based study. J Nutr Health Aging 15(1):72–77
11. Ackroyd-Stolarz S, MacKinnon NJ, Sketris I, Sabo B (2009) Potentially inappropriate prescribing of benzodiazepines for older adults and risk of falls during a hospital stay: a descriptive study. Can J Hosp Pharm 62(4):276–283
12. Pariente A, Dartigues JF, Benichou J, Letenneur L, Moore N, Fourrier-Reglat A (2008) Benzodiazepines and injurious falls in community dwelling elders. Drugs Aging 25(1):61–70
13. Allain H, Bentue-Ferrer D, Polard E, Akwa Y, Patat A (2005) Postural instability and consequent falls and hip fractures associated with use of hypnotics in the elderly: a comparative review. Drugs Aging 22(9):749–765
14. Passaro A, Volpato S, Romagnoni F, Manzoli N, Zuliani G, Fellin R (2000) Benzodiazepines with different half-life and falling in a hospitalized population: the GIFA study. Gruppo Italiano di Farmacovigilanza nell'Anziano. J Clin Epidemiol 53(12):1222–1229
15. Ray WA, Thapa PB, Gideon P (2000) Benzodiazepines and the risk of falls in nursing home residents. J Am Geriatr Soc 48(6):682–685
16. Ham AC, Swart KM, Enneman AW, van Dijk SC, Oliai AS, van Wijngaarden JP et al (2014) Medication-related fall incidents in an older, ambulant population: the B-PROOF study. Drugs Aging 31(12):917–927
17. Ensrud KE, Blackwell T, Mangione CM, Bowman PJ, Bauer DC, Schwartz A et al (2003) Central nervous system active medications and risk for fractures in older women. Arch Intern Med 163(8):949–957
18. American Geriatrics Society 2012 Beers Criteria Update Expert Panel (2012) American Geriatrics Society updated beers criteria for potentially inappropriate medication use in older adults. J Am Geriatr Soc 60(4):616–631
19. American Geriatrics Society (2015) Updated beers criteria for potentially inappropriate medication use in older adults. J Am Geriatr Soc 63(11):2227–2246

20. McLeod PJ, Huang AR, Tamblyn RM, Gayton DC (1997) Defining inappropriate practices in prescribing for elderly people: a national consensus panel. CMAJ 156(3):385–391
21. Gallagher P, Ryan C, Byrne S, Kennedy J, O'Mahony D (2008) STOPP (Screening Tool of Older Person's Prescriptions) and START (Screening Tool to Alert doctors to Right Treatment). Consensus validation. Int J Clin Pharmacol Ther 46(2):72–83
22. O'Mahony D, O'Sullivan D, Byrne S, O'Connor MN, Ryan C, Gallagher P (2015) STOPP/START criteria for potentially inappropriate prescribing in older people: version 2. Age Ageing 44(2):213–218
23. Petrovic M, Pevernagie D, Mariman A, Van MG, Afschrift M (2002) Fast withdrawal from benzodiazepines in geriatric inpatients: a randomised double-blind, placebo-controlled trial. Eur J Clin Pharmacol 57(11):759–764
24. Smith TA (2001) Type A, gamma-aminobutyric acid (GABAA) receptor subunits and benzodiazepine binding: significance to clinical syndromes and their treatment. Br J Biomed Sci 58(2):111–121
25. Stahl SM (2000) Anxiolytic and sedative – hypnotics. In: Stahl SM (ed) Essential psychopharmacology. Cambridge University Press, Cambridge, pp 297–333
26. Chouinard G, Lefko-Singh K, Teboul E (1999) Metabolism of anxiolytics and hypnotics: benzodiazepines, buspirone, zopiclone, and zolpidem. Cell Mol Neurobiol 19(4):533–552
27. Goodman LS (2011) Goodman and Gilman's the pharmacological basis of therapeutics, 12th edn. McGraw-Hill, New York. ISBN 978-0-07-162442-8
28. Bourgeois J, Elseviers MM, Van BL, Petrovic M, Vander Stichele RH (2014) One-year evolution of sleep quality in older users of benzodiazepines: a longitudinal cohort study in Belgian nursing home residents. Drugs Aging 31(9):677–682
29. Hammerlein A, Derendorf H, Lowenthal DT (1998) Pharmacokinetic and pharmacodynamic changes in the elderly. Clinical implications. Clin Pharmacokinet 35(1):49–64
30. Gray SL, LaCroix AZ, Hanlon JT, Penninx BW, Blough DK, Leveille SG et al (2006) Benzodiazepine use and physical disability in community-dwelling older adults. J Am Geriatr Soc 54(2):224–230
31. Cumming RG, Le Couteur DG (2003) Benzodiazepines and risk of hip fractures in older people: a review of the evidence. CNS Drugs 17(11):825–837
32. Leipzig RM, Cumming RG, Tinetti ME (1999) Drugs and falls in older people: a systematic review and meta-analysis: I. Psychotropic drugs. J Am Geriatr Soc 47(1):30–39
33. Woolcott JC, Richardson KJ, Wiens MO, Patel B, Marin J, Khan KM et al (2009) Meta-analysis of the impact of 9 medication classes on falls in elderly persons. Arch Intern Med 169(21):1952–1960
34. Bell CM, Fischer HD, Gill SS, Zagorski B, Sykora K, Wodchis WP et al (2007) Initiation of benzodiazepines in the elderly after hospitalization. J Gen Intern Med 22(7):1024–1029
35. Stuffken R, van Hulten RP, Heerdink ER, Movig KL, Egberts AC (2005) The impact of hospitalisation on the initiation and long-term use of benzodiazepines. Eur J Clin Pharmacol 61(4):291–295
36. Somers A, Robays H, Audenaert K, Van MG, Bogaert M, Petrovic M (2011) The use of hypnosedative drugs in a university hospital: has anything changed in 10 years? Eur J Clin Pharmacol 67(7):723–729
37. Petrovic M, Vandierendonck A, Mariman A, Van MG, Afschrift M, Pevernagie D (2002) Personality traits and socio-epidemiological status of hospitalised elderly benzodiazepine users. Int J Geriatr Psychiatry 17(8):733–738

Chapter 11
Drugs for Degenerative Neurologic Conditions: Antiparkinson Medications, Cholinesterase Inhibitors, and Memantine

Geneviève Lemay

Abstract Drugs for degenerative neurologic conditions like antiparkinson medications, cholinesterase inhibitors, and memantine are used for symptomatic treatment of Parkinson's disease and for stabilization of decline or to slow progression of dementias, respectively. Since these drugs are not curative, knowing their risks is essential. In a population at higher risk of falls, does the use of these medications further increase that risk? A literature review showed a number of studies that included cholinesterase inhibitors demonstrated mixed results on their association with falls. Studies were often retrospective in nature and failed to account for confounders, limiting their interpretation. There was paucity of studies on memantine, but the available literature failed to show an association with falls. The small number of studies on antiparkinson medication showed an association between higher levodopa dose, but it remains unclear if this could be accounted for by the underlying disease duration and severity. At present, it remains essential to address the numerous fall-related risk factors in these high-risk populations. Although some literature has suggested an association between falls and these medications, it is arguably an association influenced or directly caused by the disease itself. Further studies of higher quality are needed to clarify this issue.

Abbreviations

AD	Alzheimer's disease
CI	Cholinesterase inhibitor; confidence interval
COMT	Catechol-O-methyltransferase
HR	Hazard ratio

G. Lemay, MD, FRCPC
Internal Medicine and Geriatrics, University of Ottawa, Ottawa, ON, Canada

Division of Geriatrics, The Ottawa Hospital, Ottawa, ON, Canada

Department of Medicine, Montfort Hospital, Ottawa, ON, Canada
e-mail: gelemay@toh.ca

© Springer International Publishing Switzerland 2016

A.R. Huang, L. Mallet (eds.), *Medication-related falls in older people*,
DOI 10.1007/978-3-319-32304-6_11

LED	Levodopa equivalent dosing
MAO	Monoamine oxidase
OR	Odds ratio
PD	Parkinson's disease
RCT	Randomized controlled trial

11.1 Introduction

As the population ages, the number of individuals with neurodegenerative diseases will rise [20]. Alzheimer's disease (AD) and Parkinson's disease (PD) are two neurodegenerative conditions without a known cure. Despite the absence of a curative treatment, some pharmacologic treatment options are available for symptom management and/or for stabilization of decline. These medications are often used in a population with a higher baseline risk of falls, which is secondary to their underlying neurologic and medical conditions. For clinicians, a question remains: Are we increasing the risk of falling in these patients by using these medications for treatment of their neurodegenerative disease?

This chapter will review the drugs used for neurodegenerative conditions and their association with falls. First is a review on cognitive enhancers: cholinesterase inhibitors (which include the currently approved medications galantamine, donepezil, and rivastigmine) and memantine. Second is a review of antiparkinson medication. To conclude, a summary of current literature and clinical implications will be discussed.

11.2 Cognitive Enhancers

Older adults with dementia are at a higher risk of falling [47], with an annual incidence of approximately 60–80 % [42]. This proportion is at least twice that of cognitively normal older adults [46]. Falling ultimately leads to fractures, institutionalization, morbidity, and mortality [36]. Dementia compounds the risk of falling due to its effect on impairing judgment, gait, visual-spatial perception, and the ability to recognize and avoid hazards [44]. Patients with Alzheimer's-type dementia have a hazard ratio of 2.8 for hip fractures [6].

Since the introduction of the first cholinesterase inhibitor (CI) in 1997, most clinicians would consider the drugs donepezil, galantamine, and rivastigmine to be the first-line pharmacotherapy for mild to moderate dementia. The drugs have slightly different pharmacologic properties, but they all work by blocking the enzyme acetylcholinesterase, thus inhibiting the breakdown of acetylcholine – an important neurotransmitter associated with memory [8].

It is well known that medications with anticholinergic properties are associated with impaired balance, increased falls, and increased rates of bony fractures in the elderly [7]. Some groups have postulated that adding cholinergic drugs to one's medication regime may improve gait, effectively reducing the chance of falling. This theory was examined in a few small studies; the results suggest that CIs may reduce falls because they improve gait and balance control, possibly through their positive effects on attention and executive function [5, 34, 35].

11.2.1 Cholinesterase Inhibitors

11.2.1.1 Effects on Gait/Balance

Assal et al. [5] demonstrated an improvement in gait performance in nine subjects with mild to moderate AD after 24 weeks using galantamine. These results suggest a galantamine-associated enhancement of the ability to adapt gait patterns to unexpected situations, which results in a lower risk of falling. In addition, Montero-Odasso [35] demonstrated that people with mild AD who are treated with donepezil have a significant increase in gait velocity and a reduction in gait variability, resulting in a more stable walking pattern. These findings provided a rationale to further assess the effect of CIs on gait performance and risk of falling in a larger, controlled clinical trial; this initiative is currently underway [34, 35].

11.2.1.2 Association with Falls in Patients with Dementia

Literature of the association of CIs and falls is variable. The quality of studies is generally weak, and most studies did not specifically consider CIs, but rather focused on various medications and their association with falls. Previous studies analyzed administrative databases and were rarely able to correct for other variables and confounders. In this population, correcting for confounders is essential, as falls are generally a result of multiple factors, especially for individuals who are cognitively impaired.

In a study from 2005, French [19] examined veterans prior to their hospital admission for hip fracture, who were prescribed medications known to increase fall risk. This study found notable differences in the number of falls occurring in CI users, including a nearly twofold increase in falls and hip fractures. The relative contribution of underlying disease versus the drug remains unclear, as confounders were not controlled for.

Similarly, in a retrospective, cross-sectional, national, secondary data analysis of over 20,000 outpatients, French et al. [19] demonstrated that more patients who used CIs (5.40 %) fell compared to those who did not (2.35 %). Again, the study design made it impossible to determine the relative contribution of the disease, the medications, and other confounding factors that may contribute to the risk of an injury due to a fall.

In a population-based cohort study that analyzed healthcare databases, Gill et al. [22] found that hospital visits for syncope were more frequent in people taking CIs than those who did not (31.5 versus 18.6 events per 1000 person-years; adjusted hazard ratio 1.76; 95 % CI 1.57–1.98). Hip fractures were also more common among people receiving CIs compared with controls (22.4 versus 19.8 events per 1000 person-years; HR 1.18; 95 % CI 1.04–1.34). This analysis was limited to the variables recorded in the administrative databases.

These findings are consistent with Birks' [8] systematic review and meta-analysis of five randomized control trials (RCTs). The review established an odds ratio of 1.90 (95 % CI 1.09–3.33, $p=0.02$) for syncope in individuals who take CIs. It is important to note that falls were not listed as an adverse event, because the trials reported only adverse events suffered by more than 5 % of subjects. Interestingly this increased risk of syncope may not be secondary to bradyarrhythmias as in a case-control analysis. Huang et al. [27] found that patients with dementia taking a CI had a decreased risk of pacemaker insertion with an unadjusted HR 0.58 (0.55–0.61).

Using administrative databases from nursing homes, Olazaran [38] found an association between falls and CIs (OR 1.42; CI 1.05–1.92). Yet again, lack of access to important data, such as medical and physical conditions, gait, and balance limited their findings.

A literature review of 69 articles [9] summarized pharmaceutical concerns in the prevention of medication-related falls. This review found only one article [17] that showed a statistically significant positive association with falls and CI use ($p=0.0012$). These findings had a hazard ratio (HR) of 1.577 (95 % CI 1.197–2.078), increasing the HR by 63 %. Notable limitations include selection bias due to sampling, clinical susceptibility, medication indication, recall, the possibility of inconsistent adverse event reporting by study personnel, and lack of documentation of previous falls.

Contrary to prior studies that found positive association between CI and falls, the following six studies found a negative association.

In their retrospective study in a senior's facility, Dolgonos et al. [13] found no difference in fall rate in subjects taking CIs versus those who did not (71 % versus 65 % $p \geq 0.05$). Tamimi's [45] retrospective case-control study compared the incidence of hip fractures in a group of AD patients who either took CI treatment or not. They adjusted for possible confounders based on the information available in patient charts. Interestingly, users of CI were associated with a lower risk of hip fracture than nonusers (adjusted OR 0.44; 95 % CI 0.24–0.72), even though CI users had a higher risk of falling. In addition, patients treated with galantamine had a comparable risk of hip fracture to nonusers. Patients treated with rivastigmine and donepezil had a lower risk of hip fractures compared to nonusers – a statistic that was highly significant: a total protective adjusted OR of 0.22 (95 % CI 0.10–0.45) and 0.39 (95 % CI 0.19–0.76), respectively, compared to AD patients who did not use CIs.

Three systematic reviews were found in the literature, the first by Hartikainen et al. [25] who examined medication use as a risk factor for falls and fall-related fractures. In this review, only Kallin's [28] cross-sectional, prospective population-based study of 3304 patients addressed CIs. This study did not show any significant association between falls and use of CI (OR 0.72; 95 % CI 0.36–1.44); however, there was a lack of data about other medical diagnosis that are known to influence fall risk.

The second, a Cochrane systematic review [41], included six RCTs that examined efficacy, safety, and tolerability of CIs in 1236 patients with Parkinson's disease dementia and Lewy body dementia. This review did not find any specific difference in falls between treatment versus placebo groups (43/739 versus 16/352; OR 1.29; 95 % CI 0.72 to 2.33, $P=0.39$). The authors of the review cautioned interpretation of this data, because half of the trial data was not made available to the public.

Lastly, Kim [30] conducted a meta-analysis of 22 studies (RCTs and extension studies) to evaluate the effect of CIs on the risk of falls, syncope, and related events. They concluded that CI use was associated with greater risk of syncope (OR 1.53; 95 % CI 1.02–2.30) compared to placebo, but was not associated with other events (falls, OR 0.88; 95 % CI 0.74–1.04; fracture, OR 5 1.39; 95 % CI 5 0.75–2.56; accidental injury, OR 1.13; 95 % CI 0.87–1.45). The authors cautioned interpretation of the data because of small sample sizes, possible underreporting of events, and the possibility of small benefits or harms that could not be excluded.

11.2.1.3 Association with Falls in Patients with Parkinson's Disease (PD)

A few studies examined the use of CIs in individuals with PD. In their small study of six individuals, Kareus et al. [29] looked at the effect of donepezil using posturography. They found that cholinergic augmentation could improve integration of visual sensory information, resulting in improved balance and posture. Parashos et al. [40] had a similar finding: they were unable to associate falls and use of CIs, even after accounting for disease duration and severity of cognitive dysfunction.

More recently, Pagano et al. [39] conducted a systematic review, which including four RCTs, in order to assess efficacy and safety of CI in PD patients. The fall risk analysis failed to show any significant effect of CI (OR 1.13; CI 0.62–2.07). Only one study, an RCT by Chung et al. [10], which included 23 patients with PD at high risk of falls, found that donepezil reduced fall frequency by approximately half (0.25–0.13 falls per day) in frequent-falling subjects with PD. Absolute reduction was 0.12 falls per day with 8.3 people needing treatment to prevent a fall. The authors theorized the improvements might be attributed to the rationale that anticholinergic medications are associated with falls. Larger studies that did not assess the baseline fall risk also found a significant improvement of falling rates in patients with PD who were treated with CIs [14, 16].

11.2.1.4 Summary

There is clearly a lack of quality in the studies that examine associations between CIs and fall risk in the AD and PD populations, thus making it difficult to ascertain whether the two are related. The studies that report a possible association between CIs and falls are retrospective in nature, and they fail to account for important confounders like comorbid diseases and the presence of possible risk factors related to falling. Because of these shortcomings, the risk of falls is similar to the risk of syncope, a well-known potential side effect of the medication induced by cardiac bradyarrhythmia. Cardiac risk of cholinergic augmentation must be seriously considered in high-risk patients because fall-related syncope is well described in the literature.

The literature that reports a negative association between CIs and falls consists of stronger study designs; however, underreporting of harm may have underestimated fall frequency. Nevertheless, it is plausible – with small studies showing evidence of the benefits of cholinergic augmentation on balance measures, attention, and executive function – that CIs may decrease the risk of falls in some patients. As more literature on gait and cognition emerges, a multivariate regression model could be developed to account for all confounders and to identify whether these drugs can modify the risk of falls. At present, it is prudent to remain vigilant in prescribing CIs and to address all other fall-related risk factors, as we are yet to have strong evidence for or against the association of CIs and falls.

11.2.2 Memantine

The available literature on the association of memantine and falls is quite small with only four articles. Using nursing home administrative databases, Olazaran [38] found an association between falls and memantine, with an OR of 1.90 (95 % CI 1.32–2.74). Notable limitations include its cross-sectional design and its lack of access to data that are associated with falls, including medical and physical conditions, gait, balance, and visual acuity.

Similarly, Kim's [30] meta-analysis did not find a statistically significant effect of memantine on falls with an OR of 0.92 (95 % CI 0.72–1.18). Due to a small number and possible underreporting of events, the possibility of minor benefits or harms could not be excluded.

More recently, Epstein et al. [17] conducted a retrospective analysis using a multivariate model on data from the Alzheimer's Disease Neuroimaging Initiative. They did not find an increase in risk of falls with memantine use, even after adjusting for significant covariates of age and the Beers medications.

In McShane's [33] Cochrane review of six RCTs of memantine use in mild to severe dementia, the OR for falls was 0.96 (95 % CI 0.71–1.30), whereas in mild to moderate dementia, the OR for falls was 0.83 (95 % CI 0.41–1.67). Neither of these results indicate an increased risk of falls with the use of memantine. It is important to note that the number of falls reported in the systematic review was much lower than the rates estimated by other observational studies, suggesting that falls may have been underreported as a whole or that participants in the studies were generally healthier than the general population. If these are true, it means that there is an underestimation of the potentially important risks of fall-related adverse events associated with memantine.

11.2.3 Summary

From the limited information that is currently available, there is not a strong case for the association between memantine and falling. It is advised that physicians recommend prudence to their patients with dementia, as it is well documented that individuals with dementia have a higher risk of falling compared to the general population. There is, however, a lack of available literature – taking into account the paucity of studies and the limitations of the ones available – to be certain that memantine increases the risk of falls.

11.3 Antiparkinson Medications

Falls are highly prevalent in individuals with Parkinson's disease (PD); 33–68 % of PD patients will fall [1, 4, 49], with approximately 40 % of these falls leading to injury [23]. Both PD-related and comorbid pathologies are proposed to be potential underlying causes for falls [26].

There are several risk factors associated with falls in patients with PD. These include the severity and duration of disease, gait and balance disturbances, previous falls, fear of falling, and dementia [2]. Furthermore, it has also been shown that urinary incontinence, daily intake of alcohol, and orthostatic hypotension are associated with falling in PD patients [32]. Parkinsonism in itself has been associated with an adjusted OR of 1.2 (95 % CI 1.0–1.4) for falls [48]. Could this mean that it is important to be aware of the effects of antiparkinson medication?

11.3.1 Effect on Gait and Balance

Considering the increased baseline risk of falls in the PD population, some research has explored the effects of antiparkinson medication on gait and balance. In their cross-sectional prospective, descriptive study, D'Andrea Greve et al. [11] observed a large area of sway among patients with PD when they were under the effect of levodopa. This finding correlated with dyskinesia because the change in movement quality impaired balance reactions, thus obliging patients to make displacements over a wider area in order to remain on their feet. It was suggested that real-life situations that do not allow for this type of adaptation might contribute toward the falls that are observed among PD patients.

In contrast, Kumar's [31] observational study of 70 patients found that levodopa therapy could improve most of the gait parameters among PD patients. Furthermore, Dhall et al. [12] noted improvements in gait that were greater than improvements in balance in individuals taking levodopa. This finding may in part explain why some individuals with balance difficulty fall more frequently on levodopa: as gait speed increases, and without proportional improvement in balance, people are likely to fall.

11.3.2 Antiparkinson Medication Association with Falls

Literature on the association of antiparkinson medication and falls is variable. Eight studies on this topic were found, and the quality of these studies was generally weak. Most studies did not specifically evaluate medication and falls. These studies most often analyzed administrative databases, they were rarely able to correct for other variables and confounders, and several studies were quite small.

One study of a sample of outpatient veterans with hip fractures reported a positive association between antiparkinson medication and falls [18]; this study found a nearly fourfold increase in antiparkinson drug use. The relative contribution of underlying disease versus the drug treating the disease was unclear, considering previous evidence that fractures were significantly more common in PD patients than in a non-PD control group (PD 15 %, control 7.5 %; $p=0.007$) [21].

Similarly, in a retrospective, cross-sectional, national, secondary outpatient data analysis of more than 20,000 patients, French et al. [19] found that patients who had more previous falls used antiparkinson medications (3.67 % versus 1.32 %). Again, it was impossible to determine the relative contribution of the disease, the mediations, or other confounding factors to the risk of an injury due to a fall, which limits the study's findings.

In a population-based study of 3304 patients in a cross-sectional design that used a univariate analysis, Kallin et al. [28] found that use of levodopa (OR 1.67; 95 % CI 1.00–2.78) was associated with falls. Authors attributed this increased risk to the underlying diagnosis rather than the medication itself, because PD leads to mobility disturbances and orthostatic hypotension.

Shuto et al. [43] conducted a similar analysis in an acute hospital setting. This study was a case-crossover study that examined administrative databases of 349 patients who had inhospital falls. The initial use of antiparkinson medication (within 3 days of the fall) was significantly associated with falls (OR 4.18; CI 1.75–10.02). The contribution of comorbid disease, medication dose, and other fall risk factors were not included in the analysis, which limited attribution of the fall to the medication itself.

Only one systematic review [9] on fall risk and medication included antiparkinson medications. After reviewing 69 articles on multifaceted pharmaceutical concerns in the prevention of medication-related falls, anti-Parkinson's medication were found to be significantly associated with inpatient falls with an OR of approximately 4–5 [17].

In their case-control study, Vestergaard et al. [48] found a dose-response relationship with risk of fracture for levodopa alone or combined with carbidopa and/or catechol-O-methyltransferase (COMT) inhibitors. No excess fracture risk was associated with anticholinergic drugs, monoamine oxidase (MAO)-B inhibitors, or dopamine agonists after adjusting for numerous covariates. It is important to note that the doses of these drugs were low. The increased risk of fracture associated with levodopa and correlated with the dose may be due to confounding by indication, where increased drug use may be due to increased disease severity. An additional noteworthy point is that this study did not specifically evaluate falls or other injuries due to falls.

Similarly, Parashos [40] found that the levodopa equivalent dosing (LED) was significantly associated with presence ($p=0.014$), number of falls ($p=0.032$), and total events ($p=0.033$). When accounting for disease duration, LED was no longer a significant predictor for any of the outcomes.

Furthermore, in their multivariate analysis, Almeida et al. [3] found that LED was an independent risk factor ($p=<0.05$) for recurrent falls (two or more falls per year) with an OR of 1.283 per 100 mg increase (95 % CI 1.092–1.507). This finding may be explained by LED's relationship to longer PD, which may be characterized by disease severity and postural instability.

In their 1-year prospective study, Allcock et al. [1] found that fallers were taking more dopaminergic replacement medication than non-fallers (LED fallers 400 mg, non-fallers 300 mg, $p<0.03$). There was no difference in the proportion taking dopamine agonists when falls were dichotomized in this way ($p=0.18$).

Grubb et al. [24] examined administrative databases for the number of hospitalizations, emergency room visits, fractures, and falls among patients diagnosed with PD who initiated therapy with either selegiline or rasagiline. After controlling for patient characteristics, general health, disability status, comorbid diagnoses, and index prescription characteristics, logistic regression found that rasagiline was associated with a significantly lower likelihood of falls (OR 0.552; CI 0.335–0.909) compared to patients starting on selegiline therapy.

In their 2-year prospective study that evaluated 125 PD patients, Matinolli et al. [32] found that the daily levodopa dose was significantly higher ($P=0.002$) among those who were recurring fallers. The recurrent fallers had a longer PD duration and a more severe disease than the nonrecurrent fallers (7.5 years versus 4.8 years, $p=0.010$), but there was no difference in the proportion of patients using levodopa, dopamine agonists, selegiline, or entacapone. This finding also indicates an association between falls, disease duration, and severity, rather than medication alone.

Lastly, during the 6-year open-label study of rotigotine transdermal system, Elmer et al. [15] found that 16.5 % of patients experienced falls. It is unclear if these falls were due to the drug itself, because about 74 % of patients were on concomitant use of levodopa and other antiparkinson drugs. In a later study [37], patients who were younger than 65 years old experienced fewer falls with rotigotine treatment than placebo, which may have been the results of a reduction in "off-time." In the over 65 cohort, falls increased in a similar fashion in people taking treatment and placebo, but falls were higher than those under the age of 65; this is expected due to increased frailty in older age.

11.3.3 Summary

This review on antiparkinson medications ascertained that there are only a small number of studies addressing this important issue. The available literature reports an increase in falls in patients using antiparkinson medication, particularly those using levodopa. It is important to note that the increase in the number of falls was also due to a longer disease duration and disease severity. It is unclear if this increased risk can be attributed solely to the disease itself and not due to a positive or negative influence of the medication. In addition, falls were seen more frequently in patients on higher doses of dopaminergic drugs. This finding suggests that either higher doses increase fall risk or increased fall risk can be attributed solely to more severe and advanced disease, as this is a well-documented phenomenon. With this in mind, small studies that demonstrate evidence of the benefits of dopaminergic augmentation on balance and gait may be an indication that these medications improve movement and ambulation with a subsequent increase in risk of falling.

At present, it remains essential to address the numerous fall-related risk factors in this high-risk population. It is imperative that physicians treat the disease to improve mobility, freeness of movement, and quality of life. Although some literature has suggested an association between falls and antiparkinson medication, it is arguably an association influenced or directly caused by the disease itself. Further studies of higher quality are needed to clarify this issue.

References

1. Allcock LM, Rowan EN, Steen IN, Wesnes K, Kenny RA, Burn DJ (2009) Impaired attention predicts falling in Parkinson's disease. Parkinsonism Relat Disord 15(2):110–115
2. Allen NE, Schwarzel AK, Canning CG (2013) Recurrent falls in Parkinson's disease: a systematic review. Park Dis 2013:906274. doi:10.1155/2013/906274
3. Almeida LRS, Valença GT, Negreiros NN, Pinto EB, and Oliveira-Filho J (2014) Recurrent falls in people with Parkinson's disease without cognitive impairment: focusing on modifiable risk factors. Park Dis. Article ID 432924. doi:10.1155/2014/432924
4. Ashburn A, Stack E, Pickering RM, Ward CD (2001) A community-dwelling sample of people with Parkinson's disease characteristics of fallers and non-fallers. Age Ageing 30:47–52
5. Assal F, Allali G, Kressig RW et al (2008) Galantamine improves gait performance in patients with Alzheimer's disease. J Am Geriatr Soc 56:946–947
6. Baker NL, Cook MN, Arrighi HM, Bullock R (2011) Hip fracture risk and subsequent mortality among Alzheimer's disease patients in the United Kingdom, 1988–2007. Age Ageing 40(1):49–54
7. Berdot S, Bertrand M, Dartigues JF et al (2009) Inappropriate medication use and risk of falls: a prospective study in a large community-dwelling elderly cohort. BMC Geriatr 9:30
8. Birks J (2006) Cholinesterase inhibitors for Alzheimer's disease. Cochrane Database Syst Rev Jan 25;(1):CD005593
9. Chen Y, Zhu LL, Zhou Q (2014) Effects of drug pharmacokinetic/pharmacodynamic properties, characteristics of medication use, and relevant pharmacological interventions on fall risk in elderly patients. Ther Clin Risk Manag 10:437–448
10. Chung KA, Lobb BM, Nutt JG, Horak FB (2010) Effects of a central cholinesterase inhibitor on reducing falls in Parkinson disease. Neurology 75(14):1263–1269
11. D'Andrea Greve JM, Luna NM, de Siqueira JP, Prota C, Alonso AC (2014) Assessment of postural balance among individuals with Parkinson disease with and without effects from dopaminergic medications. Am J Phys Med Rehabil 93(5):365–371
12. Dhall R, Krishnamurthi N, Lieberman A, Dhanani S, Pan D (2013) Why levodopa may increase falls in parkinson's disease. Neurology 80(Meeting Abstract)
13. Dolgonos O, Tam S, Golshan S, Sargent J, Daly JW, Sewell D (2011) Impact of acetylcholinesterase inhibitors on fall risk in later stages of dementia. J Am Geriatr Soc 59:S45

14. Dubois B, Tolosa E, Katzenschlager R et al (2012) Donepezil in Parkinson's disease dementia: a randomized, double-blind efficacy and safety study. Mov Disord 27:1230–1238
15. Elmer LW, Surmann E, Boroojerdi B, Jankovic J (2012) Long-term safety and tolerability of rotigotine transdermal system in patients with early-stage idiopathic Parkinson's disease: a prospective, open-label extension study. Parkinsonism Relat Disord 18(5):488–493
16. Emre M, Aarsland D, Albanese A et al (2004) Rivastigmine for dementia associated with Parkinson's disease. N Engl J Med 351:2509–2518
17. Epstein NU, Guo R, Farlow MR, Singh JP, Fisher M (2014) Medication for Alzheimer's disease and associated fall hazard: a retrospective cohort study from the Alzheimer's disease neuroimaging initiative. Drugs Aging 31(2):125–129
18. French DD, Campbell R, Spehar A, Cunningham F, Foulis P (2005) Outpatient medications and hip fractures in the US: a national veterans study. Drugs Aging 22(10):877–885
19. French DD, Campbell R, Spehar A, Cunningham F, Bulat T, Luther SL (2006) Drugs and falls in community-dwelling older people: a national veterans study. Clin Ther 28(4):619–630
20. Gammon K (2014) Neurodegenerative disease: brain windfall. Nature 515:299–300
21. Genever RW, Downes TW, Medcalf P (2005) Fracture rate in Parkinson's disease compared with age and gender matched controls: a retrospective cohort study. Age Ageing 34: 21–24
22. Gill SS, Anderson GM, Fischer HD, Bell CM, Li P, Normand SL, Rochon PA (2009) Syncope and its consequences in patients with dementia receiving cholinesterase inhibitors: a population-based cohort study. Arch Intern Med 169(9):867–873. doi:10.1001/archinternmed.2009.43
23. Gray P, Hildebrand K (2000) Fall risk factors in Parkinson's disease. J Neurosci Nurs 32:222–228
24. Grubb E, Treglia M, Lage M, Castelli-Haley J (2013) Comparison of hospitalizations, emergency room visits, fractures, and falls among parkinson disease patients who initiated therapy with selegiline or rasagiline: a retrospective study. Value Health 16(3):A105
25. Hartikainen S, Lönnroos E, Louhivuori K (2007) Medication as a risk factor for falls: critical systematic review. J Gerontol A Biol Sci Med Sci 62(10):1172–1181
26. Hiorth YH, Larsen JP, Lode K, Pedersen KF (2014) Natural history of falls in a population-based cohort of patients with Parkinson's disease: an 8-year prospective study. Parkinsonism Relat Disord 20(10):1059–1064
27. Huang A, Redpath C, Van Walraven C (2015) The influence of cholinesterase therapy for dementia on risk of cardiac pacemaker insertion: a retrospective, population-based, health administrative databases study in Ontario, Canada. BMC Neurol 15:66
28. Kallin K, Gustafson Y, Sandman PO, Karlsson S (2004) Drugs and falls in older people in geriatric care settings. Aging Clin Exp Res 16(4):270–276
29. Kareus SA, Lai A, Horak FB, Nutt JG, Chung KA (2012) The effect of donepezil on a quantitative measure of balance in Parkinson's disease. Mov Disord 27:S123
30. Kim DH, Brown RT, Ding EL, Diel DP, Berry SD (2011) Dementia Medications and Risk of Falls, Syncope and Related Advserse Events: Meta-Analysis of Randomized Controlled Trials. JAGS. 59(6):1019–31. doi:10.1111/j.1532-5415.2011.03450.x. Epub 2011 Jun 7
31. Kumar H, Mondal B, Sen S, Chatterjee P, Choudhury S, Anand SS et al (2014) Objective gait analysis in Parkinson's disease reflecting the effect of levodopa. Ann Indian Acad Neurol 17:S175
32. Matinolli M, Korpelainen JT, Sotaniemi KA, Myllyla VV, Korpelainen R (2011) Recurrent falls and mortality in Parkinson's disease: a prospective two-year follow-up study. Acta Neurol Scand 123(3):193–200
33. McShane R, Areosa Sastre A, Minakaran N (2006) Memantine for dementia. Cochrane Database Syst Rev (2):CD003154
34. Montero-Odasso M, Wells J, Borrie M (2009) Can cognitive enhancers reduce the risk of falls in people with dementia? An open-label study with controls. J Am Geriatr Soc 57(2):359–360
35. Montero-Odasso M, Borrie J, Wells M, Speechley M (2009) Can cognitive enhancers reduce the risk of falls in older people with mild cognitive impairment? A protocol for a randomised controlled double blind trial. BMC Neurol 9:42. doi:10.1186/1471-2377-9-42

36. Morris JC, Rubin EH, Morris E (1987) Senile dementia of the Alzheimer's type: an important risk factor for serious falls. J Gerontol 42:412–417
37. Oertel W, LeWitt P, Giladi N, Ghys L, Grieger F, Boroojerdi B (2013) Treatment of patients with early and advanced Parkinson's disease with rotigotine transdermal system: age-relationship to safety and tolerability. Parkinsonism Relat Disord 19(1):37–42
38. Olazaran J, Valle D, Serra JA, Cano P, Muniz R (2013) Psychotropic medications and falls in nursing homes: a cross-sectional study. J Am Med Dir Assoc 14(3):213–217
39. Pagano G, Rengo G, Pasqualetti G, Femminella GD, Monzani F, Ferrara N, Tagliati M (2014) Cholinesterase inhibitors for Parkinson's disease: a systematic review and meta-analysis. J Neurol Neurosurg Psychiatry. pii: jnnp-2014-308764; 767–73. doi:10.1136/jnnp-2014-308764. [Epub ahead of print]
40. Parashos S, Wielinski C, Nance M (2013) Lack of association between central anticholinesterase treatment and falls in Parkinson disease. J Park Dis 3:129
41. Rolinski M, Fox C, Maidment I, McShane R (2012) Cholinesterase inhibitors for dementia with Lewy bodies, Parkinson's disease dementia and cognitive impairment in Parkinson's disease. Cochrane Database Syst Rev (3):CD006504. doi:10.1002/14651858.CD006504.pub2
42. Shaw FE (2007) Prevention of falls in older people with dementia. J Neural Transm 114:1259–1264
43. Shuto H, Imakyure O, Matsumoto J, Egawa T, Jiang Y, Hirakawa M et al (2010) Medication use as a risk factor for inpatient falls in an acute care hospital: a case-crossover study. Br J Clin Pharmacol 69(5):535–542
44. Suttanon P, Hill KD, Said CM, Logiudice D, Lautenschlager NT, Dodd KJ (2012) Balance and mobility dysfunction and falls risk in older people with mild to moderate Alzheimer disease. Am J Phys Med Rehabil 91(1):12–23
45. Tamimi I, Ojea T, Sanchez-Siles JM, Rojas F, Martin I, Gormaz I, Perez A, Dawid-Milner MS, Mendez L, Tamimi F (2012) Acetylcholinesterase inhibitors and the risk of hip fracture in Alzheimer's disease patients: a case-control study. J Bone Miner Res 27(7):1518–1527. doi:10.1002/jbmr.1616
46. Tinetti ME, Speechley M, Ginter SF (1988) Risk factors for falls among elderly persons living in the community. N Engl J Med 319:1701–1707
47. Van DC, Gruber-Baldini AL, Zimmerman S et al (2003) Dementia as a risk factor for falls and fall injuries among nursing home residents. J Am Geriatr Soc 51:1213–1218
48. Vestergaard P, Rejnmark L, Mosekilde L (2007) Fracture risk associated with parkinsonism and anti-parkinson drugs. Calcif Tissue Int 81:153–161
49. Wood BH, Bilclough JA, Bowron A, Walker RW (2002) Incidence and prediction of falls in Parkinson's disease: a prospective multidisciplinary study. J Neurol Neurosurg Psychiatry 72:721–725

Chapter 12
Antihypertensives and Cardiovascular Medications

Rebecca L. Salbu, Rosanne M. Leipzig, and Fred C. Ko

Abstract The use of antihypertensive drugs in the elderly population places patients at an increased risk of adverse drug events in both the inpatient and outpatient setting. The setting of appropriate blood pressure goals and using antihypertensive medications is complex and no consensus exists. Hypertension treatment goals need to be individualized. Well-known trials have described the risks of falls and fall-related injuries in older adults taking antihypertensive medications. The results from these studies may not be directly applicable to the population of frail older patients. In three meta-analyses conducted in 1999, 2009, and 2013, there was no clear statistically significant evidence indicating that antihypertensive medications increase the risk of falls, but the clinician still needs to be aware of the impact of drug therapies and fall-related injuries. Although the adverse relationship between cardiovascular medications and falls and fall-related injuries in older adults is supported by high-quality and well-conducted observational studies, only thiazide diuretics have been singled out. The safe and effective use of cardiovascular medications in physically frail older patients requires deliberate and thoughtful considerations. Managing polypharmacy, performing medication reconciliation and review, and employing deprescribing strategies will result in an appropriate cardiovascular medication regimen while minimizing adverse effects and reducing the risk for falls in older patients.

R.L. Salbu, PharmD, CGP (✉)
Department of Pharmacy Practice, Touro College of Pharmacy, New York, NY, USA

Mount Sinai Hospital, New York, NY, USA
e-mail: Rebecca.Salbu@touro.edu

R.M. Leipzig, MD, PhD
Brookdale Department of Geriatrics and Palliative Medicine, Icahn School of Medicine at Mount Sinai, New York, NY, USA

F.C. Ko, MD, MS
Brookdale Department of Geriatrics and Palliative Medicine, Icahn School of Medicine at Mount Sinai, New York, NY, USA

Geriatric Research, Education, and Clinical Center (GRECC), James J. Peters VA Medical Center, Bronx, NY, USA

© Springer International Publishing Switzerland 2016

A.R. Huang, L. Mallet (eds.), *Medication-related falls in older people*,
DOI 10.1007/978-3-319-32304-6_12

Abbreviations

ACCF	American College of Cardiology Foundation
ACCORD	Action to Control Cardiovascular Risk in Diabetes
ACE	Angiotensin-converting enzyme
ADA	The American Diabetes Association
AGS	American Geriatrics Society
ALLHAT	Antihypertensive and Lipid-Lowering Treatment to Prevent Heart Attack Trial
ARB	Angiotensin II receptor blockers
ASH/ISH	The American Society of Hypertension and The International Society of Hypertension
BBs	Beta-blockers
CCBs	Calcium channel blockers
CHEP	The Canadian Hypertension Education Program
CI	Confidence interval
ESH/ESC	The European Society of Hypertension and The European Society of Cardiology
HR	Hazard ratio
HYVET	Hypertension in the Very Elderly Trial
JNC	Joint National Committee
KDIGO	The Kidney Disease Improving Global Outcomes workgroup
OR	Odds ratio
SBP	Systolic blood pressure
SHEP	Systolic Hypertension in the Elderly Program
SPRINT	Systolic Blood Pressure Intervention Trial

12.1 Introduction

The use of antihypertensives in the elderly population places patients at an increased risk of adverse drug events in both the inpatient and outpatient setting [1, 2]. These adverse drug events, including balance and gait impairment, dizziness, and autonomic dysregulation contributing to orthostatic hypotension, are among the most common and place a patient at an increased risk for fall and fracture [3, 4]. Before reviewing specific cardiovascular medications that may contribute to falls, it is imperative to discuss blood pressure goals in the elderly population, to ensure we are treating the patients appropriately, while not placing them at increased risk for adverse events.

12.2 Hypertension Treatment Goals in Older Adults

The management of hypertension in the elderly including setting blood pressure goals and using antihypertensive medications is complex. These complex clinical decisions stem from the need to consider patient-centered factors such as multiple chronic conditions, physical frailty, and polypharmacy required to achieve these goals. The use of multiple cardiovascular medications to achieve blood pressure goals was discussed in the well-known Antihypertensive and Lipid-Lowering Treatment to Prevent Heart Attack Trial (ALLHAT). The authors of this trial concluded that 60 % of patients (mean age 66.9 years old) with a controlled blood pressure of <140/90 mmHg required two or more antihypertensive medications and only 30 % of patients were controlled on one drug and suggested that for individuals with even lower blood pressure goals, three or more medications may be required [5, 6]. This need for three or more medications to reach a lower blood pressure goal raises concern as it is well known that increasing numbers of medications places elderly patients at increased risk for adverse events [7].

Thus, hypertension treatment goals in older adults need to be decided on an individualized basis. Professional medical societies frequently differ when stating an ideal blood pressure goal in an elderly patient. In general, these societies often recommend higher blood pressure goals in the older population compared to younger healthier adults. However, the rationales attributing to different age-related blood pressure goals are rarely discussed, and the recommendations are seldom absolute in the older population. This lack of a definitive recommendation for hypertension treatment goals is reflective of an absence of randomized clinical trial data on the treatment of hypertension in physically frail elderly patients [4].

In 2011, the American College of Cardiology Foundation (ACCF) published an expert consensus document on hypertension in the elderly, in collaboration with various professional organizations including the American Geriatrics Society (AGS) [4]. The Expert Consensus Document on Hypertension in the Elderly Recommendations are as follows: (1) systolic blood pressure (SBP) values <140 mmHg are appropriate goals for most patients 60–79 years of age, and (2) for those 80 years of age and older, SBP values 140–145 mmHg, if tolerated, can be acceptable. The ACCF's consensus statement expresses specific concerns with each antihypertensive medication class in the elderly population, which may help to guide clinicians in making treatment decisions. For instance, the ACCF describes the benefits, but also the risks of diuretics, dihydropyridines, and centrally acting antihypertensives with regard to falls, stating that these medications may be doing more harm than good [4]. Diuretics may cause sodium and water depletion and increase risk for orthostatic hypotension and dehydration thus potentially leading to falls. Dihydropyridines have vasodilatory effects which can result in postural hypotension leading to dizziness and falls. Lastly, centrally acting agents, such as clonidine, increase risk of sedation and bradycardia and should not be considered first-line treatment for hypertension [4].

Blood pressure goals in the elderly patient have been recommended by a number of other professional medical societies. These include the Eighth Joint National Committee (JNC), European Society of Hypertension and European Society of Cardiology (ESH/ESC), American Society of Hypertension and International Society of Hypertension (ASH/ISH), Canadian Hypertension Education Program (CHEP), American Diabetes Association (ADA), and Kidney Disease Improving Global Outcomes (KDIGO) workgroup [8–13] (Table 12.1). Because of the differing blood pressure goals recommended by these professional societies, the management of hypertension in the elderly can become a confusing task for clinicians.

Table 12.1 Blood pressure goals in older patients recommended by professional medical societies [8–13]

Society (year)	Goal Systolic Blood Pressure (SBP) and Diastolic Blood Pressure (DBP)		Comments
	60–79 years old	≥80 years old	
ASH/ISH (2014)	SBP <140 mmHg	SBP <150 mmHg	States SBP <150 mmHg associated with strong cardiovascular and stroke protection
ESH/ESC (2013)	SBP <140 mmHg	SBP 140–150 mmHg	Recommendations provided for patients in good physical and mental conditions only
ACCF (2011)	SBP <140 mmHg	SBP 140–145 mmHg if tolerated	Discusses risks with specific classes of medications and how they may lead to falls
CHEP (2015)	SBP <140 mmHg and DBP <90 mmHg	SBP <150 mmHg	Notes caution should be exercised in elderly patients when initiating combination therapy, as this may be poorly tolerated
ADA (2015)	SBP of <140 mmHg and DBP of <90 mmHg for patients with both diabetes and hypertension, regardless of age		Does not recommend goal based on age States lower blood pressure goals may be appropriate for younger patients
JNC 8 (2014)	For individuals >60 years old, SBP <150 mmHg and DBP <90 mmHg		More conservative than JNC 7 recommendations
KDIGO (2012)	SBP <140 and DBP <90 mmHg in non-albuminuric patients, unable to recommend specific blood pressure goals in the elderly, and even harder to make recommendations in individuals >80 years old		Notes that blood pressure goals may be difficult to achieve without adverse effects Suggests asking older patients being treated for high blood pressure about dizziness and to measure blood pressure while sitting and standing to assess for orthostatic hypotension

ASH/ISH American Society of Hypertension and International Society of Hypertension, *ESH/ESC* European Society of Hypertension and European Society of Cardiology, *ACCF* American College of Cardiology Foundation, *CHEP* Canadian Hypertension Education Program, *ADA* American Diabetes Association, *JNC 8* Eighth Joint National Committee, *KDIGO* Kidney Disease Improving Global Outcomes workgroup

12.3 Associations Between Cardiovascular Medications and Falls: The Evidence

There is compelling evidence that pharmacologic treatment of hypertension in elderly patients decreases the risk of adverse cardiovascular disease outcomes. However, less is known about the optimal blood pressure threshold and risk of falls and fall-related injuries due to hypertension treatment in older adults. This gap in knowledge may be directly attributed to a number of reasons including the absence of falls and fall-related adverse events as primary outcomes and exclusion of physically frail older adults in hypertension clinical trials. Thus, it is likely that cardiovascular medication-associated adverse events are suboptimally reported in physically frail older adults who are at higher risk for falls. Furthermore, this deficit in knowledge has significant implications in the clinical care of older adults. As an illustration, when a clinician is presented with a physically frail elderly patient with elevated blood pressure, what should the treatment goal be for this patient, to which professional society treatment guideline should the clinician adhere, and would stringent therapy lead to increased falls and adverse events such as hip fractures, functional impairments, and long-term care placement?

In this section, we will review evidence that supports or refutes associations between antihypertensive and cardiovascular medications and falls and fall-related injuries. The evidence is derived from clinical studies of older adults and is grouped by study design (i.e., randomized controlled trials, observational studies, and systematic reviews).

12.3.1 Randomized Controlled Trials

Well-known, notable randomized controlled trials have described the risks of falls and fall-related injuries in older adults taking antihypertensive medications [14–17]. Although the Systolic Hypertension in the Elderly Program (SHEP), the Hypertension in the Very Elderly Trial (HYVET), the Action to Control Cardiovascular Risk in Diabetes (ACCORD), and the Systolic Blood Pressure Intervention Trial (SPRINT) reported relatively low risks of falls and fall-related injuries in older adults taking antihypertensive medications, it is important to remember that these reported low risks were either observed in trials of relatively healthy older adults or younger geriatric patients (Table 12.2). These trials did not always have falls and fractures as their primary outcome and did not include patients residing in nursing homes or assisted living facilities, and falls were often self-reported. It is critical to recognize that many older adults have multiple comorbidities, physical frailty, and disability, all of which could increase their vulnerability to adverse outcomes. Thus, findings from these trials may not be directly applicable to the clinical management of hypertension in frail older patients who are at higher risk for poor clinical outcomes and may experience higher rates of harmful medication effects than the average trial participant.

12.3.2 Observational Studies

The associations between antihypertensive and cardiovascular medications and falls and fall-related injuries have been examined by a number of observational studies. Because randomized controlled trials do not ascertain falls and fall-related injuries

Table 12.2 Randomized controlled trials describing risks of falls and fall-related injuries in older adults taking antihypertensives [14–17]

	Primary objective	Patient population	Interventions	Outcomes	Comments
SHEP	Nonfatal and fatal stroke in persons with isolated systolic hypertension	4,700 community-dwelling persons ≥60 years old (mean age 72 years)	Placebo vs. stepped-care antihypertensive treatment Step 1: chlorthalidone 12.5 mg/day [dose 1] or 25 mg/day [dose 2] Step 2: atenolol 25 mg/day [dose 1] or 50 mg/day [dose 2]	Antihypertensive medications resulted in lower SBP (143 mmHg vs. 155 mmHg) and lower risk of all stroke (RR 0.64, $p=0.0003$)	Active treatment group had nonsignificant, but higher prevalence of falls (12.8 % vs. 10.4 %), fractures (2.4 % vs. 2.0 %), and cardiopulmonary symptoms such as faintness on standing (12.8 % vs. 10.6 %), feelings of unsteadiness or imbalance (33.7 % vs. 32.9 %), and loss of consciousness (2.2 % vs. 1.3 %)
HYVET	Nonfatal and fatal stroke in persons aged ≥80 years old treated with antihypertensives	3,845 persons ≥80 years old with sustained SBP ≥160 mmHg (Mean age 84 years)	Placebo vs. thiazide-diuretic (indapamide 1.5 mg) In addition, perindopril (2 or 4 mg) was added if necessary to achieve a target blood pressure of 150/80 mmHg	At 2 years follow-up, the mean SBP in the active treatment group (145 mmHg) was 15 mmHg lower compared to the placebo group (160 mmHg) and the treatment group trended toward lower risk of all stroke ($p=0.06$)	Fewer serious events were reported in the active treatment group compared to the placebo group, including fractures (38 vs. 52; HR 0.58, $p=0.05$)
ACCORD	Falls and non-spine fractures with intensive control of blood pressure to lower thresholds (SBP target <120 mmHg)	3,099 person subsample of the ACCORD trial (mean age 62 years)	Intensive control (SBP <120 mmHg) vs. standard blood pressure control (SBP <140 mmHg)	Patient-reported annual falls was slightly lower in intensive control group vs. standard group but did not differ when adjusted (RR = 0.84, $p=0.43$)	In the intensive control group, there was a trend toward reduction of non-spine fractures (HR 0.79, $p=0.06$)

SPRINT	First occurrence of myocardial infarction, acute coronary syndrome, stroke, heart failure, or death with standard blood pressure control vs. intensive control	>9,300 persons >50 years old (mean age 67.9; 28.2% ≥75) with elevated SBP and at least one additional risk factor	Intensive control (SBP <120 mmHg) vs. standard blood pressure control (SBP <140 mmHg)	Intervention stopped early at median 3.26 years due to significantly lower rate of primary outcome in intensive treatment group vs. standard treatment group ($p<0.001$)	Intensive treatment group with higher prevalence of serious adverse event or emergency department visit due to hypotension ($p<0.001$), syncope ($p=0.003$), electrolyte abnormalities ($p=0.006$). Injurious fall, defined as fall resulting in emergency department visit or hospital admission occurred in 7.1 % of patients in either treatment group ($p=0.97$)

as their primary outcomes, well-conducted prospective or retrospective studies exploring these associations may provide better insight into this clinically important question.

A meta-analysis performed by Leipzig and colleagues critically evaluated the evidence linking specific classes of cardiovascular medications to falls in older adults. All studies included in this meta-analysis provided data on the number of fallers and non-fallers using medications from the following classes: any diuretic, loop diuretics, thiazide diuretics, beta-blockers (BBs), centrally acting antihypertensives, calcium channel blockers (CCBs), angiotensin-converting enzyme (ACE) inhibitors, type IA antiarrhythmic agents, and digoxin. The authors concluded that diuretic use (pooled OR 1.08; 95 % CI 1.02–1.16), digoxin (pooled OR 1.22; 95 % CI 1.05–1.42), and type IA antiarrhythmics (pooled OR 1.59; 95 % CI 1.02–2.48) were weakly associated with an increase in the risk of one or more falls of older adults. The risk of falls was greater with thiazide diuretics than with loop diuretics (pooled OR 1.06 vs. 0.90). The authors also concluded that patients taking more than three to four medications and those taking more than one antihypertensive medication were at increased odd of falling [18].

A quantitative update to the meta-analysis described above was published in 2009 by Woolcott and colleagues, providing new data for medications previously assessed by Leipzig and colleagues as well as new medication classes. This meta-analysis did not show an association between falls and diuretics (Bayesian adjusted OR 0.99; 95 % CI 0.78–1.25) or with BBs (Bayesian OR 1.01; 95 % CI 0.86–1.17) [19]. Given the divergent results, the authors reiterated the need for caution when prescribing antihypertensive and cardiovascular medications to older adults. This comment was supported in a recent review of meta-analyses performed by Zang which attempted to determine whether the administration of thiazide diuretics, ACE inhibitors, angiotensin II receptor blockers (ARB), CCBs, and/or BBs affected the risk of fall-related injuries in elderly patients aged ≥60 years old. The author concluded that there was no clear, statistically significant evidence indicating antihypertensive medications increase the risk of falls, but that the clinician needs to be aware of the impact of drug therapies and fall-related injuries [20].

The studies described below are high-quality observational studies that are either not included in, or published since, the latest meta-analysis on this topic [19]. A number of observational studies support the notion that antihypertensive and cardiovascular medications are associated with increased falls and fall-related injuries. Using a representative sample of older adults in the United States, Tinetti and colleagues reported a well-conducted prospective study that demonstrated the association of antihypertensive medication use and serious fall-related injuries including hip and other major fractures, traumatic brain injuries, and joint dislocations [21]. The participants included 4,961 community-dwelling adults aged 70 years old and above with hypertension who were followed for 3 years. Competing risk analyses were performed with propensity score using a cumulative logit regression model with adjustment and matching in the US representative Medicare Current Beneficiary Survey cohort. The antihypertensive medication classes examined included diuretics, renin-angiotensin system blockers (ACE inhibitors and ARBs), BBs (selective, nonselective, and α-β-blocker agents), CCBs (nondihydropyridines and dihydropyridines), centrally acting antiadrenergic agents, and others (peripheral acting antiadrenergic agents or vasodilators). Antihypertensive medication intensity was then calculated based on the standardized daily dose for each antihypertensive medication class that participants used. Of these participants, 14.1 % received no antihypertensive medications, 54.6 % were in the moderate-intensity group, and 31.3 % were in the high-intensity group. During follow-up, 446 participants (9 %) experienced serious fall-related injuries and 837 (17 %) died. The risks for serious fall-related injury calculated by Cox proportional hazards regression were higher in the moderate-intensity (HR 1.40; 95 % CI 1.03–1.90) and high-intensity (HR 1.28; 95 % CI 0.91–1.80) antihypertensive groups compared with nonusers. Interestingly, no individual class of antihypertensive was associated with an increased risk of serious fall-related injuries. Moreover, in the 503 participants who had a previous fall-related injury, the risks for serious fall injury were even higher in both the moderate-intensity (HR 2.17; 95 % CI 0.98–4.80) and high-intensity (HR 2.31; 95 % CI 1.01–5.29) antihypertensive groups. Thus, the authors concluded that antihypertensive medications were associated with an increased risk of serious fall-related injuries, particularly among those with previous fall injuries [21].

The findings from Tinetti and colleagues are supported by several smaller observational studies that investigated risk factors for falls among older adults living in the community [21–23]. In a retrospective study of 2,793 respondents aged 65 years old and above in North East England, Prudham and colleagues found that the annual prevalence rate of self-reported falls was 28.0 %. The fallers, compared with non-fallers, showed higher prevalence of problems with mobility and daily living, vertigo, double vision, fainting, and episodes of weakness or numbness. In addition, the proportion of fallers using diuretics was higher than that in non-fallers (22.6 % vs. 17.6 %, $p<0.01$, *chi-square*) [22]. In a separate prospective study of 336 participants aged 75 years old and above, Tinetti and colleagues reported that 108 participants (32 %) fell at least once and 24 % of those who fell had serious injuries and 6 % had fractures during 1 year of follow-up. Predisposing factors for falls identified by multiple regression models included disability of the lower extremities (OR 3.8; 95 % CI 2.2–6.7) and abnormalities of balance and gait (OR 1.9; 95 % CI 1.0–3.7). Moreover, fallers compared to non-fallers were more likely to use diuretics, antihypertensive agents, and cardiovascular medications (adjusted RR 1.5; 95 % CI 1.1–2.1) [23].

Although studies suggest that antihypertensive medications increase falls in some elderly patients, the size of medication class-specific adverse effects remains unclear. Gribbin and colleagues explored the effect size of antihypertensive medications on falls in a large case-control study of participants over 60 years of age utilizing the Health Improvement Network primary care database in the United Kingdom [24]. Participants with a recorded fall in primary care practices were selected as cases (9,682 cases) and were matched by age, gender, and general practice to controls. Medication classes studied included thiazide diuretics, ACE inhibitors, ARBs,

BBs, and CCBs. Using conditional logistic regression models, the risk of first fall for participants ever prescribed thiazides was 25 % higher than for those never prescribed (OR 1.25; 95 % CI 1.15–1.36). Moreover, this medication class-specific adverse effect was stronger in the 3 weeks after the first thiazide prescription (OR 4.28; 95 % CI 1.19–15.42). In contrast, the prescribing of BBs reduced risk for fall (OR 0.90; 95 % CI 0.85–0.96). The prescribing of any other class of antihypertensive medications was not associated with falls [24].

12.3.3 Systematic Reviews

A review conducted by Darowski and Whiting specifically focused on cardiovascular medications and falls. The authors recognized that while it is widely known that cardiovascular medications cause syncope, the data showing that these medications cause falls is inconclusive [25]. They commented specifically on the mechanisms of cardiovascular-related falls, stating a sudden cessation of cerebral blood flow for 6–8 s and/or a decrease in SBP to 60 mmHg was significant enough to cause complete loss of consciousness. The drop in blood pressure caused by cardiovascular medications may be insufficient to cause loss of consciousness on its own, but may cause a feeling of faintness or unsteadiness sufficient enough to make a person prone to falling [25]. Darowski described correlations between falls with lower standing SBPs, orthostatic hypotension, cardiac arrhythmias leading to syncope, carotid sinus hypersensitivity, and neurally mediated syncope. All of these conditions described above can be further exacerbated, and fall risk increased, when cardiovascular medications are added. The authors concluded that although studies may report a weak relationship between cardiovascular medications and falls, these studies are contrary to expert opinions and experiences in fall clinics and suggested that well-conducted studies are needed to better reflect the older frail patients on multiple medications who often seek care in these specialized services.

Howard and colleagues published a systematic review aiming to estimate the percentages of preventable hospital admissions and the most common underlying causes of preventable medication-related admissions. Of the hospital admissions (n = 1,263) due to adverse medication reactions and overtreatment in all patients, diuretics accounted for 16 % (n = 202). These preventable hospital admissions were a result of prescribing problems (30.6 %, range 11.1–41.8), adherence problems (33.3 %, range 20.9–41.7), and monitoring problems (22.2 %, range 0–31.3) [26]. Although the authors did not provide additional detail regarding the reason for hospital admission due to diuretic use, common side effects of diuretics including dizziness, vertigo, and diuresis leading to urgent need for voiding may have been potential inducers of falls. In addition, the overtreatment with diuretics may have led to hypotension and dehydration, thus potentially placing a patient at higher risk for falls.

12.4 Other Common Adverse Effects of Cardiovascular Medications

Our own review of the adverse effects that may occur with various classes of cardiovascular medications reveals a variety of potential mechanisms that may predispose an older patient to falling. Table 12.3 lists potential adverse effects associated with a variety of cardiovascular medications, many of which are often used in combination to achieve a therapeutic endpoint. Dizziness, fatigue, hypotension, orthostatic hypotension, and weakness are most frequently listed within the classes of medications. These adverse effects are particularly concerning in physically frail older adults, especially if they are concurrently receiving medications in more than one class, resulting in additive adverse effects.

12.5 Conclusions

The adverse relationship between cardiovascular medications and falls and fall-related injuries in older adults is supported by high-quality and well-conducted observational studies. However, aside from thiazide diuretics, there is limited evidence to clearly delineate these associations between individual antihypertensive or cardiovascular medications and falls and fall-related injuries in older adults due to limitations of hypertension clinical trials described in this chapter. This gap in knowledge poses a significant challenge to clinicians in the treatment of hypertension in frail older adults who are at particularly high risk for falls. Thus, in the absence of a consensus blood pressure goal, along with unanswered questions regarding the desired intensity of treatment in older patients with hypertension, clinicians should exercise care and use their best clinical judgment to optimize cardiovascular outcomes while minimizing treatment-associated adverse events in these vulnerable patients.

The safe and effective use of cardiovascular medications in physically frail older patients requires deliberate and thoughtful considerations. Other key areas of emphasis need to include polypharmacy assessment, medication reconciliation and review, and deprescribing (medication debridement) strategies as discussed in other chapters of this book. Increased pill burden in older patients may result in poor adherence of cardiovascular medication regimens and subsequent inaccurate blood pressure assessment by clinicians. This in turn may lead to uncontrolled blood pressure that is followed by a dangerous and unnecessary prescribing cascade of additional classes of antihypertensive medications in order to achieve blood pressure goals. Furthermore, modification of medication regimens along with the ever-changing appearances of generic medications and increasing production of combination pills create additional sources of confusion for older patient. Importantly, medication

Table 12.3 Adverse effects of cardiovascular medications [27]

Cardiovascular medication class	Adverse effects associated with falls		
ACE inhibitors	Dizziness	Hypotension	Syncope
	Fatigue	Orthostatic hypotension	Weakness
ARBs	Dizziness	Hypotension	Vertigo
	Fatigue	Orthostatic hypotension	
BBs	Arthralgia	Dizziness	Orthostatic hypotension
	Arthritis	Fatigue	Paresthesia
	Bradycardia	Hypotension	Peripheral edema
	Decreased mental acuity	Lethargy	
		Muscle cramps	
CCBs	Bradycardia	Fatigue	Paresthesia
	Dizziness	Hypotension	Peripheral edema
	Drowsiness	Muscle cramps	Weakness
		Myalgia	
Diuretics	Dehydration	Light-headedness	Vertigo
	Dizziness	Orthostatic hypotension	Weakness
	Hypotension	Paresthesia	
Vasodilators	Dizziness	Light-headedness	Weakness
	Edema	Orthostatic hypotension	
	Hypotension	Tremor	
Aldosterone antagonists	Dizziness	Fatigue	
	Drowsiness	Lethargy	
Alpha agonists	Arthralgia	Edema	Numbness
	Blurred vision	Fatigue	Paresthesia
	Bradycardia	Leg cramps	Sedation
	Delirium	Lethargy	Syncope
	Dizziness	Malaise	Tremor
	Drowsiness	Myalgia	Weakness
Alpha-blockers	Dizziness	Hypotension	Orthostatic hypotension
	Drowsiness	Malaise	Vertigo
	Edema	Muscle cramps	Weakness
	Fatigue	Myalgia	
Antiarrhythmics – classes Ia, Ib, Ic	Arthralgia	Incoordination	Syncope
	Blurred vision	Light-headedness	Tremor/trembling
	Dizziness	Numbness of fingers/toes	Unsteady gait
	Fatigue	Paresthesia	Weakness

Table 12.3 (continued)

Cardiovascular medication class	Adverse effects associated with falls		
Antiarrhythmics – class III	Abnormal gait	Edema	Peripheral neuropathy
	Ataxia	Fatigue	Tremor
	Bradycardia	Hypotension	Visual disturbances
	Dizziness	Malaise	
Antianginal	Blurred vision	Hypotension	Peripheral edema
	Bradycardia	Orthostatic hypotension	Weakness
	Dizziness		
Inotropes	Delirium	Visual disturbances	
	Dizziness	Weakness	

ACE angiotensin-converting enzyme, *BB* beta-blocker, *ARB* angiotensin II receptor blocker, *CCB* calcium channel blocker

adherence counseling along with continual medication reconciliation needs to be a part of the prescribing process in order to determine the appropriate cardiovascular medication regimen while minimizing adverse effects and reducing the risk for falls in older patients.

References

1. Gray SL, Sager M, Lestico MR et al (1998) Adverse drug events in hospitalized elderly. J Gerontol A Biol Sci Med Sci 53(1):M59–M63
2. Field TS, Gurwitz JH, Harrold LR et al (2004) Risk factors for adverse drug events among older adults in the ambulatory setting. J Am Geriatr Soc 52(8):1349–1354
3. Tinetti ME, McAvay GJ, Fried TR et al (2008) Health outcome priorities among competing cardiovascular, fall injury, and medication related symptom outcomes. J Am Geriatr Soc 56:1409–1416
4. Aronow WS, Fleg JL, Pepine CJ et al (2011) ACCF/AHA expert consensus document on hypertension in the elderly: a report of the American College of Cardiology Foundation Task Force on Clinical Expert Consensus documents developed in collaboration with the American Academy of Neurology, American Geriatrics Society, American Society for Preventive Cardiology, American Society of Hypertension, American Society of Nephrology, Association of Black Cardiologists, and European Society of Hypertension. J Am Coll Cardiol 57:2037–2114
5. Cushman WC, Ford CE, Cutler JA et al (2002) Success and predictors of blood pressure control in diverse North American settings: the Antihypertensive and Lipid-Lowering Treatment to Prevent Heart Attack Trial (ALLHAT). J Clin Hypertens (Greenwich) 4:393–404
6. Chobanian AV, Bakris GL, Black HR, National Heart, Lung, and Blood Institute Joint National Committee on Prevention, Detection, Evaluation, and Treatment of High Blood Pressure; National High Blood Pressure Education Program Coordinating Committee et al (2003) The seventh report of the Joint National Committee on Prevention, Detection, Evaluation, and Treatment of High Blood Pressure: the JNC 7 report. JAMA 289(19):2560–2572
7. Runganga M, Peel NM (2014) Hubbard RE Multiple medication use in older patients in post-acute transitional care: a prospective cohort study. Clin Interv Aging 9:1453–1462

8. James PA, Oparil S, Carter BL et al (2014) 2014 evidence-based guideline for the management of high blood pressure in adults: report from the panel members appointed to the Eighth Joint National Committee (JNC 8). JAMA 311:507–520
9. Mancia G, Fagard R, Narkiewicz K et al (2014) 2013 ESH/ESC practice guidelines for the management of arterial hypertension. Blood Press 23(1):3–16
10. Weber MA, Schiffrin EL, White WB et al (2014) Clinical practice guidelines for the management of hypertension in the community a statement by the American Society of Hypertension and the International Society of Hypertension. J Hypertens 32(1):3–15
11. Daskalopoulou SS, Rabi DM, Zarnke KB et al (2015) The 2015 Canadian Hypertension Education Program recommendations for blood pressure measurement, diagnosis, assessment of risk, prevention, and treatment of hypertension. Can J Cardiol 31(5):549–568
12. American Diabetes Association (2015) Cardiovascular disease and risk management. Sec. 8. In standards of medical care in diabetes – 2015. Diabetes Care 38(uppl. 1):S49–S57
13. Kidney Disease: Improving Global Outcomes (KDIGO) Blood Pressure Work Group (2012) KDIGO clinical practice guideline for the management of blood pressure in chronic kidney disease. Kidney Inter Suppl 2:337–414
14. [No authors listed]. Prevention of stroke by antihypertensive drug treatment in older persons with isolated systolic hypertension. Final results of the Systolic Hypertension in the Elderly Program (SHEP). SHEP Cooperative Research Group (1991) JAMA 265:3255–3264
15. Beckett NS, Peters R, Fletcher AE et al (2008) Treatment of hypertension in patients 80 years of age or older. N Engl J Med 358(18):1887–1898
16. Margolis KL, Palermo L, Vittinghoff E et al (2014) Intensive blood pressure control, falls, and fractures in patients with type 2 diabetes: the ACCORD trial. J Gen Intern Med 29(12):1599–1606
17. SPRINT Research Group (2015) A randomized trial of intensive versus standard blood-pressure control. N Engl J Med 373(22):2103–2116
18. Leipzig RM, Cumming RG, Tinetti ME (1999) Drugs and falls in older people: a systemic review and meta-analysis: II. Cardiac and analgesic drugs. J Am Geriatr Soc 47:40–50
19. Woolcott JC, Richardson KJ, Wiens MO et al (2009) Meta-analysis of the impact of 9 medication classes on falls in elderly persons. Arch Intern Med 169(21):1952–1960
20. Zang G (2013) Antihypertensive drugs and the risk of fall injuries: a systematic review and meta-analysis. J Int Med Res 41(5):1408–1417
21. Tinetti ME, Han L, Lee DS et al (2014) Antihypertensive medications and serious fall injuries in a nationally representative sample of older adults. JAMA Intern Med 174(4):588–595
22. Prudham D, Evans JG (1981) Factors associated with falls in the elderly: a community study. Age Ageing 10(3):141–146
23. Tinetti ME, Speechley M, Ginter SF (1988) Risk factors for falls among elderly persons living in the community. N Engl J Med 319(26):1701–1707
24. Gribbin J, Hubbard R, Gladman JR et al (2010) Risk of falls associated with antihypertensive medication: population-based case-control study. Age Ageing 39(5):592–597
25. Darowski A, Whiting R (2011) Cardiovascular medication and falls. Rev Clin Gerontol 21:170–179
26. Howard RL, Avery AJ, Slavenburg S et al (2007) Which drugs cause preventable admissions to hospital? A systematic review. Br J Clin Pharmacol 63(2):136–147, Epub 2006 Jun 26
27. Lexi-Comp Online™, Lexi-Drugs Online™, Hudson, Ohio: Lexi-Comp, Inc., 2015; September 21, 2015

Chapter 13
Glucose Control Medications

Louise Mallet

Abstract Elderly patients with diabetes are at risk of falls. Various neuropathies, nephropathy, orthostatic hypotension (OH), and retinopathy may contribute to fall risk in this population. The dosage of renally excreted oral hypoglycemic agents needs to be carefully adjusted to avoid hypoglycemia. Long-acting sulfonylureas such as glyburide and glimepiride should be avoided in older individuals. Metformin has a low risk of hypoglycemia, but when used in the situation of decreased renal function, there is an elevated risk of lactic acidosis. New dipeptidyl peptidase-4 (DPP4) inhibitors are excreted renally and their dosage should be adjusted. Patients with type 2 diabetes are 1.6 times more likely to have a fracture and 2.8 times more likely to have a hip fracture than patients without diabetes. The use of thiazolidinediones doubles the risk of fractures in women when compared to other oral hypoglycemia agents. Metformin can cause vitamin B12 deficiency which can be associated with neuropathy and increase the risk of falls. The literature studying the use of antidiabetic medications and the risk of falls is limited. Trials were not originally designed to evaluate the risk of falls or fractures, and some studies were done over short periods of time. Information on the risk of falls with the use of newer antidiabetic medications such as glucagon-like peptide 1 receptor agonists are lacking.

Abbreviations

CI	Confidence interval
DM	Diabetes mellitus
DN	Diabetic nephropathy
DPP4	Dipeptidyl peptidase-4
DPN	Distal polyneuropathy
DR	Diabetic retinopathy

L. Mallet, BScPharm, PharmD, CGP, FESCP
Faculty of Pharmacy, University of Montréal, Montréal, QC, Canada

Department of Pharmacy, McGill University Health Center, Montréal, QC, Canada
e-mail: Louise.mallet@umontreal.ca

© Springer International Publishing Switzerland 2016

A.R. Huang, L. Mallet (eds.), *Medication-related falls in older people*,
DOI 10.1007/978-3-319-32304-6_13

DSPN	Distal symmetric polyneuropathy
eGFR	Estimated glomerular filtration rate
OH	Orthostatic hypotension
OR	Odds ratio

13.1 Introduction

Falls represent a major health burden in older adults with diabetes mellitus (DM) [1]. The annual incidence of falls in elderly adults with DM has been reported to be 39 % [2]. Different factors may contribute to falls among older diabetic patients including microvascular-related complications such as neuropathy, retinopathy and nephropathy, foot and body pain, poor balance, impaired vision, arthritis, history of cardiovascular disease, depression, and the use of multiple medications [2, 3]. This chapter will discuss the different factors associated with falls in diabetic patients.

13.2 Falls, Fractures, and Diabetes Mellitus

13.2.1 Neuropathies

Neuropathies can present in different forms in diabetic patients and can have a significant impact on the quality of life of these patients. Diabetic neuropathies include mononeuropathies, polyneuropathy, and autonomic neuropathy. Distal symmetric polyneuropathy (DSPN) is a common chronic complication of diabetes mellitus in older adults. The pathogenesis of DSPN is not fully understood, but it is multifactorial in nature, related to chronic hyperglycemia, duration of diabetes, and cardiovascular risk factors [4]. DSPN predisposes patients to the development of neuropathic foot ulcers, pain syndromes, and unsteadiness. Neuropathic foot ulcers are the leading cause of foot amputation in the United States [5]. Patients suffering from DSPN often have impaired mobility.

Proximal motor neuropathy is primarily found in elderly diabetic patients. Patients present with proximal muscle weakness and muscle wasting. The onset may be acute or gradual. It may start on one side and then progress to involve both sides. Pain is reported in the thighs, hips, or buttocks [6].

Chronic sensorimotor distal polyneuropathy (DPN) is a common form of diabetic neuropathy. DPN involves small and large sensory nerve fibers. Patients present with a "glove and stocking" distribution of sensation loss. Patients report a sensation of "walking on cotton," "floors feeling strange," inability to turn the pages of a book and inability to discriminate between different types of coins. Severe distal muscle weakness may also develop with this syndrome and contribute to an inability to stand on one's toes or on one's heels [6]. Data from the Women's Health and Aging study reported that diabetic women had more difficulties performing activities of daily living tasks such as walking two to three blocks, using a telephone, bathing, and lifting objects weighing 10 lb [7]. Patients with neuropathy have slow walking speed, reduced step length when walking on irregular surfaces, impaired peripheral sensation, increased reaction time, impaired balance, and falls [8].

Orthostatic hypotension (OH) is an important risk factor for falls and can be a consequence of a diabetic autonomic neuropathy. It is defined as a drop in systolic blood pressure of more than 20 mmHg or diastolic blood pressure of more than 10 mmHg within 3 min after assuming the standing position from supine [9]. Orthostatic hypotension is frequently found in older individuals as well as in frail elderly adults [9]. Low et al. reported a prevalence of orthostatic hypotension in 8.4 % and 7.4 % of type 1 and type 2 diabetic patients, respectively [10]. Orthostatic hypotension increases the risk of syncope, falls, and injury. Common symptoms reported by patients are dizziness, light-headedness when standing, fainting, or darkening or clouding of vision.

13.2.2 Retinopathy and Visual Impairments

Diabetic retinopathy (DR), a microvascular complication of diabetes, represents the leading cause of blindness in the United States [11]. DR is classified as being nonproliferative or proliferative. Signs of nonproliferative DR are microaneurysms and retinal hemorrhages with the presence of cotton-wool spots, venous bleeding, and intraretinal microvascular abnormalities. Proliferative DR is characterized by the growth of new blood vessels which are present on the surface of the retina or the optic disc. These abnormal vessels can bleed resulting in vitreous hemorrhage, fibrosis, and retinal detachment. Diabetic macular edema can appear at any stage of DR, caused by increased vascular permeability, leading to hemorrhages and the presence of hard exudates in the central retina [11, 12].

Diabetics older than 65 years also have twice the risk of developing cataracts and three times the risk of presenting with glaucoma than those without diabetes [13]. Vision loss associated with DM results in an increased risk of falls and accidents due to impaired visual acuity, depth perception, and contrast sensitivity [14].

13.2.3 Nephropathy and Oral Hypoglycemic Agents

Diabetic nephropathy (DN) is the cause for more than 50 % of all cases of end-stage renal disease in people over the age of 65 years worldwide [15]. DN causes a decline in glomerular filtration rate and albuminuria. Medications and/or their metabolites that are renally excreted can accumulate with DN. Dosages of oral hypoglycemic agents and insulin need to be carefully selected to avoid hypoglycemia which can lead to increased risk of falls and fall-related morbidity in the elderly.

The first-generation sulfonylureas (e.g., chlorpropamide) are contraindicated in the elderly since they are exclusively cleared by the kidneys [16]. These medications should no longer be prescribed. Long-acting sulfonylureas such as glyburide and glimepiride have been associated with an increased risk of hypoglycemia in elderly patients [16]. Glyburide is eliminated renally, has an active metabolite with a long half-life, and should be avoided in older diabetic patients [17–19]. Reductions in renal functioning can lead to reduced renal catabolism of insulin and renal gluconeogenesis resulting in lower insulin requirements in the elderly [19].

Metformin is well tolerated in the elderly with low risk of hypoglycemia. However, in patients with renal insufficiency, the risk of lactic acidosis is increased; renal function should be monitored before and during metformin therapy [16]. Dosage adjustment is necessary for metformin in the presence of renal impairment, and it is recommended not to prescribe metformin when the estimated glomerular filtration rate (eGFR) falls below 30 ml/min per 1.73 m^2 [20]. Sitagliptin, a DPP4 inhibitor, is excreted mostly unchanged in the urine. The terminal half-life of sitagliptin in patients with mild, moderate, severe, and end-stage renal disease increased to 16.1, 19.1, 22.5, and 28.4 h, respectively [16]. Saxagliptin has an active metabolite (5-hydroxy-saxagliptin) that is also renally excreted. The serum concentrations (area under the curves) of saxagliptin and its metabolites are 2.1- and 4.5-fold higher in the presence of severe renal impairment (eGFR less than 30 ml/min) [16]. Therefore, the dose of saxagliptin needs to be adjusted in patients with chronic renal disease stages 3 to 5D [16].

Incretin mimetic agents such as exenatide is primarily excreted and converted into inactive peptide fragments by the kidney. In patients with end-stage renal disease, eGFR less than 30 ml/min, toxic blood levels of exenatide have been detected [16]. Limited data are available for the safe use of liraglutide with a creatinine clearance of less than 60 ml/min [16].

Renal impairment and decreased vitamin D metabolism can also decrease muscle strength and bone mineral density and increase fall and fracture risk.

13.2.4 Bone Fragility

Fractures and diabetes are prevalent in older adults and the relation between diabetes and osteoporosis is complex. Studies have reported a higher risk of fractures in both type 1 and type 2 diabetes even though bone mineral density is unchanged or moderately increased in type 2 diabetes [21]. Patients with type 2 diabetes are 1.6 times more likely to have a fracture than patients without diabetes and 2.8 times more likely to have a hip fracture [14, 21]. The quality of the bone has been questioned. Diabetic nephropathy can also lead to renal osteodystrophy. Renal impairment and decreased vitamin D metabolism can also decrease muscle strength and bone mineral density and increase fall and fracture risk.

Visceral fat accumulation and loss of lean body mass may also contribute to poor bone quality. Poor glycemic control can lead to the accumulation of nonenzymatic glycation end products which can interfere with the collagen metabolism within the bone [22].

The A Diabetes Outcome Progression Trial (ADOPT) reported an increased risk of peripheral fractures in women on rosiglitazone but no increase in the risk of falls [23]. Thiazolidinediones have been found to double the risk of distal upper and lower limb fractures in women when compared to other oral hypoglycemic agents [23, 24]. This class of drug should be avoided in diabetic patients at risk for falls. The pathophysiologic mechanism has been postulated that this class of drug causes an increase in adipocyte differentiation, which in turn leads to a decrease in osteoblast formation resulting in decreased new bone formation [25].

13.3 Oral Hypoglycemic Medications and Risk of Falls

13.3.1 Sulfonylureas

Lapane reported in 2013 the results of a systematic review that included 9 randomized trials and 12 nonexperimental studies to assess the association between sulfonylurea medications and falls or fall-related fractures among diabetic older adults. The studies included community-dwelling patients or those living in nursing homes [26]. Frail elderly patients were excluded from these trials. Furthermore, these trials were not designed to evaluate the risk of falls or fractures with sulfonylurea. Fractures or falls were not included as primary outcomes. Some of the studies were performed over a short period of time with few fracture events to provide meaningful results. Comparison groups or definition of medication exposure was unclear. This systematic review did not find an increased risk of falls or fractures with sulfonylureas [26]. Further studies are needed to clarify the effect of sulfonylureas on falls or fall-related fractures in older adults at risk of hypoglycemia.

13.3.2 Metformin

Metformin is the drug of choice for the first-line management of type 2 diabetes mellitus in older adults. It is not directly associated with an increased risk of falls and fractures. Metformin has been shown to cause vitamin B12 deficiency, which is associated with neuropathy and an increased risk of falls [25]. This risk is associated with increasing age of the patient, metformin dose, and the duration of use [27]. In a nested case control study, Ting et al. compared 155 Chinese diabetic patients on metformin with 310 matched controls. For each 1 g/day increase in the metformin dose, an odds ratio of 2.88 (95 % CI 2.25–3.87; $p<0.001$) was found for developing vitamin B12 deficiency. In patients using metformin for ≥3 years, the adjusted OR was 2.4 (95 % CI 1.46–3.91) compared with patients who used metformin for less than 3 years [28]. Normally, vitamin B12 binds to an intrinsic factor complex, via a calcium-dependent process, in the gastrointestinal tract. It is postulated that metformin competes with these calcium-binding sites resulting in vitamin B12 malabsorption [25, 27]. Elderly patients on metformin should have periodic screening for vitamin B12 deficiency and given oral vitamin B12 supplements if necessary.

13.3.3 Other Agents

Limited date is available regarding an increased risk of falls or fractures with other classes of diabetes medications. Studies of DPP4 inhibitors have not been associated with an increased risk of falls. These agents also have a low risk of hypoglycemia. As previously mentioned, these agents need to be adjusted for reduced renal function [25].

Alpha-glucosidase inhibitors are oral antidiabetic medications that prevent the digestion of carbohydrates. These agents do not increase the risk of falls. A study of four patients evaluated the effects of acarbose on postprandial hypotension. Acarbose significantly improved postprandial fall in systolic and diastolic blood pressures [29].

13.4 Conclusion

Few studies are available regarding the risk of falls and diabetes medications. Some sulfonylureas are contraindicated in elderly patients or their dosage needs to be adjusted for decreases in renal function. Due to poor study design, falls have not been conclusively associated with antidiabetic agents. Prolonged hypoglycemia has been reported with glyburide. Further high-quality studies are needed to evaluate the risk of falls and fractures with diabetes medications in the elderly.

References

1. Crews RT, Yalla SV, Fleischer AE, Wu SC (2013) A growing troubling triad: diabetes, aging, and falls. J Aging Res 2013:342650
2. Tilling LM, Darawil K, Britton M (2006) Falls as a complication of diabetes mellitus in older adults. J Diabetes Complicat 28:158–162
3. Schwartz AV, Hillier TA, Sellmeyer DE, Resnick HE, Gregg E, Ensrud KE et al (2002) Older women with diabetes have a higher risk o falls: a prospective study. Diabetes Care 25:1749–1754
4. Kasznicki J (2014) Advances in the diagnosis and management of diabetic distal symmetric polyneuropathy. Arch Med Sci 10:345–354
5. Bild DE, Selby JV, Sinnock P, Browner WS, Braveman P, Showstack JA (1989) Low-extremity amputation in people with diabetes. Epidemiology and prevention. Diabetes Care 12:24–31
6. Vinik AI, Strotmeyer ES, Nakave AA, Patel CV (2008) Diabetic neuropathy in older adults. Clin Geriatr Med 24:407–435

7. Maty SC, Fried LP, Volpato S, Williamson J, Brancati FL, Blaum CS (2004) Patterns of disability related to diabetes mellitus in older women. J Gerontol A Biol Sci Med Sci 59: 148–153
8. Menz HB, Lord SR, St George R, Fitzpatrick RC (2004) Walking stability and sensorimotor function in older people with diabetic peripheral neuropathy. Arch Phys Med Rehabil 85: 245–252
9. Lanier EF, Mote MB, Clay EC (2011) Evaluation and management of orthostatic hypotension. Am Fam Physician 84:527–536
10. Low PA, Benrud-Larson LM, Sletten DM, Opfer-Gehrking L, Weigand SD, O'Brian PC et al (2004) Autonomic symptoms and diabetic neuropathy: a population-based study. Diabetes Care 27:2942–2947
11. Mohamed O, Gillies MC, Wong TY (2007) Management of diabetic retinopathy: a systematic review. JAMA 298:902–916
12. Hornick T, Aron DC (2008) Preventing and managing diabetic complications in elderly patients. Clev Clin J Med 75:153–158
13. Antonetti D, Klein R, Gardner TW (2012) Diabetic retinopathy. N Engl J Med 366: 1227–1239
14. Mayne D, Stout NR, Aspray TJ (2010) Diabetes, falls and fractures. Age Aging 39:522–525
15. Abdel-Rahman EM, Alhamad T, Reeves W, Awad AS (2012) Management of diabetic nephropathy in the elderly: special considerations. J Nephrol Ther 2: pii: 124
16. Lalau JD, Arnouts P, Sharif A, De Broe ME (2015) Metformin and other antidiabetic agents in renal failure patients. Kidney Int 87:308–322
17. Shorr RI, Ray WA, Daugherty JR, Griffin MR (1996) Individual sulfonylureas and serious hypoglycemia in older people. J Am Geriatr Soc 44:751–755
18. American Geriatrics Society 2015 Beers Criteria Update Expert Panel (2015) American Geriatrics Society 2015 updated beers criteria for potentially inappropriate medication use in older adults. J Am Geriatr Soc 63:2227–2246
19. van Staa T, Abenhaim L, Monette J (1997) Rates of hypoglycemia in users of sulfonylureas. J Clin Epidemiol 50:735–741
20. Inzucchi SE, Lipska KJ, Mayo H, Bailey CJ, McGuire DK (2014) Metformin in patients with type 2 diabetes and kidney disease: a systematic review. JAMA 312:2668–2675
21. Rakel A, Sheehy O, Rahme E, LeLorier J (2008) Osteoporosis among patients with type 1 and type 2 diabetes. Diabetes Metab 34:193–205
22. Yamagishi S, Nakamura K, Inoue H (2005) Possible participation of advanced glycation end products in the pathogenesis of osteoporosis in diabetic patients. Med Hypotheses 65:1013–1015
23. Kahn SE, Zinman B, Lachin JM, Haffner SM, Herman WH, Holman RR et al (2008) Thiazolidinedione use and bone loss in type 2 diabetes: an analysis form A Diabetes Outcome Progression Trial (ADOPT). Diabetes Care 21:845–851
24. Schwartz AV, Sellmeyer DE, Vittinghoff E, Palermo L, Lecka-Czernik B, Feingold KR et al (2006) Thiazolidinedione use and bone loss in older diabetic adults. J Clin Endocrinol Metab 91:3349–3354
25. Berlie HD, Garwood CL (2010) Diabetes medications related to an increased risk of falls and fall-related morbidity in the elderly. Ann Pharmacother 44:712–717
26. Lapane KL, Yang S, Brown MJ, Jawahar R, Pagliasotti C, Rajpathak S (2013) Sulfonylureas and risk of falls and fractures: a systematic review. Drugs Aging 30:527–547
27. Kibirige D, Mwebaze R (2013) Vitamin B12 deficiency among patients with diabetes mellitus: is routine screening and supplementation justified ? J Diabetes Metab Disord 12:12–17
28. Ting R, Szeto C, Chan M, Ma K, Chow K (2006) Risk factors of vitamin B12 deficiency in patients receiving metformin. Arch Intern Med 166:1975–1979
29. Shibao C, Gamboa A, Diedrich A, Dossett C, Choi L, Farley G et al (2007) Acarbose, an alpha-glucosidase inhibitor, attenuates postprandial hypotension in autonomic failure. Hypertension 50:54–61

Part IV
Management of Medication-Related Falls

Chapter 14
Inappropriate Medications and Risk of Falls in Older Adults

Jennifer Greene Naples, Joseph T. Hanlon, Christine M. Ruby, and Susan L. Greenspan

Abstract Among older adults, potentially inappropriate medications have been associated with an increased risk of falls and hip fractures (a proxy measure for serious falls). In addition to the medications listed in other chapters in this book, skeletal muscle relaxants (SMR), antiepileptic drugs (AED), opioids, and combinations of medications affecting the central nervous system (CNS) have been shown to increase the risk of serious falls. Moreover, this increased risk is even more pronounced among older adults with a previous history of falls and hip fractures. This chapter will summarize literature highlighting the specific risks of these medications, with an emphasis on rigorously designed observational studies.

Abbreviations

AED	Antiepileptic drug
ARR	Adjusted risk ratio
AOR	Adjusted odds ratio
CI	Confidence interval
CNS	Central nervous system
CYP	Cytochrome P450
IRR	Incident risk ratio
NCQA	National Committee for Quality Assurance
OR	Odds ratio

J.G. Naples, PharmD (✉) • J.T. Hanlon, MS, PharmD • S.L. Greenspan, MD
Department of Medicine, Geriatrics and Gerontology, University of Pittsburgh School of Medicine, 3471 Fifth Avenue, Suite 500, Kaufmann Medical Building, Pittsburgh, PA 15213, USA
e-mail: jennifer.naples@pitt.edu; jth14@pitt.edu; greenspn@pitt.edu

C.M. Ruby, PharmD, BCPS
Department of Pharmacy and Therapeutics, University of Pittsburgh School of Pharmacy, Salk Hall, Room 727, 3501 Terrace Street, Pittsburgh, PA 15213, USA
e-mail: cms101@pitt.edu

© Springer International Publishing Switzerland 2016

A.R. Huang, L. Mallet (eds.), *Medication-related falls in older people*,
DOI 10.1007/978-3-319-32304-6_14

PIM	Potentially inappropriate medications
RR	Relative risk
SMR	Skeletal muscle relaxants
US	United States

14.1 Introduction

Potentially inappropriate medications (PIM) in older adults are those where the possible risks associated with their use outweigh potential benefits [1]. Alternatively, PIM may be defined as the use of medications in a manner that does not align with generally accepted medical standards [2]. Evidence-based explicit criteria have been developed through consensus by expert panels to categorize PIM in several ways, including drugs to avoid in the elderly, excessive dose, therapeutic duplication, prolonged duration, and drug-drug and drug-disease interactions [3, 4].

Other chapters in this textbook have focused on drug classes to avoid based on their ability to increase fall risk (e.g., benzodiazepines, antidepressants, and antipsychotics). This chapter will expand discussion to four additional topics that represent one of the explicit criteria included in the 2015 American Geriatrics Society Beers criteria: (1) skeletal muscle relaxants (SMR) (drugs to avoid), (2) concomitant use of multiple central nervous system drugs (pharmacodynamic drug-drug interaction), and (3) use of antiepileptic drugs (AED) or (4) opioid analgesics in those with a history of falls or fracture (drug-disease interactions) [3]. Additionally, only the findings from rigorously conducted observational studies such as nested case-control and cohort studies that focus on adults 65 years of age and older in which falls were expanded to include hip fractures as per National Committee for Quality Assurance (NCQA) specifications will be reported [5].

14.2 Skeletal Muscle Relaxants

SMR are classified as drugs to avoid in the elderly due to their unfavorable risk-benefit profile: the efficacy of SMR for musculoskeletal pain is questionable, but their adverse effects are well-documented. Orphenadrine and cyclobenzaprine are highly anticholinergic, and all SMR are highly sedative, two properties that may increase the risk of falls [6]. Despite these risks, approximately 2 % of older adults use SMR [3, 7].

Although three studies have been published examining the risk of injury associated with the use of SMR, the rate of falls versus hip fractures were not independently calculated and the risk attributable to SMR was not quantified [7–9]. Recently, however, a large new-user cohort study of older Veterans from the United States (US) evaluated falls and hip fractures using NCQA specifications [10]. After matching on propensity scores, over 27,000 individuals with new prescriptions for SMR (i.e., methocarbamol, cyclobenzaprine, carisoprodol, chlorzoxazone, metaxalone, orphenadrine) were more than two times as likely to experience falls or fractures requiring an emergency room visit (adjusted odds ratio [AOR] 2.20, 95 % confidence interval [CI] 1.84–2.63) within 1 year. Data on drug-specific associations were not collected.

14.3 Multiple Central Nervous System Medications

The use of individual medication classes that affect the CNS, such as opioids, benzodiazepines, antidepressants, and antipsychotics, are common in older adults. This is especially true in older nursing home patients where chronic pain and dementia with behavioral and psychological sequelae are common. Indeed, one study using national nursing home data found that 60 % of older nursing home residents used two or more psychotropic medications [11].

Few studies have examined the risk associated with the concomitant use of multiple CNS medications and falls or fractures in older adults. In one prospective cohort study of 305 older US Veteran outpatients, the risk of any falls (measured via patient diary and monthly telephone surveillance) was examined in relation to exposure to CNS medications [12]. Nearly 10 % of participants took two or more medications from these classes. After controlling for age, depression, cognition, and mobility, the investigators found the risk of falls increased with increasing number of CNS medications, from an AOR of 1.54 (95 % CI 1.07–2.22) with one drug to an AOR of 2.37 (95 % CI 1.14–4.94) with two or more.

Another prospective study from the US examined the risk of recurrent falls in well-functioning community-dwelling elders taking opioids, benzodiazepine receptor agonists, antidepressants, or antipsychotics [13]. Exposure to CNS medications was determined using both absolute number of medications and categorical level of exposure (low or high) calculated using standardized daily doses (i.e., the sum of reported daily dose divided by the minimum effective geriatric daily dose). Over the 5 years follow-up period, as many as 24.1 % of CNS medication users took at least two CNS agents, whereas as no more than 18.9 % took high doses (i.e., $\geq$ 3 standardized daily doses) annually. In multivariable analyses, individuals taking $\geq$ 2 CNS medications and those taking higher doses had an increased risk of recurrent falls (AOR 1.95, 95 % CI 1.35–2.81 and AOR 2.89, 95 % CI 1.96–4.25, respectively).

A third prospective cohort study of older Australian Veterans examined the risk of multiple psychoactive drugs (defined as AED, sedative hypnotics, opioids, benzodiazepines, antiparkinson agents, antidepressants, and antipsychotics) and falls leading to hospitalization (determined by ICD-10 codes) [14]. Again, there was increasing risk of falls associated with increasing number of CNS medications. The adjusted incident risk ratio (IRR) rose from 1.70 (95 % CI 1.45–1.99) with 2 drugs to 1.96 (95 % CI 1.58–2.43) with 3–4 drugs to 3.15 (95 % CI 1.90–5.23) with 5 or more drugs. Moreover, there was also a dose-response relationship between psychoactive medications and falls.

Finally, a prospective study in Finland evaluated the risk of fracture in older adults using two CNS medications simultaneously [15]. In men, the combination of an opioid and antipsychotic or an opioid and a benzodiazepine was associated with an increased risk of fractures (adjusted risk ratio (ARR) 21.1, 95 % CI 1.7–256.9 and ARR 5.0, 95 % CI 1.0–25.2, respectively). This suggests that the combined burden of medications sharing the same CNS adverse effect profile may further increase the risk of falls in older adults.

14.4 Antiepileptic Drugs

AED use is common, ranging from 2 % among community-dwelling older adults to 10 % among institutionalized older adults [16]. In addition to epilepsy (which is prevalent in 1 % of older adults), AEDs are increasingly used to treat non-seizure conditions such as neuropathic pain and mood disorders [17].

An important potentially harmful drug-disease interaction is the use of AED in those with a previous history of falls. A recent meta-analysis pooled the results from four studies of these medications in older adults and found that AED use nearly doubled the risk of any fall (OR 1.9, 95 % CI 1.02–3.49) [18]. Furthermore, the risk associated with AED use was more pronounced when the outcome was recurrent falls (OR 2.7, 95 % CI 1.83–3.92). An additional study examined the association between AED use and recurrent falls over more than 7 years follow-up using data collected as part of the Women's Health Initiative [19]. For the analysis, 138,667 women aged 50–79 were included; of those, 1,385 women used AED. In adjusted analyses, AEDs were associated with recurrent falls (hazard ratio 1.62, 95 % CI 1.50–1.74).

In older adults, nontraumatic hip fractures may also serve as a proxy indicator for serious falls requiring emergency room visits or hospitalizations. A number of rigorously conducted observational studies have shown an increased risk of fractures with AED use in the elderly. One large case-control study of Danish older adults evaluated the relationship between AED use and hip fracture using registry data [20]. Any use of AED was associated with a 30 % increased likelihood of hip fracture (OR 1.31, 95 % CI 1.16–1.48). In another cohort study following older US Veterans with an underlying history of bipolar disorder for 4–5 years, individuals using AED were 2.35 times as likely to experience a hip fracture compared with propensity-matched controls [21]. A third study using information from an Italian primary care database reported that over the 5-year follow-up, AED use increased the risk of hip fracture in both older men (IRR 2.07, 95 % CI 1.45–2.96) and older women (IRR 1.61, 95 % CI 1.28–2.01) [22]. Using data from eight studies (including the three previously described), a recent meta-analysis found the risk of hip fracture nearly doubled (RR 1.90) with exposure to AED [23]. Currently, it is unclear as to whether the risk of hip fractures is greater for enzyme-inducing AEDs (i.e., phenobarbital, phenytoin, carbamazepine, oxcarbazepine) versus those do not affect the cytochrome (CYP) P450 system [20, 24].

14.5 Opioids

More than seven million older adults use prescription opioids to manage chronic pain [25]. Furthermore, over 70 % of nursing home patients with pain are prescribed an opioid, either alone or in combination with another analgesic [26]. However, a new addition to the 2015 American Geriatrics Society Beers criteria is a drug-disease interaction regarding the use of opioids in individuals with a previous history of falls [3]. A 2007 meta-analysis using pooled data from six observational studies reported that individuals exposed to opioids had a 38 % increased risk of fractures (OR 1.38, 95 % CI 1.15–1.66) [27]. Since then, only one study evaluating the risk of falls has been published [28]. Analyzing data from an integrated health system in rural Pennsylvania for 13,300 elderly patients with arthritis, the authors found that opioid users were at an increased risk of falls and fractures compared with individuals using nonsteroidal anti-inflammatory drugs (OR 4.1, 95 % CI 3.7–4.5) and cyclooxygenase-2 inhibitors (OR 3.3, 95 % CI 2.5–4.3). Unfortunately, four other recent studies used a composite endpoint for fractures and did not isolate the risk of hip fracture as a potential proxy for serious falls [29–32].

Additionally, drugs that inhibit hepatic isoenzymes by which certain opioids are metabolized may result in further increased risk of falls. Using participant data from the Swedish National Patient Registry in a case-crossover design, one study looked at the association between opioids with or without concomitantly prescribed CYP2D6 inhibitors and fall-related injury [33]. Again, the use of any opioid was associated with an increased risk of falls. As expected, the risk of fall-related injury associated with opioids metabolized via 3A4 (e.g., oxycodone, fentanyl) did not change when a CYP2D6 inhibitor was also prescribed. However, for the prodrugs codeine and tramadol that require transformation by CYP2D6 to the active form, a lower risk of falls was noted.

14.6 Conclusion

The use of potentially inappropriate medications is especially concerning given their ability to induce or exacerbate falls in older adults. SMR, AED, and opioids have been shown to increase the risk of falls and hip fractures in older adults. Moreover, use of these medications may further increase risk in older adults with a previous history of falls or fractures. Additional evidence suggests that beyond specific medication classes, the overall burden of drugs that may affect the CNS is an important risk factor for falls. Strategies for mitigating these risks in older adults include applying evidence-based criteria to help identify PIM, assessing the necessity of each medication, selecting alternatives to problematic medications when they exist, and using the lowest effective dose of each centrally acting medication when no other option is available.

References

1. Spinewine A, Schmader KE, Barber N et al (2007) Appropriate prescribing in elderly people: how can it be measured and optimized? Lancet 370:173–184
2. Hanlon JT, Schmader KE (2013) The medication appropriateness index at 20: where it started, where it has been and where it may be going. Drugs Aging 30:893–900
3. The American Geriatrics Society 2015 Beers Criteria Update Expert Panel (2015) AGS Updated Beers Criteria for potentially inappropriate medication use in older adults. J Am Geriatr Soc 63(11):2227–2246
4. O'Mahony D, O'Sullivan D, Byrne S, O'Connor MN, Ryan C, Gallagher P (2015) STOPP/START criteria for potentially inappropriate prescribing in older people: version 2. Age Aging 44:213–218
5. National Committee on Quality Assurance. http://www.ncqa.org/HEDISQualityMeasurement/HEDISMeasures/HEDIS2015.aspx. Accessed 24 Aug 2015
6. See S, Ginzburg R (2008) Skeletal muscle relaxants. Pharmacotherapy 28:207–213
7. Spence MM, Shin PJ, Lee EA, Gibbs NE (2013) Risk of injury associated with skeletal muscle relaxant use in older adults. Ann Pharmacother 47:993–998
8. Golden AG, Ma Q, Nair V, Florez HJ, Roos BA (2010) Risk for fractures with centrally acting muscle relaxants: an analysis of a national Medicare advantage claims database. Ann Pharmacother 44:1369–1375
9. Billups SJ, Delate T, Hoover B (2011) Injury in an elderly population before and after initiating a skeletal muscle relaxant. Ann Pharmacother 45:485–491
10. Alvarez CA, Mortensen EM, Makris UE et al (2015) Association of skeletal muscle relaxers and antihistamines on mortality, hospitalizations, and emergency department visits in elderly patients: a nationwide retrospective cohort study. BMC Geriatr 15:2
11. Simoni-Wastila L, Wei YJ, Luong M et al (2014) Quality of psychopharmacological medication use in nursing home residents. Res Soc Admin Pharm 10:494–507
12. Weiner D, Hanlon JT, Studenski S (1998) CNS drug-related falls liability in community dwelling elderly. Gerontology 44:217–221
13. Hanlon JT, Boudreau RM, Roumani YF et al (2009) Number and dosage of central nervous system medications on recurrent falls in community elders: the health, aging and body composition study. J Gerontol Med Sci 64A:492–498
14. Pratt NL, Ramsay EN, Kalisch Ellet LM, Nguyen TA, Barratt JD, Roughead EE (2014) Association between use of multiple psychoactive medicines and hospitalization for falls: retrospective analysis of a large healthcare claim database. Drug Saf 37:529–535
15. Nurminen J, Puustinen J, Piirtola M, Vahlberg T, Lyles A, Kivelä SL (2013) Opioids, antiepileptic and anticholinergic drugs and the risk of fractures in patients 65 years of age and older: a prospective population-based study. Age Ageing 42:318–324
16. Johnell K, Fastbom J (2011) Antiepileptic drug use in community-dwelling and institutionalized elderly: a nationwide study of over 1,300,000 older people. Eur J Clin Pharmacol 67: 1069–1075
17. Garrard J, Harms S, Hardie N et al (2003) Antiepileptic drug use in nursing home admissions. Ann Neurol 54:75–85
18. Deandrea S, Lucenteforte E, Bravi F et al (2010) Risk factors for falls in community-dwelling older people: a systematic review and meta-analysis. Epidemiology 21:658–668

19. Carbone LD, Johnson KC, Robbins J, Larson JC, Curb JD, Watson K, Gass M, Lacroix AZ (2010) Antiepileptic drug use, falls, fractures, and BMD in postmenopausal women: findings from the women's health initiative (WHI). J Bone Miner Res 25:873–881
20. Tsiropoulos I, Andersen M, Nymark T, Lauritsen J, Gaist D, Hallas J (2008) Exposure to antiepileptic drugs and the risk of hip fracture: a case-control study. Epilepsia 49:2092–2099
21. Mezuk B, Morden NE, Ganoczy D, Post EP, Kilbourne AM (2010) Anticonvulsant use, bipolar disorder, and risk of fracture among older adults in the veterans health administration. Am J Geriatr Psychiatry 18(3):245–255
22. Lapi F, Simonetti M, Michieli R, Pasqua A, Brandi ML, Frediani B, Cricelli C, Mazzaglia G (2012) Assessing 5-year incidence rates and determinants of osteoporotic fractures in primary care. Bone 50:85–90
23. Shen C, Chen F, Zhang Y, Guo Y, Ding M (2014) Association between use of antiepileptic drugs and fracture risk: a systematic review and meta-analysis. Bone 64:246–253
24. Schelleman H, Pollard JR, Newcomb C et al (2011) Exposure to CYP3A4-inducing and CYP3A4-non-inducing antiepileptic agents and the risk of fractures. Pharmacoepidemiol Drug Saf 20(6):619–625
25. Williams RE, Sampson TJ, Kalilani L et al (2008) Epidemiology of opioid pharmacy claims in the United States. J Opioid Manag 4:145–152
26. Lapane KL, Quilliam BJ, Chow W, Kim MS (2013) Pharmacologic management of non-cancer pain among nursing home residents. J Pain Symptom Manage 45:33–42
27. Takkouche B, Montes-Martínez A, Gill SS, Etminan M (2007) Psychotropic medications and the risk of fracture: a meta-analysis. Drug Saf 30:171–184
28. Rolita L, Spegman A, Tang X, Cronstein BN (2013) Greater number of narcotic analgesic prescriptions for osteoarthritis is associated with falls and fractures in elderly adults. J Am Geriatr Soc 61:335–340
29. Buckeridge D, Huang A, Hanley J et al (2010) Risk of injury associated with opioid use in older adults. J Amer Geriatr Soc 58:1664–1670
30. Saunders KW, Dunn KM, Merrill JO et al (2010) Relationship of opioid use and dosage levels to fractures in older chronic pain patients. J Gen Intern Med 25:310–315
31. Solomon DH, Rassen JA, Glynn RJ et al (2010) The comparative safety of opioids for nonmalignant pain in older adults. Arch Intern Med 170:1979–1986
32. Miller M, Stürmer T, Azrael D, Levin R, Solomon DH (2011) Opioid analgesics and the risk of fractures in older adults with arthritis. J Am Geriatr Soc 59:430–438
33. Möller J, Laflamme L, Söderberg LK (2015) CYP2D6-inhibiting drugs and the increased risk of fall-related injuries due to newly initiated opioid treatment – a Swedish, register-based case-crossover study. Basic Clin Pharmacol Toxicol 116:134–139

Chapter 15
Identifying Explicit Criteria for the Prevention of Falls

Denis Curtin, Stephen Byrne, and Denis O'Mahony

Abstract Over the last 25 years, several lists of potentially inappropriate medications (PIMs) for older patients have been validated and published with a view to using them as screening tools in clinical practice. Explicit criteria were developed as a guide for avoidance of PIMs and to supplement the physician's clinical knowledge and expertise in routine clinical practice. These explicit criteria typically do not require detailed or specialist knowledge to be used effectively. Most lists have been developed using the Delphi process. Beers criteria, developed in the United States and updated in 2015, include 88 medications and medication classes, which are divided into 5 categories. Screening Tool of Older Person's potentially inappropriate Prescriptions (STOPP) and the Screening Tool to Alert doctors to the Right Treatments (START) were developed in Ireland in 2008 and most recently updated in 2014. STOPP includes 80 criteria and there are 34 START criteria. Norwegian General Practice (NORGEP) criteria were developed in 2009 and include 36 criteria based on the Beers list. PRISCUS list medications are listed by pharmacological category rather than by physiological system, along with details of their potential danger as well as alternative medications that are likely safer. The combination of the Beers criteria and STOPP criteria may offer a more complete list. None of the published explicit criteria sets was designed specifically as a fall prevention tool.

Abbreviations

ADE	Adverse drug event
ADR	Adverse drug reaction
CI	Confidence interval
CMS	Centers for Medicare and Medicaid Services

D. Curtin, MB, MRCPI • D. O'Mahony, MD, FRCPI (✉)
Department of Medicine (Geriatrics), University College Cork & Cork University Hospital, Wilton, Cork, Ireland
e-mail: denis.omahony@ucc.ie

S. Byrne, BSc Pharmacy, PhD
School of Pharmacy, University College Cork, Cork, Ireland

© Springer International Publishing Switzerland 2016

A.R. Huang, L. Mallet (eds.), *Medication-related falls in older people*,
DOI 10.1007/978-3-319-32304-6_15

NICE	National Institutes of Clinical Excellence
NORGEP	Norwegian General Practice
OR	Odds ratio
PIM	Potentially inappropriate medication
PIP	Potentially inappropriate prescribing
PPO	Potential prescribing omission
START	Screening Tool to Alert doctors to the Right Treatments
STOPP	Screening Tool of Older Person's potentially inappropriate Prescriptions
TCA	Tricyclic antidepressants

15.1 Introduction

The prescribing of multiple medications to treat several concurrent comorbidities is considered a fundamental component of care of an older person. In the modern era, polypharmacy, i.e., the need for five or more daily drugs has become highly prevalent in both developed and developing countries, where rapid expansion of the population of older people is now happening and expected to continue over the next four decades. There is a direct causal relationship between multi-morbidity of late life and polypharmacy. Polypharmacy, in turn, is the principal risk factor for inappropriate prescribing and associated adverse drug reactions (ADRs) and adverse drug events (ADEs) [1]. Inappropriate prescribing in older adults is common and expensive, often leads to poor clinical outcomes, and is wasteful of resources.

Achieving an optimal balance between benefits and risks of a drug regime in frailer older patients with multi-morbidity is often very challenging. This is further complicated by the fact that advancing age is associated with an increased risk of both potentially inappropriate prescribing (PIP) and ADRs/ADEs [1]. Despite this, PIP and related ADRs/ADEs are often preventable.

Over the last 25 years, several PIP criteria sets have been validated and published with a view to using them as screening tools in clinical practice. The various tools mostly use explicit PIP criteria (as distinct from implicit PIP criteria), which are usually clearly defined statements indicating the potentially inappropriate use of certain drugs in older people in particular clinical circumstances. The explicit criteria sets are intended to be a guide for avoidance of potentially inappropriate medications (PIMs) and to supplement the physician's clinical knowledge and expertise in routine clinical practice. Explicit PIP criteria typically do not require detailed or specialist knowledge to be used effectively. They are generally easy to deploy and exhibit high levels of interrater reliability [2–4]. On the other hand, explicit PIP criteria do not take all aspects of a patient's care into consideration, nor do they consider patient preference, previously unsuccessful treatment regimens, or issues relating to multimorbidity [5, 6]. It is generally acknowledged that PIP is a common clinical problem in older people. Recent studies applying STOPP criteria and Beers criteria show high rates of PIM prescriptions in a variety of clinical settings, i.e., primary care, hospital care, and long-term nursing care [7–9].

Many older people present to hospital with falls and associated injuries. Falls are common in older people, particularly in frailer elders with multi-morbidity. Falls are commonly the result of adverse reactions to psychotropic medication. Falls may also be a nonspecific presentation of acute illness in older people, such as acute sepsis with delirium. Another common emergency department presentation in older people is falls resulting from syncope or pre-syncope where the cause of the syncopal symptoms is often drug related. Therefore, when considering the clinical relevance of any set of PIP explicit criteria, it is important that it includes common and important drug causes of falls in older people.

15.2 Development of Explicit Criteria

Despite being the greatest consumers of medication, older people are commonly excluded from well-designed clinical trials [10]. Evidence-based criteria, to guide prescribing in this population, are therefore problematic. To overcome this, most explicit criteria have been developed using the Delphi process, a survey technique used to find consensus among a panel of experts when existing knowledge is uncertain or incomplete [11]. Firstly, following a review of the scientific literature, a preliminary set of criteria are developed. These criteria are then disseminated to the expert panelists accompanied by a questionnaire. After each round, an anonymous summary of the experts' responses is fed back to the panel experts. The experts are then encouraged to review their answers to each item for consideration in light of the responses of other members of the group. Consensus is usually reached after two to three iterations. The anonymity of the process has been highlighted as both an advantage and a weakness. While the process prevents the authority or reputation of some participants from dominating others, accountability for individual responses may be diminished [12, 13]. Expert consensus is no substitution for sound scientific evidence, and the quality of criteria depends on the level of expertise among the panel members involved in the validation process. It has been suggested that an interdisciplinary panel will reduce the potential for skewed results while fewer rounds in the process minimize potential bias due to response fatigue [13, 14]. There is no guidance on the optimal number of expert panelists or the number of validation rounds [12, 13].

15.3 Explicit PIP Criteria and Fall Prevention

The various sets of explicit PIP criteria guiding prescribing in older adults were developed to detect potentially inappropriate prescribing and, in some cases, potential prescribing omissions (PPOs); they were not designed specifically to prevent falls. To date, there is only one randomized controlled clinical trial showing that prospective clinical application of PIP criteria reduces the risk of falls in older people. In that trial, intervention patients' medication lists were reviewed at baseline, 6 months and 12 months, applying STOPP/START criteria [4] to detect PIMs and PPOs. During the 12 months post-randomization follow-up period, the average number of falls in the intervention group dropped significantly while there was no significant drop in fall incidence in the control group [15].

Some of the commonly used sets of explicit PIP criteria and how they pertain to falls are described below and illustrated in Table 15.1. PIMs that are directly linked to falls and common to both Beers criteria and STOPP criteria (the most widely used explicit PIP criteria internationally) are illustrated in Table 15.2.

15.3.1 Beers Criteria

Beers criteria are the most widely used criteria to evaluate inappropriate prescribing in the United States. The criteria have been adopted by the American Geriatrics Society and form part of policy and practice in the Centers for Medicare and Medicaid Services (CMS) regulations [16, 17]. The first set of criteria was published in 1991 and has been updated four times since then. The most recent version in 2015 was developed following an extensive literature review, and consensus opinion of a 13-member expert panel was reached using modified Delphi methodology [18]. The interdisciplinary panel had expertise in geriatric medicine, nursing, pharmacotherapy, quality measures, and research. After an initial meeting examining new articles relevant to the previous 2012 criteria set, the panelists were divided into four working groups and were assigned to evaluate specific criteria related to their own area of expertise. Each group presented their findings to the full panel for consensus. Conference calls or face-to-face meetings were used to work through differences until a final consensus was reached.

The final criteria include 88 medications and medication classes, which are divided into 5 categories: (i) criteria for potentially inappropriate medications and classes to avoid in older adults – independent of diagnosis or condition, (ii) criteria for PIMs and drug classes to avoid in older adults with certain diseases and conditions, (iii) criteria for potentially inappropriate medication use in older adults that should be used with caution, (iv) criteria for potentially clinically important non-anti-infective drug-drug interactions to avoid in older adults, and (v) criteria for non-anti-infective medications that should be avoided or have their dosage reduced with varying levels of kidney function. Quality of evidence and strength of recommendation are qualified for each criterion. The first category includes 37 medications or medication classes, many of which contribute indirectly to the risk of falls through various pharmacological mechanisms, such as orthostatic hypotension, extrapyramidal symptoms, impaired cognition, and sedation. The second category specifically lists PIMs to be avoided in older adults with a history of falls or fractures as well as those with a history of syncope (Table 15.1). In addition, a list of medications with strong anticholinergic properties is included.

Table 15.1 Commonly used explicit criteria and their application to older patients at risk of falls

Criteria, publication year	Validation method	Structure of criteria	Medications directly linked to falls	Medications indirectly linked to falls	Potential prescribing omissions in patients at risk of falls
Beers criteria, 2015	Modified Delphi consensus; 13 panelists	88 criteria; 5 categories: 1. PIMs to be avoided for all older adults 2. PIMs to be avoided in older adults with specific conditions (including those with history of falls and syncope) 3. PIMs to be used with caution in older adults 4. Drug-drug interactions to be avoided in older adults 5. Medications to be avoided or have their dosage reduced in older adults with impaired kidney function	Anticonvulsants Neuroleptics Benzodiazepines Non-benzodiazepine hypnotics TCAs SSRIs Opioids	*Anticholinergic effects*: First-generation antihistamines, antispasmodics, skeletal muscle relaxants, disopyramide, benztropine, prochlorperazine *OH*: Dipyridamole, central alpha-blockers, nifedipine, peripheral alpha-blockers, e.g., doxazosin, prazosin, terazosin *Syncope*: AChEIs *Extrapyramidal side effects*: Metoclopramide, trimethobenzamide *Sedation*: Meprobamate	Not included

(continued)

Table 15.1 (continued)

Criteria, publication year	Validation method	Structure of criteria	Medications directly linked to falls	Medications indirectly linked to falls	Potential prescribing omissions in patients at risk of falls
Screening Tool of Older Person's potentially inappropriate Prescriptions (STOPP) and Screening Tool to Alert doctors to the Right Treatments (START), 2014	Delphi consensus; 19 panelists	STOPP: 80 criteria START: 34 criteria	Benzodiazepines Neuroleptics Vasodilator drugs (alpha-1 receptor blockers, calcium channel blockers, long-acting nitrates, ACE inhibitors, angiotensin I receptor blockers) with persistent OH Non-benzodiazepine hypnotics	Beta-blockers with bradycardia AChEIs with a known history of persistent bradycardia Prochlorperazine or metoclopramide with parkinsonism Concomitant use of two or more drugs with anticholinergic properties Phosphodiesterase type-5 inhibitors in severe heart failure characterized by hypotension	Vitamin D supplements Vitamin D and calcium supplements in patients with previous fragility fracture(s) Bone antiresorptive or anabolic therapy in patients with history of fragility fracture(s) where no contraindication exists
Norwegian General Practice (NORGEP) criteria, 2009	Delphi consensus; 47 panelists	36 criteria: 21 PIMs and dosages 15 drug-drug interactions	Diazepam Oxazepam Concomitant prescription of three or more drugs within the groups centrally acting analgesics, antipsychotics, antidepressants, and/or benzodiazepines	*Anticholinergic effects*: Amitriptyline, carisoprodol, dexchlorpheniramine *Extrapyramidal side effects*: Chlorpromazine	Not included

Criteria, publication year	Validation method	Structure of criteria	Medications directly linked to falls	Medications indirectly linked to falls	Potential prescribing omissions in patients at risk of falls
PRISCUS list, 2010	Modified Delphi consensus; 38 panelists	83 criteria	Benzodiazepines Neuroleptics Non-benzodiazepine hypnotics TCAs Pethidine Baclofen	*Anticholinergic effects*: Hydroxyzine, chlorpheniramine, diphenhydramine, doxylamine, oxybutynin, tolterodine (nonsustained release), solifenacin *Hypotension*: Clonidine, alpha-blockers, methyldopa, reserpine, nifedipine *Sedation*: Phenobarbitone, SSRIs, chloral hydrate	Not included

PIMs potentially inappropriate medications, *TCAs* tricyclic antidepressants, *SSRIs* selective serotonin reuptake inhibitors, *AChEIs* acetylcholine esterase inhibitors, *OH* orthostatic hypotension

Table 15.2 Fall-related PIMs included in both Beers criteria (version 5) and STOPP criteria (version 2)

Drug-drug class	Rationale
Benzodiazepines	Reduced sensorium, impaired balance
Non-benzodiazepine hypnotics	Reduced sensorium, impaired balance
Neuroleptic major tranquilizers	Gait apraxia, parkinsonism
Alpha-1 receptor blockers	Orthostatic hypotension
Acetylcholine esterase inhibitors	May cause syncope in patients with persistent bradycardia

A multicenter prospective cohort study conducted in France, involving 6,343 participants with a mean age of 74 years with 4 years of follow-up, evaluated the association between PIMs as defined by Beers criteria (third iteration [19]) and the French Consensus Panel criteria for PIMs in older people [20] and the risk of falls [21]. The study identified three categories of commonly prescribed drugs which were significantly associated with incident falls during the prospective 4-year follow-up interval. These included regular use of long-acting benzodiazepines (adjusted odds ratio (OR) = 1.4, 95 % CI 1.1–1.8); other psychotropics, i.e., anticholinergic antidepressants, antipsychotic drugs, and anticholinergic hypnotic drugs (adjusted OR = 1.7, 95 % confidence interval 1.7–2.7); or medication with anticholinergic properties (adjusted OR = 1.6, 95 % CI 1.2–2.1) [21].

15.3.2 STOPP/START Criteria

The Screening Tool of Older Person's potentially inappropriate Prescriptions (STOPP) and the Screening Tool to Alert doctors to the Right Treatments (START) were developed in Ireland in 2008 and most recently updated in 2014 [22]. The most recent version was developed following an extensive literature review and two rounds of Delphi validation with 19 panel members across 13 European countries, with recognized expertise in geriatric medicine and pharmacotherapy in older adults. The tool forms part of the National Institutes of Clinical Excellence (NICE) guidelines on medication optimization in the United Kingdom [23]. STOPP includes 80 PIP criteria outlining clinical circumstances where certain medications or medication classes would be considered potentially inappropriate in older individuals across all settings of care. The criteria are organized according to the physiological system to which each criterion relates. In addition, there is a section that lists medication classes that predictably increase the risk of falls in older people (Table 15.1).

The START criteria are also an explicit set of criteria designed to assess for PPOs in older individuals in any care setting. Thirty-four START criteria are included in the most recent iteration [22]. STOPP and START are intended to be used concomitantly, and herein lies an advantage of this PIP criteria set. As well as identifying medications that could be potentially harmful to older adults with a history of falls, potentially *beneficial* medications are also identified. Examples include calcium and vitamin D supplementation as well as antiresorptive or anabolic therapy in patients with known osteoporosis and/or fragility fractures (Table 15.1).

15.3.3 NORGEP Criteria

The Norwegian General Practice (NORGEP) criteria were developed in 2009 and include 36 explicit criteria based on Beers criteria, an extensive literature review, and the clinical practices of the lead authors [24]. The criteria underwent three rounds of Delphi validation by 47 Norwegian-based panelists with expertise in pharmacology, geriatric medicine, and general practice. Twenty-one of the 36 criteria relate to single drugs and doses considered potentially inappropriate in older people while 15 criteria relate to drug-drug interactions. Most, but not all, of the single drug criteria are accompanied by an explanatory statement. Unlike Beers criteria and STOPP/START, the NORGEP criteria are not structured in ways that highlight PIMs to be avoided in older adults at risk of falls. Only individual benzodiazepines, i.e., diazepam and oxazepam, as well as the use of three or more psychotropic medications are specifically linked with an increased risk of falls. Other medications are indirectly associated with an increased risk of falls through various mechanisms including sedation, extrapyramidal symptoms, and anticholinergic effects (Table 15.1).

15.3.4 PRISCUS Criteria

The PRISCUS PIM list was developed by Holt et al. in 2010 and was developed for specific use in Germany across all settings of care [25]. Initially, a preliminary PIM list intended for the German market was created following a literature review and an analysis of published international PIM lists. The final list was established following two rounds of a modified Delphi process involving 38 German-speaking panelists with expertise in geriatric medicine, clinical pharmacology, general practice, internal medicine, pain therapy, neurology, psychiatry, and clinical pharmacy. PRISCUS includes 83 criteria that are categorized according to medication class. Each potentially inappropriate medication class is accompanied by an explanation highlighting the main concerns associated with use in older adults, and safer alternative medications are suggested. If it is deemed necessary to prescribe the PIM, precautionary advice is offered. Benzodiazepines, non-benzodiazepine hypnotics, neuroleptics, tricyclic antidepressants (TCAs), and pethidine and baclofen are directly linked to an increased risk of falls. Several other medications are indirectly linked through a variety of mechanisms (Table 15.1). Once again, unlike Beers criteria and STOPP/START, PIMs for older adults at risk of falls are not grouped together in PRISCUS.

15.4 Conclusion

The aging process is associated with an increased risk of ADRs and ADEs. Inappropriate prescribing leading to ADEs, including falls and fractures, is common, expensive, and potentially avoidable. Several PIP criteria sets have been developed to reduce ADEs in older adults. These criteria sets were developed using an evidence-based approach and, when evidence was incomplete, expert consensus. While they do not always comprehensively address the care needs of an individual patient, PIP criteria may guide decision-making and prove particularly beneficial to the physician who is not attuned to the nuances of care of the older adult.

None of the published PIP criteria sets was designed specifically as a fall prevention tool. Used alone, they do not represent comprehensive, complete lists of medications to be avoided in older adults at risk of falls. The combination of Beers criteria and STOPP criteria (Table 15.2) may offer a more complete list drugs and medication classes to be avoided or at least used with caution in older people who fall or are at risk of falls. Future iterations of these criteria sets should attempt to include more complete lists of PIMs that heighten risk of falls in older adults.

References

1. Hamilton HJ, Gallagher P, O'Mahony D (2009) Inappropriate prescribing and adverse drug events in older people. BMC Geriatr 9:5
2. Dimitrow MS, Airaksinen MS, Kivelä SL, Lyles A, Leikola SN (2011) Comparison of prescribing criteria to evaluate the appropriateness of drug treatment in individuals aged 65 and older: a systematic review. J Am Geriatr Soc 59(8):1521–1530
3. Spinewine A, Schmader KE, Barber N, Hughes C, Lapane KL, Swine C, Hanlon JT (2007) Appropriate prescribing in elderly people: how well can it be measured and optimised? Lancet 370(9582):173–184
4. Gallagher P, Ryan C, Byrne S, Kennedy J, O'Mahony D (2008) Screening Tool of Older Person's Prescriptions (STOPP) and Screening Tool to Alert doctors to Right Treatment (START). Consensus validation. Int J Clin Pharmacol Ther 46:72–83
5. O'Connor MN, Gallagher P, O'Mahony D (2012) Inappropriate prescribing: criteria, detection and prevention. Drugs Aging 29(6):437–452
6. Page RL, Linnebur SA, Bryant LL, Ruscin JM (2010) Inappropriate prescribing in the hospitalized elderly patient: defining the problem, evaluation tools, and possible solutions. Clin Interv Aging 5:75–87
7. Gallagher P, O'Mahony D (2008) Screening Tool of Older Persons' potentially inappropriate Prescriptions (STOPP): application to acutely ill elderly patients and comparison with Beers' criteria. Age Ageing 37:673–679
8. Ryan C, O'Mahony D, Kennedy J, Weedle P, Byrne S (2009) Potentially inappropriate prescribing in an Irish elderly population in primary care. Br J Clin Pharmacol 68(6):936–47.
9. O'Mahony D, Gallagher P, Ryan C, Byrne S, Hamilton H, Barry P, O'Connor M, Kennedy J (2010) STOPP & START criteria: a new approach to detecting potentially inappropriate prescribing in old age. Eur Geriatr Med 1(1):45–51
10. Van Spall HGC, Toren A et al (2007) Eligibility criteria of randomized controlled trials published in high-impact general medical journals. JAMA 297:1233–1240

11. Williams PL, Webb C (1994) The Delphi technique: a methodological discussion. Aust J Adv Nurs 19:180–186
12. Marriott J, Stehlik P (2012) A critical analysis of the methods used to develop explicit clinical criteria for use in older people. Age Ageing 41(4):441–450
13. Goodman CM (1987) The Delphi technique: a critique. Aust J Adv Nurs 12:729–734
14. Keeney S, Hasson F, McKenna H (2006) Consulting the oracle: ten lessons from using the Delphi technique in nursing research. Aust J Adv Nurs 53:205–212
15. Frankenthal D, Lerman Y, Kalendaryev E, Lerman Y (2014) Intervention with the screening tool of older persons potentially inappropriate prescriptions/screening tool to alert doctors to right treatment criteria in elderly residents of a chronic geriatric facility: a randomized clinical trial. J Am Geriatr Soc 62(9):1658–1665
16. Blackwell S, Montgomery M, Baugh D, Ciborowski G, Riley G (2012) Applying the 2003 Beers update to elderly Medicare enrollees in the part D program. MMRR 2:2
17. American Geriatrics Society 2012 Beers Criteria Update Expert Panel (2012) American Geriatrics Society updated Beers criteria for potentially inappropriate medication use in older adults. J Am Geriatr Soc 60(4):616–631
18. American Geriatrics Society 2015 Beers Criteria Update Expert Panel (2015) American Geriatrics Society 2015 updated Beers criteria for potentially inappropriate medication use in older adults. J Am Geriatr Soc 63(11):2227–2246
19. Fick DM, Cooper JW, Wade WE, Waller JL, Maclean JR, Beers MH (2003) Updating the Beers criteria for potentially inappropriate medication use in older adults: results of a US consensus panel of experts. Arch Intern Med 163(22):2716–2724
20. Laroche ML, Charmes JP, Merle L (2007) Potentially inappropriate medications in the elderly: a French consensus panel list. Eur J Clin Pharmacol 63(8):725–731
21. Berdot S, Bertrand M, Dartigues JF, Fourrier A, Tavernier B, Ritchie K, et al (2009) Inappropriate medication use and risk of falls–a prospective study in a large community-dwelling elderly cohort. BMC Geriatr 9:30; doi:10.1186/1471-2318-9-30
22. O'Mahony D, O'Sullivan D, Byrne S, O'Connor MN, Ryan C, Gallagher P (2015) STOPP/START criteria for potentially inappropriate prescribing in older people: version 2. Age Ageing 44(2):213–218
23. National Institute for Health and Care Excellence (NICE). Medicines optimisation: the safe and effective use of medicines to enable the best possible outcomes. 2015. http://www.nice.org.uk/guidance/ng5/chapter/1-Recommendations
24. Rognstad S, Brekke M, Fetveit A, Spigset O, Wyller TB, Straand J (2009) The Norwegian General Practice (NORGEP) criteria for assessing potentially inappropriate prescriptions to elderly patients. A modified Delphi study. Scand J Prim Health Care 27(3):153–159
25. Holt S, Schmiedl S, Thürmann PA (2010) Potentially inappropriate medications in the elderly: the PRISCUS list. Dtsch Arztebl Int 107(31–32):543–551

Chapter 16
Approach to Medication Reviews in Older Adults

Derek Dyks

Abstract The terms medication review and medication reconciliation refer to two different activities and should not be used interchangeably. *Medication review* is the process of evaluating current medication treatment to manage the risk and optimize the outcomes of medication treatment by detecting, solving, and preventing medication-related problems. *Medication reconciliation* is the process of obtaining and documenting a complete and accurate list of current patient medications and comparing this list with medication orders at each point of care transition to identify and rectify any discrepancies. Medication review is especially valuable for older adults who tend to take more medications, have more comorbid illnesses, and consequently suffer more adverse drug reactions. ARMOR is an acronym for *A*ssess, *R*eview, *M*inimize, *O*ptimize, *R*eassess and represents an example mnemonic for a structured process used to conduct a medication review. It is important to note that intentional nonadherence is common. The Medication Appropriateness Index (MAI) is a tool that can facilitate the analysis of patient's medication profile. Engaging patients in their medication review and possible deprescribing process will dramatically increase the chance of success in decreasing polypharmacy, stopping inappropriate medications, and lowering the incidence of adverse events such as falls.

Abbreviations

AGS	American Geriatrics Society
ARMOR	Acronym for *A*ssess, *R*eview, *M*inimize, *O*ptimize, *R*eassess
BPMH	Best possible medication history
MAI	Medication appropriateness index
OTC	Over the counter
PIM	Potentially inappropriate medications (PIMs)
RaR	Rate ratio

D. Dyks, BScPhm, RPh, CGP
Clinical Pharmacist, Geriatric Medicine Unit, The Ottawa Hospital, Ottawa, ON, Canada
e-mail: ddyks@toh.ca

© Springer International Publishing Switzerland 2016

A.R. Huang, L. Mallet (eds.), *Medication-related falls in older people*,
DOI 10.1007/978-3-319-32304-6_16

Medications are common and potentially modifiable contributors to falls in older persons across the continuum of care, from private residence to acute care hospitalization. Previous studies have shown that discontinuation of unnecessary medications can lower fall risk. Accordingly, medication review has been incorporated into the American Geriatrics Society's (AGS) recommendations as part of a multipronged approach to fall prevention [1]. This chapter will cover medication review, including integral components, tips on performing medication reviews, and pitfalls to avoid.

16.1 Medication Review vs. Medication Reconciliation

There is often confusion surrounding the differences between the terms medication review and medication reconciliation. These are two different activities and the terms should not be used interchangeably.

Medication review is the process of evaluating current medication treatment to manage the risk and optimize the outcomes of medication treatment by detecting, solving, and preventing medication-related problems [2]. Medication review has also been defined as "a structured, critical examination of a person's medicines with the objective of reaching an agreement with the person about treatment, optimizing the impact of medicines, minimizing the number of medication-related problems and reducing waste" [3].

Medication reconciliation is the process of obtaining and documenting a complete and accurate list of current patient medications and comparing this list with medication orders at each point of care transition to identify and rectify any discrepancies [2]. It is a required organizational practice within Accreditation Canada standards.

Both medication reconciliation and medication review are important aspects of medication safety, especially in vulnerable elderly patients. This chapter will focus on the activity of medication review and its role in fall prevention.

16.2 Rationale for Conducting Medication Reviews

As mentioned previously, medications are well recognized as a contribution factor to falls in older adults [4, 5]. Fall risk increases with the number of medications a person takes. Additionally, numerous classes of medication have consistently been associated with and increased risk of falling [5–7]. Mechanisms by which medications increase the risk of falling include impaired muscle strength, motor retardation, postural hypotension, impaired judgment, and cognition [6, 8]. In a 2012, Cochrane review which looked at interventions to reduce falls, multifactorial interventions, which include medication review, were shown to decrease the rate of falls Rate Ratio (RaR) 0.76 (0.67–0.86) but not the risk of falling RaR 0.93 (0.86–1.02) [9]. In the same review, gradual psychotropic withdrawal specifically was also shown to decrease the rate of falls RaR 0.34 (0.16–0.73) but not fall risk. Tools to help identify these and other fall risk medications are covered in other chapters of this book.

Medication review is especially valuable for older adults who tend to take more medications, have more comorbid illnesses, and consequently suffer more adverse drug reactions. Medication review has been shown to reduce the risk of falls and should be a part of a multipronged approach to fall prevention [1, 4, 9, 10]. This includes patients who have fallen as well as those who have not yet fallen but are at risk of falling. Medication review should be performed for patients with complicated medication regimens, following hospital admission, when there is a documented or suspected adverse drug event, a transition of level of care (e.g., move to a retirement home/nursing home), and otherwise on a yearly basis [11].

16.3 Principles of Medication Review

To facilitate optimal efficiency and effectiveness, the medication review process can be conceptualized into structure, process, and outcomes [12].

16.3.1 Structure

A medication review that is structured using standardized forms for collection of patient information is recommended to support organization and efficiency. Standardized forms will ensure that the appropriate information is being gathered and will minimize the effect of interviewer variability.

16.3.2 Process

Similarly, the process of the medication review should be standardized as well. The elements to the review should occur in the same manner and sequence each time to minimize the risk of information being missed.

16.3.3 Outcome

The goal (or outcome) of the medication review should be the detection and/or prevention of potential or current adverse drug effects, such as falls. A systematic approach to medication review will maximize the likelihood of achieving this outcome and maximize the benefit to the patient.

A tool developed to facilitate a stepwise approach to medication review is ARMOR, which is an acronym for *A*ssess, *R*eview, *M*inimize, *O*ptimize, *R*eassess [13].

Assess – the individual for polypharmacy and potentially inappropriate medications.
Review – for possible drug-drug interactions, drug-disease interactions, subclinical adverse drug reactions, and impact on functional status.
Minimize – nonessential medications and those that the risk outweighs the potential benefit.
Optimize – address duplication and redundancy, adjust dosages based on renal function, drug levels, and other monitoring parameters (e.g., blood pressure, heart rate, blood glucose levels, etc.).
Reassess – once changes have been made, evaluate monitoring parameters for beneficial (or harmful) effects and readjust medications if warranted.

The ARMOR tool encompasses the medication history, evaluation of the appropriateness of each medication, and the deprescribing process. Deprescribing is the process of tapering, stopping, discontinuing, or withdrawing drugs, with the goal of managing polypharmacy and improving outcomes [14]. ARMOR also highlights the importance of following up/monitoring the changes made to the patient's medication. This not only minimizes the risk of adverse events such as withdrawal, but it also allows the patient to feel supported as an active participant in the deprescribing process and provides an opportunity for him or her to voice their concerns. In other words, it minimizes the risk of the patient feeling as if he or she is worse off without their medication that was potentially causing them harm.

16.4 Medication History

The first step in the medication review process is accurately determining which medications your older patient is taking. This is often referred to as generating the Best Possible Medication History (BPMH). Errors in medication histories are common. One study found that the frequency of at least one error in the medication history ranged from 27 to 83 % [15]. Another study determined that medication history discrepancies can have significant clinical impact; 38.6 % of the discrepancies found had the potential to cause moderate or serious harm to patients [16].

Barriers to obtaining accurate medication histories include time required to obtain an accurate complete history, inadequate training in the skill of obtaining medication histories, lack of patient knowledge of his or her medications, as well as patient illness (including cognitive status) [17]. Awareness of these barriers helps minimize their impact in collecting medication information and minimizes the risk of basing therapeutic decisions on inaccurate information.

Potential sources of information used in obtaining an accurate medication history include the patient himself or herself, medication profiles from their pharmacy, family members, and the patient's medication bottle labels. If the patient's cognitive status is poor or questionable, then having family members, caregivers, or substitute decision-maker present can be valuable in obtaining accurate information.

If the medication history is being taken in the ambulatory clinic setting, it is ideal to have the patients bring all their medication with them. Having the patient's bottles of medication at the interview (as opposed to a medication list) is helpful in confirming medication adherence. Pill counts and dates of previous refills give clues as to how well the patients adhere to their medication regimen. It is important to specify that they bring in all prescription, nonprescription over-the-counter (OTC) medications, vitamins, herbal supplements, and other alternative therapy. It is not uncommon for patients to bring only their prescription medication as they feel the other classes "don't count" because they were not prescribed by a physician. The false sense that nonprescription medications are benign further adds to their danger. Additive sedative or anticholinergic effects with prescription and nonprescription medications can often be misdiagnosed due to the lack of awareness of the patient's self-medication, in addition to the underestimation of potential adverse effects associated with some classes of these readily available medications.

Performing the medication history in the patient's home may give you a more accurate picture of what the patient is actually taking and the patient's medication adherence compared to medication histories taken in the ambulatory clinic setting. Keeping medications in multiple locations in the home may indicate poor adherence due to poor organization or inadvertently forgetting to take important medications.

It has been well documented that medication adherence decreases with the number of medications prescribed [18]. This is especially true for classes of medication where the benefit of therapy is not apparent to the patient (e.g., antihypertensives). If medication adherence is poor and the clinician assumes that the medication is being taken by the patient as prescribed and therapeutic endpoints are not being met, this scenario may be misinterpreted as requiring additional therapy or dosage increases, which may result in excessive or duplication of therapy. This situation can result in additional unnecessary cost to the patient and the health-care system. If the patient becomes adherent to his or her regimen, as during an admission to hospital or initiation of compliance packaging such as blister packs or dosette boxes, there is a significant risk of adverse drug events. Adverse events, such as hypotension for antihypertensives and confusion or excess sedation for psychotropic medications or narcotic analgesics, can lead to falls.

It is important to note that intentional nonadherence is common [19]. Compliance packaging is unlikely to be of benefit if the patient does not see the value in taking the medication or is not taking it due to self-observed adverse effects. Education regarding the rationale for medication and including the patients in decisions regarding their medication is a more effective strategy to minimize nonadherence in these cases.

16.5 Analyzing Medication History

Once it has been determined which medications the patient is actually taking, the next step is to analyze and assess the appropriateness of each medication. In general, a common approach is to match a patient's medications with his or her comorbidities to identify extraneous medications. Subsequently, the remaining medication can be reviewed to assess if it is the most appropriate for that particular patient's situation.

If the patient is experiencing falls or near falls, a problem-based medication review may be the most practical method to attempt to identify any medication-related causes for the falls. It is helpful to determine the time frame of when falls commenced as it may be possible to correlate this with the initiation of certain medications, which could impair balance, cause muscle weakness, slow reaction time, as well as interact or have additive effects with preexisting medication.

A change in dosage of a preexisting medication can also explain new-onset falls. Acute illness can change the way in which the patient reacts to his or her medication which was previously well tolerated.

An algorithm for a problem-based medication review is presented below (Fig. 16.1).

If no *new* medications have been identified as potential causes of falls, it is possible that the onset of difficulties with adverse drug events leading to falls may be more subtle and more difficult to identify. In this case, addressing *longer-standing* potentially inappropriate medications (PIMs) and those known to cause falls is the next step. Gradual changes in pharmacodynamics and pharmacokinetics may lead to gradual increases in medication intolerances leading to falls. Tools to identify and address PIMs are covered elsewhere in this book (see chapters "Inappropriate Medications and Risk of Falls in Older Adults" and "Identifying Explicit Criteria for the Prevention of Falls").

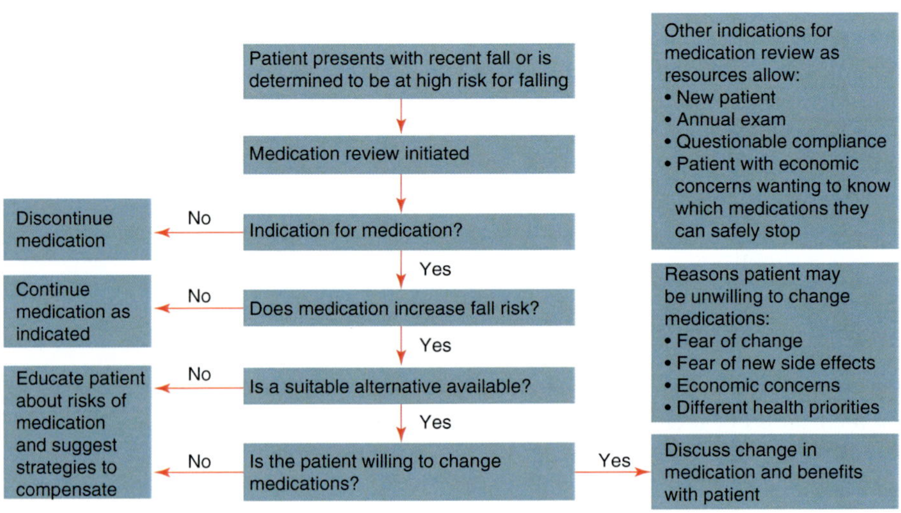

Fig. 16.1 Medication review algorithm [4]

A more comprehensive approach to medication review (as opposed to problem-based medication review) is to review each medication with the patient and to classify each medication by purpose and its importance [20]. Doing this with the patient involves the patient in the decision-making process as well as allows you to assess the patient's understanding of his or her medication. When a medication is deemed optional or not indicated, discontinuation should be considered, especially if it is known to cause adverse effects such as falls. If therapy is required but known to increase fall risk, then exploring safer alternatives or dose reductions should occur.

Systematically evaluating each medication is time consuming but minimizes the risk of missing potential culprits in causing adverse drug reactions such as falls. The Medication Appropriateness Index (MAI) is a tool to facilitate such a process [21].

The reviewer is intended to look at each medication individually and ask the following questions:

1. Is there an indication for the drug?
2. Is the medication effective for the condition?
3. Is the dosage correct?
4. Are the directions correct?
5. Are the directions practical?
6. Are there clinically significant drug-drug interactions?
7. Are there clinically significant drug-disease/condition interactions?
8. Is there unnecessary duplication with other drugs?
9. Is the duration of therapy acceptable?
10. Is this drug the least expensive alternative compared with others of equal usefulness?

Practically speaking, it is not often possible to apply this strategy to all medications for all patients. However, the principle of critically evaluating each medication for appropriateness for a particular patient is an ideal to strive toward to reduce inappropriate medication use and consequences of polypharmacy, one of which being falls.

16.6 Conclusion

Many medications are known to increase fall risk. Medication reviews are an integral part of a multipronged approach to addressing falls in the elderly. An accurate medication history is the first step in performing a medication review. Ideally performed in the patient's home, care should be taken to assess medication adherence and to include prescription, nonprescription, herbals, supplements, alcohol, and recreational drug use. In cases where the patient has experienced a fall or repeated falls, special attention should be paid to medications that were added or dose adjusted at the same time that the patient's falls started. In the case of a patient who is taking a previously well-tolerated medication, acute illness can also increase the risk of falls. Targeting medications that are known to increase fall risk should be considered in the interest of time efficiency. Patient's "buy-in" to the medication review and deprescribing process will dramatically increase the chance of success in decreasing polypharmacy, stopping inappropriate medications, and lowering the incidence of adverse events such as falls.

References

1. AGSguidelines – http://www.americangeriatrics.org/health_care_professionals/clinical_practice/clinical_guidelines_recommendations/prevention_of_falls_summary_of_recommendations. Accessed 12 Sept 2015
2. Lehnbom EC, Stewart MJ, Manas E, Westbrook JI (2014) Impact of medication reconcilliation and review on clinical outcomes. Ann Pharmacother 48(10):1298–312
3. NICE guidelines – medicines optimisation: the safe and effective use of medicines to enable the best possible outcomes. http://www.nice.org.uk/guidance/NG5/chapter/1-recommendations#medication-review. Accessed 5 Sept 2015
4. Kelly D, Frick E, Hale L (2011) How the medication review can help to reduce risk of falls in older patients. JAAPA 24(4):30–34
5. Huang A, Mallet L, Rochefort C et al (2012) Medication-related falls in the elderly–causative factors and preventive strategies. Drugs Aging 29:359–376
6. Dyks D, Sadowski C (2015) Interventions to reduce medication-related falls. CGS J CME 5(1):23–31
7. Boyle N, Naganathan V, Cummings RG (2010) Medications and Falls:risk and optimization. Clin geriatr Med 26:583–605
8. Walker P et al (2005) Medication use as a risk factor for falls among hospitalized elderly patients. Am J Health Syst Pharm 62:2495–2499
9. Gillespie LD, Gillespie WJ, Robertson MC et al (2003) Interventions for preventing falls in elderly people. Cochrane Database Syst Rev 4:CD000340. doi:10.1002/14651846.CD000340
10. van der Velde N, Stricker BHC, Pols HAP, van der Cammen TJM (2006) Risk of falls after withdrawal of fall-risk-increasing drugs: a prospective cohort study. Br J of Clin Pharmacol 63(2):232–237
11. Grindrod K et al (2013) Living MedsCheck: learning how to deliver MedsCheck in community practice in Ontario. CPJ 146(1):33–38
12. Barnette DJ, PharmD, BCPS, CDE (2003) A pharmacist's guide to medication review. J Am Pharm Assoc 42:131–132
13. Haque R (2009) ARMOR: a tool to evaluate polypharmacy in elderly persons. Ann Longterm Care 17(6):26–30
14. Thompson W et al (2013) Deprescribing: what is it and what does the evidence tell us? Can J Hosp Pharm 66(3):201–202
15. Tam VC, Knowles SR, Cornish PL, Fine N, Marchesano R, Etchells EE (2005) Frequency, type and clinical importance of medication history errors at admission to hospital: a systematic review. CMAJ 173(5):510–515
16. Cornish PL, Knowles SR, Marchesano R, Tam V, Shadowitz S, Juurlink DN et al (2005) Unintended medication discrepancies at the time of hospital admission. Arch Intern Med 165(4):424–429
17. Halapy H, Kertland H (2013) Ascertaining problems with medication histories. Can J Hosp Pharm 65(5):360–367
18. Hajjar ER, Cariero AC, Hanlon JT (2007) Polypharmacy in elderly patients. Am J Ger Pharmacol 5:345–351
19. Dore N et al (2011) Intentional medication nonadherence in a geriatric day hospital. CPJ 144(6):260–264
20. Courtney DL (1996) Medication reduction strategies. Comp Ther 22(5):318–323
21. Hanlon JT, Schmader KE, Samsa GP et al (1992) A method for assessing drug therapy appropriateness. J Clin Epidemiol 45:1045–1051

Chapter 17
Withdrawal of Fall Risk-Increasing Drugs

Nathalie van der Velde and Tischa J.M. van der Cammen

Abstract Falls are among the most serious problems faced by older persons and are associated with considerable morbidity and mortality.

Falls are multifactorial in origin. Hence, assessment of falls and fall risk is a complex task. An important risk factor for falls is the use of certain drugs, i.e., fall risk-increasing drugs (FRIDs). The exact contribution of FRIDs use to fall risk is not known. To date, information about the effects and effectiveness of FRIDs withdrawal on falls in older persons is scarce.

There is evidence that withdrawal of psychotropics reduces rate of falls and that a prescribing modification program for primary care physicians can reduce risk of falling.

Withdrawal of all FRIDs, including cardiovascular and psychotropic drugs, appears to be an effective intervention for lowering fall incidence and can lead to improvement of mobility tests and cardiovascular end points. Withdrawal of psychotropics, especially benzodiazepines (BZD), was an important factor in lowering risk of falls requiring medical treatment during the first year after a 12-month multifactorial intervention. BZD withdrawal has also been shown to result in a significant improvement in the stability of the body, a recovery of cognitive functions, and improvement of handgrip strength and balance.

N. van der Velde, MD, PhD
Section of Geriatric Medicine, Department of Internal Medicine, Academic Medical Center, Meibergdreef 9, Amsterdam 1100 DD, The Netherlands
e-mail: n.vandervelde@amc.uva.nl

T.J.M. van der Cammen, MD, PhD (✉)
Faculty of Industrial Design Engineering, Delft University of Technology, Landbergstraat 15, Delft 2628 CE, The Netherlands

Section of Geriatric Medicine, Department of Internal Medicine, Erasmus MC, University Medical Center Rotterdam, s-Gravendijkwal 230, Rotterdam 3015 CE, The Netherlands
e-mail: T.J.M.vanderCammen@tudelft.nl

© Springer International Publishing Switzerland 2016

A.R. Huang, L. Mallet (eds.), *Medication-related falls in older people*,
DOI 10.1007/978-3-319-32304-6_17

Pharmacological interventions, including withdrawal of FRIDs, pharmacist-conducted clinical medication review, and computerized drug alerts, are effective in reducing fall risk and should be incorporated in the care of older persons.

Abbreviations

BZD/BZDRD	Benzodiazepines or related drug
CG	Control group
DDI	Drug–drug interaction
FRIDs	Fall risk-increasing drugs
IG	Intervention group
IQR	Interquartile range
NSAID	Nonsteroidal anti-inflammatory drugs
RCT	Randomized controlled trial
SD	Standard deviation
TUG	Timed up and Go
US	United States

17.1 Introduction

One of the main challenges in geriatric medicine is to correctly diagnose and treat a patient presenting with vague or atypical symptoms. With increasing age, disease presentation becomes more atypical, with less than 50 % of older patients fitting the classical medical model of illness. There are four main reasons why disease presentation in this age category is often atypical: comorbidity may be present which may mask the presentation of another disease, a causal chain of problems may lead to a certain complaint, patients and physicians may attribute symptoms of a new disease to a chronic problem, or longstanding, unrecognized morbidity may be unmasked by a certain event [1].

Falls are among the most common "atypical" presenting symptoms in older persons. They are also among the most serious problems facing older persons and are associated with considerable morbidity and mortality [2]. Falls can be caused by many different factors and many of these factors are interrelated. Hence, assessment of falls and fall risk is a complex task. An important risk factor for falls is the use of certain drugs. Since the late 1990s, drugs associated with falls in the elderly have been identified (see Part 3: Medications Associated with Falls in the Elderly). General opinion is growing that drug cessation in complex older patients is warranted in the clinical situation of falls [3]. However, to date, little information is available about the effects and effectiveness of drug cessation on falls in older persons.

17.2 Effects and Effectiveness of Interventions Aimed at Withdrawal of Fall Risk-Increasing Drugs

Can withdrawal of FRIDs reduce falls?
The evidence

17.2.1 Randomized Controlled Trials of Withdrawal of Fall Risk-Increasing Drugs

Available randomized trials of interventions to reduce falls in older people living in the community, summarized in the Cochrane Database in 2012 [4], have shown that there is evidence that withdrawal of psychotropics is effective in reducing the rate of falls [5] and that a prescribing modification program for primary care physicians can reduce risk of falling [6]. The prescribing modification program included a major educational component for family physicians, with a face-to-face education session with a clinical pharmacist and feedback on prescribing practices, as well as financial rewards. The primary outcome measure was a composite score reflecting use of benzodiazepines (BZD), nonsteroidal anti-inflammatory drugs (NSAIDs), and thiazide diuretics; secondary measures were use of medication reviews, occurrence of falls, and quality of life as assessed by Short Form-12 and EuroQol-5D survey scores. Compared with the control group, participants in the intervention group had increased odds of having an improved medication use composite score at 4-month follow-up but not at 12 months.

At the 4-month follow-up, the intervention group had reduced odds of using NSAIDs and showed a nonsignificant reduction in use of benzodiazepines and thiazide diuretics. Changes in drug use were not significant at 12-month follow-up. At 12 months, intervention group participants had a significantly reduced risk of falling. Quality-of-life scores were unaffected by the intervention. It is important to note that the prescribing physician (i.e., the family physician) was the lead person in the medication review and advising the patients about the medication modifications [6]. Two recent reviews further confirmed that withdrawal of psychotropics is effective in reducing the rate of falls [7, 8].

Recruitment and randomization of older patients to drug withdrawal intervention trials is difficult. A randomized controlled trial (RCT) of 217 cognitively intact community-dwelling Dutch patients older than 65 years at high risk for recurrent falls failed to show an effect on fall rate. A multifactorial intervention which included a medication review and appropriate withdrawal of fall risk-increasing drugs was used. In the follow-up year, no significant treatment effect was demonstrated between the 106 intervention participants and 111 usual care (control) participants, for the time to first fall (hazard ratio, 0.96; 95 % confidence interval, 0.67–1.37) or the time to second fall (1.13; 0.71–1.80) [9].

A new RCT on the (cost)-effectiveness of withdrawal of fall risk-increasing drugs versus conservative treatment in older fallers is the IMPROveFALL study

[10]. This prospective, multicenter RCT is being conducted in hospitals in the Netherlands. Persons 65 years and older who visit the emergency department due to a fall are invited to participate in this trial. All patients receive a full geriatric assessment at the research outpatient clinic. Patients are randomized between a structured medication assessment including withdrawal of fall risk-increasing drugs and "care as usual." A 3-monthly fall calendar is used for assessing the number of falls, the fallers, and associated injuries over a 1-year follow-up period. Measurements will be at 3, 6, 9, and 12 months and include functional outcomes, healthcare utilization, sociodemographic characteristics, and clinical information. After 12 months a second visit to the research outpatient clinic will be performed, and adherence to the new medication regimen in the intervention group will be measured. The primary outcome will be the incidence of new falls. Secondary outcome measurements are possible health effects of medication withdrawal, health-related quality of life (Short Form-12 and EuroQol-5D), costs, and cost-effectiveness of the intervention. Data will be analyzed using an intention-to-treat analysis. The results of this trial are pending [10].

17.2.2 Non-randomized Trials of Withdrawal of Fall Risk-Increasing Drugs

Smaller studies of medication withdrawal in geriatric patients have shown beneficial effects of withdrawal of FRIDs on fall risk. In a prospective cohort study of 139 fallers visiting the geriatric outpatient clinic of a university hospital in the Netherlands, withdrawal of FRIDs was possible and successful in 75 participants. Withdrawal of all FRIDs, including cardiovascular and psychotropic drugs, appeared an effective intervention for lowering the incidence of falls. The effect appeared to be highest for withdrawal of cardiovascular drugs. In all fallers FRIDs were stopped if considered redundant or otherwise, if safely possible, reduced in dose over a 1-month period. During follow-up, no other interventions were performed [11]. This study also demonstrated a net cost savings of €1,691 (2008 value) per patient in the cohort, with an estimated reduction of €60 million in healthcare expenditures in the Netherlands (i.e., 15 % of fall-related health costs) [12].

A non-randomized, controlled trial by Salonoja et al. assessed the effects of stopping FRIDs (psychotropics, opiates, or potent anticholinergics) on the risk of falls requiring medical treatment as a sub-analysis of a randomized, controlled multifactorial fall prevention study. Five hundred and twelve community-dwelling people 65 years and older who had a history of at least one fall were enrolled. The subjects were divided retrospectively into three groups: (1) those using any FRIDs, (2) those using any psychotropic drug, and (3) those using any benzodiazepine or related drugs (BZDs/BZDRDs). Falls were recorded from the medical records. During the 1-year follow-up period after the 12-month intervention, the relative risk ratio for falls in the control group (CG) participants compared with intervention group (IG) participants was 8.26 (1.07–63.73) among the users of psychotropics and 8.11 (1.03–63.60) among the users of BZDs/BZDRDs. The authors conclude that withdrawal of psychotropics, especially BZDs/BZDRDs, may have played an important role by lowering the risk of falls requiring medical treatment during the year after the 12-month multifactorial intervention [13].

17.2.3 Effects of Multiple Pharmacotherapy-Related Interventions

In a review on the effects of drug pharmacokinetic/pharmacodynamic properties, characteristics of medication use, and relevant pharmacological interventions on fall risk in elderly patients, Chen et al. found that the degree of medication-related fall risk was dependent on one or some of the following factors: drug pharmacokinetic/pharmacodynamic properties (e.g., elimination half-life, metabolic pathway, genetic polymorphism, risk rating of medications despite belonging to the same therapeutic class) and/or characteristics of medication use (e.g., number of medications and drug–drug interactions, dose strength, duration of medication use and time since stopping, medication change, prescribing appropriateness, and medication adherence).

The FRIDs they included in the review were central nervous system-acting agents, cough preparations, nonsteroidal anti-inflammatory drugs, anti-Alzheimer's agents, antiplatelet agents, calcium antagonists, diuretics, α-blockers, digoxin, hypoglycemic drugs, neurotoxic chemotherapeutic agents, nasal preparations, and antiglaucoma ophthalmic preparations.

The authors conclude with the following list of practical recommendations:

- Make a list of FRIDs.
- Establish a computerized alert system for when to e-prescribe FRIDs.
- Seek an alternative drug with lower fall risk.
- Withdraw FRIDs if clinically indicated.
- Prescribe cautiously when the use of FRIDs cannot be avoidable.
- Pay attention to prescribing appropriateness.
- Simplify the medication regimen.
- Encourage and enable pharmacist-conducted clinical medication review.
- Ensure the label of each FRID dispensed contains a corresponding warning sign.
- Be vigilant when medication change occurs.
- Enhance medication adherence.
- Mandate for periodic reassessment of potential risk associated with the patient's medication regimen.

Pharmacological interventions, including withdrawal of FRIDs, pharmacist-conducted clinical medication review, and computerized drug alerts, were effective in reducing fall risk [14].

17.2.4 Pharmacist-Led Medication Review

This topic is presented in detail in Chapter 16. Evidence for the effectiveness of this process in reducing falls comes from the following studies. An RCT by Zermansky reported that at the end of a 6-month intervention period, in 661 elderly care home residents, the mean number of medication changes per patient was 3.1 for intervention and 2.4 for the control group ($p=0.0001$), and there were 0.8 and 1.3 falls per patient, respectively ($p=0.0001$) [15]. Ferreri et al. published a methodology of a randomized controlled trial to prevent falls through enhanced pharmaceutical care [16]. Individuals in the intervention group were invited to attend a face-to-face medication consultation provided by a community pharmacy resident (i.e., identification of drug–therapy problems and therapeutic recommendations), whereas those in the control group did not. All participants were followed up for 24 months. The primary study end points included time to first fall and proportion of participants who experienced one or more falls during the first year of follow-up. Although there was no significant reduction in the rate of recurrent falls, injurious falls, or overall use of high-risk medications, individuals in the intervention group were more likely to discontinue use of a high-risk medication or have the dosage reduced during the 1-year follow-up period compared with those in the control group [17]. Haumschild et al. described the effects of a 1-year fall-focused pharmaceutical intervention program on the clinical and economic outcomes of elderly patients in a rehabilitation center. Two hundred patients were randomly selected from the preintervention phase and postintervention phase. The pharmaceutical intervention included a complete review of all medications by a consultant pharmacist. Any medications identified as causing a particular adverse effect (e.g., dizziness) or clinical condition (e.g., falls and fractures) were listed in table format for review by the pharmacist, nurse, and physician. Written recommendations for dosage reduction and frequency adjustment were made. Precautions for drug administration were given to nursing personnel and attached to the patients' medication administration records within 24 h of admission to the rehabilitation center. The consultant pharmacist and nurse immediately implemented the pharmaceutical interventions in the patient's plan of care after collaborating with the physician to obtain medical orders relevant to the interventions. The number of falls was reduced in the postintervention group by 47 %, resulting in future savings of $7.74 US dollars (2003 value) per patient per day. The use of the following drug classes decreased in the postintervention period: cardiovascular agents, 10.7 %; analgesics, 6.3 %; psychoactive drugs, 18.2 %; and sedatives and hypnotics, 13.9 % [18].

17.2.5 Physician-Led Medication Review

In an RCT on the effects of a physician-led medication review on FRIDs use, Sjoberg et al. investigated whether medication reviews increased treatment with fracture-preventing drugs and decreased treatment with FRIDs. One hundred ninety-nine consecutive individuals with hip fracture aged 65 and older participated. The intervention consisted of medication reviews, performed by a physician and communicated to hospital physicians during the hospital stay and to general practitioners after discharge. Primary outcomes were changes in treatment with fracture preventing drugs and FRIDs 12 months after discharge. Secondary outcomes were falls, fractures, deaths, and physicians' attitudes toward the intervention. At admission, 26 % of intervention and 29 % of control participants were taking FRIDs, and 12 % and 11 %, respectively, were taking bone-active drugs. After 12 months, 77 % of intervention and 58 % of control participants were taking fracture-preventing drugs ($p=0.01$), and 29 % and 15 %, respectively, were taking bone-active drugs ($p=0.04$). Mean number of FRIDs per participant was 3.1 (intervention) and 3.1 (control) at admission and 2.9 (intervention) and 3.1 (control) at 12 months ($p=0.62$). No significant differences were found. The 65 responding physicians appreciated the intervention with a median score of 5 (1 = very bad, 6 = very good). The authors conclude that medication reviews performed and conveyed by a physician increased treatment with fracture-preventing drugs but did not significantly decrease treatment with FRIDs in older adults with hip fracture [19].

17.2.6 Computerized Systems

In the review by Chen et al., computerized drug alerts were effective in reducing fall risk [14].

Computerized drug alerts are expected to reduce fall-related injuries in older patients.

In a first of its kind intervention trial, Tamblyn et al. showed that a creative, individualized computer-assisted prescribing alert which focused on FRIDs was successful in reducing the risk of injury by 1.7 injuries per 1,000 patients (95 % CI 0.2/1,000–3.2/1,000, $p=0.02$). The effect of the intervention was greater for patients with higher baseline risks of injury ($p=0.03$) [20]. Details of the concepts and design behind this study can be found in Chapter 20.

A study by Tzeng et al. determined the correlations between hospital-acquired injurious fall rates in US acute care hospitals and these institutions' implementation levels of computerized systems. The results showed that computerized decision support systems for drug–drug interaction (DDI) alerts, drug allergy alerts, and drug–laboratory interaction alerts were effective to inform practice for better interventions to reduce fall risk [21].

17.3 Mechanisms of Drug-Related Falls and Mechanisms of Withdrawal Effects

17.3.1 How Can Drugs Increase Fall Risk? Possible Mechanisms of Drug-Related Falls

Falls can be caused by almost any drug that acts on the brain or on the circulation. Usually the mechanism leading to a fall is one or more of the following: *sedation*, with slowing of reaction times and impaired balance; *hypotension*, including the three syndromes of paroxysmal hypotension –i.e., orthostatic hypotension, vasovagal syndrome, and vasodepressor carotid sinus hypersensitivity; and *bradycardia, tachycardia, or periods of asystole*. Falls may be the consequence of recent medication changes but are usually caused by medicines that have been given for some time [22].

In a literature review by De Groot et al., on the effects of FRIDs on postural control, electronic databases and reference lists of identified papers were searched until June 2013. Only controlled research studies were included. The FRIDs included were antidepressants, neuroleptics, benzodiazepines, antiepileptic drugs, digoxin, type IA antiarrhythmics, and diuretics. Ninety-four papers were included. Postural control was assessed with a variety of instruments, mainly evaluating aspects of body sway during quiet standing. Psychotropic drug use was associated with an increase in body sway, and the effects were more pronounced with older age, use at higher daily doses, drugs with longer half-lives, and drugs administered for a longer period. The authors concluded that psychotropic drugs cause impairments in postural control, which is probably one of the mediating factors for the increased fall risk. The sedative effects of these drugs on postural control are reversible, as was proven in intervention studies where psychotropic FRIDs were withdrawn. The findings of the present literature review highlight the importance of using psychotropic drugs in the older population only at the lowest effective dose and for a limited period of time [23].

17.3.2 How Can Drug Withdrawal Lead to a Reduction of Fall Risk? Mechanisms of Withdrawal Effects: Possible Pathways

17.3.2.1 Literature Review

From the literature review by De Groot et al. it was concluded that the sedative effects of psychotropic drugs on postural control are reversible [23]. The authors conclude that their findings highlight the importance of using psychotropic drugs in the older population only at the lowest effective dose and for a limited period of time [23]. In the same literature review, the authors found only two intervention studies which examined the effects of discontinuation of FRIDs on postural control, i.e., the studies by Van der Velde et al. and by Tsunoda et al. [24, 25].

17.3.2.2 Intervention Studies

In the prospective cohort study of geriatric outpatients by Van der Velde et al. [11], withdrawal of all fall risk-increasing drugs, including cardiovascular and psychotropic drugs, had positive effects on mobility tests and cardiovascular end points.

In the group of fallers with FRIDs withdrawal ($n=65$ out of 137), all mobility tests improved, as opposed to non-fallers and fallers without FRID withdrawal. Specifically, the 10 m-walking test (adjusted OR 0.14; 95 % CI, 0.03–0.59) and timed up and go (TUG) test (adjusted OR 0.19; 95 % CI, 0.04–0.86) significantly improved during the 6.7 months of follow-up. For the subgroup of psychotropic FRIDs withdrawal (e.g., sedatives, neuroleptics, and antidepressants), the improvement in the 10 m-walking test (adjusted OR 0.27; 95 % CI 0.10–0.75) and TUG test (adjusted OR 0.23; 95 % CI 0.08–0.65) were also significant. Effect size of cardiovascular FRIDs withdrawal was similar but did not reach significance [24]. The results of Tsunoda et al. are in line with these results, that is, they found that discontinuation of benzodiazepine hypnotics was feasible in a majority of older persons. In an 8-week open-label study, 26 subjects 60 years and older living in a nursing home were recruited. Benzodiazepine withdrawal resulted in a significant improvement in the stability of the body (total distance and range of trunk motion with eyes closed) and recovery of daytime cognitive functions as measured by the critical flicker fusion test and the Repeatable Battery for the Assessment of Neuropsychological Status subsets of immediate memory, language, and attention index scores. Subjective worsening in sleep, as assessed by the Leeds sleep evaluation questionnaire, was not reported [25]. In a recent intervention study on the effects of withdrawal of benzodiazepines, Nurminen et al. studied handgrip strength and balance in older outpatients following withdrawal from long-term use of temazepam, zopiclone, or zolpidem as hypnotics.

Eighty-nine chronic users (59 women, 30 men) 55 years and older participated in this study.

Individual physician-directed withdrawal was done gradually over a 1-month period and participants were followed up to 6 months. Within 3 weeks after initiating withdrawal, handgrip strength improved significantly ($P \leq 0.005$) compared to baseline values. This improvement was more durable in women. Improvements in balance testing were also apparent from the first week after withdrawal initiation. However there was only a borderline difference ($P=0.054$) in balance improvement at long-term follow-up. Of note, there was improvement in handgrip strength and balance compared to baseline values, in participants who reduced but were unable to discontinue their benzodiazepine use. The results encourage discontinuing benzodiazepine hypnotics, particularly in older women who are at a high risk of falling and sustaining fractures [26]. In a prospective study of geriatric outpatients, Van der Velde et al. [11, 27] also assessed the cardiovascular effects of FRIDs withdrawal. They performed tilt-table testing in all participants at baseline. Subsequently, FRIDs were withdrawn in all fallers, in whom this was safely possible. At a mean follow-up of 6.7 months, tilt-table testing was repeated in 137 participants. Tilt-table testing addressed carotid sinus hypersensitivity, orthostatic hypotension, and vasovagal collapse. Orthostatic hypotension improved significantly after withdrawal of FRIDs (adjusted OR 0.35; 95 % CI = 0.13–0.99). Subgroup analysis of cardiovascular FRIDs withdrawal showed a significant reduction in both orthostatic hypotension (adjusted OR 0.44; 95 % CI = 0.18–1.0) and carotid sinus hypersensitivity (adjusted OR 0.13; 95 % CI = 0.03–0.59). These results imply that FRID withdrawal can result in substantial improvement of cardiovascular homeostasis [27].

17.4 Drug Withdrawal, How to Do It, and Safety and Feasibility

Optimizing the drug regimen for the individual older faller means that besides possible withdrawal (cessation or dose reduction) of certain drugs, adding new drugs may be necessary, in order to reach a maximum reduction of fall risk and other possible adverse events. Withdrawal can be done by immediate cessation of a drug or in a stepwise fashion, i.e., by dose reduction. Withdrawal can be done according to guidelines if available for the specific drug, by following the instructions of the national formulary for withdrawing the specific drug [28, 29].

17.4.1 Safety and Feasibility

Iyer et al. conducted a systematic review to assess the benefits and risks of medication withdrawal in people 65 years and older as documented in trials of medication withdrawal published between 1966 and 2007. Only trials that focused on the withdrawal of specific classes of medication were included. Withdrawal of diuretics was maintained in 51–100 % of subjects and was unsuccessful primarily when heart failure was present. Adverse effects were infrequently encountered. After withdrawal of antihypertensive therapy, many subjects (20–85 %) remained normotensive or did not require reinstatement of therapy for between 6 months and 5 years, and there was no increase in mortality. Withdrawal of psychotropic medications was associated with a reduction in falls and improved cognition [7].

Garfinkel et al. designed an approach, called the Good Palliative–Geriatric Practice algorithm, for medication discontinuation in community-dwelling older patients. When no evidence existed to support the use of a particular drug, clinical judgment was used and the balance of risks and benefits of the drug for the individual were presented to the participants and their families. Success rates of drug discontinuation, morbidity, mortality, and changes in health status were recorded. The mean ± SD age of the 70 participants was 82.8 ± 6.9 years. Forty-three patients (61 %) had three or more and 26 % had five or more comorbidities. The mean follow-up was 19 months. Participants were using 7.7 ± 3.7 medications. Discontinuation was recommended for 311 medications in 64 patients (58 % of all drugs representing 4.4 ± 2.5 drugs per patient overall). Of the discontinued drug therapies, 2 % were restarted because of recurrence of the original indication. Taking non-consent and failures together, successful discontinuation was achieved in 81 % of the targeted drugs. Ten elderly patients (14 %) died after a mean follow-up of 13 months, with the mean age at death of 89 years. No significant adverse events were reported, and 88 % of patients reported a global improvement in health. The authors concluded that it is feasible to decrease medication burden in community-dwelling elderly patients and that their tool is suitable for use in randomized controlled trials in different clinical settings [30].

17.5 Discussion

Falls in older adults are not a disease but a symptom. Falls can be caused by many different interrelated factors. The majority of the studies regarding falls have used a multifactorial approach. Fall risk-increasing drugs have been identified, but the exact contribution of these medications to fall risk is not completely known. Literature on the effects and effectiveness of withdrawal of FRIDs is scarce. There is evidence that withdrawal of psychotropics is effective in reducing rate of falls [5] and that a prescribing modification program for primary care physicians can reduce risk of falling [6]. Smaller intervention trials have also shown beneficial effects of FRIDs withdrawal on fall risk and on cardiovascular end points [24, 25, 27].

Discontinuing benzodiazepine hypnotics has been shown to improve handgrip strength and balance [26].

The results of the currently available literature encourage FRIDs withdrawal whenever possible, in older non-fallers, first fallers, and frequent fallers, especially as withdrawal has been shown to be feasible and safe in the majority of cases [7, 30].

17.6 Conclusions

Withdrawal of FRIDs can reduce fall risk and fall rates and can improve handgrip strength, balance, mobility tests, and cardiovascular end points. Withdrawal or dose reduction of FRIDs can be done safely and should be attempted in older persons, especially in those at risk of falls.

References

1. Fried LP, Storer DJ, King DE, Lodder F (1991) Diagnosis of illness presentation in the elderly. JAGS 39(2):117–228
2. American Geriatrics Society, British Geriatrics Society, and American Academy of Orthopaedic Surgeons Panel on falls prevention (2001) guideline for the prevention of falls in older persons. J Am Geriatr Soc 49:664–672
3. Van der Cammen TJ, Rajkumar C, Onder G, Sterke CS, Petrovic M (2014) Drug cessation in complex older adults: time for action. Age Ageing 43(1):20–25. doi:10.1093/ageing/aft166, Epub 2013 Nov 12
4. Gillespie LD, Robertson MC, Gillespie WJ, Sherrington C, Gates S, Clemson LM, Lamb SE (2012) Interventions for preventing falls in older people living in the community. Cochrane Database Syst Rev 9:CD007146, Epub 2012 Sep 12
5. Campbell AJ, Robertson MC, Gardner MM, Norton RN, Buchner DM (1999) Psychotropic medication withdrawal and a home-based exercise program to prevent falls: a randomized, controlled trial. J Am Geriatr Soc 47:850–853
6. Pit SW, Byles JE, Henry DA, Holt L, Hansen V, Bowman DA (2007) A quality use of medicines program for general practitioners and older people: a cluster randomized controlled trial. Med J Aust 187:23–30

7. Iyer S, Naganathan V, McLachlan AJ, Le Couteur DG (2008) Medication withdrawal trials in people aged 65 years and older: a systematic review. Drugs Aging 25:1021–1031
8. Hill KD, Wee R (2012) Psychotropic drug-induced falls in older people: a review of interventions aimed at reducing the problem. Drugs Aging 29:15–30
9. de Vries OJ, Peeters GM, Elders PJ, Muller M, Knol DL, Danner SA, Bouter LM, Lips P (2010) Multifactorial intervention to reduce falls in older people at high risk of recurrent falls: a randomized controlled trial. Arch Intern Med 170(13):1110–1117. doi:10.1001/archinternmed.2010.169
10. Hartholt KA, Boyé ND, Van der Velde N, Van Lieshout EM, Polinder S, De Vries OJ, Kerver AJ, Ziere G, Bruijninckx MM, De Vries MR, Mattace-Raso FU, Uitterlinden AG, Van Beeck EF, Lips P, Patka P, Van der Cammen TJ (2011) [Cost]-effectiveness of withdrawal of fall-risk increasing drugs versus conservative treatment in older fallers: design of a multicenter randomized controlled trial (IMPROveFALL-study). BMC Geriatr 11:48. doi:10.1186/1471-2318-11-48
11. Van der Velde N, Stricker BHC, Pols HAP, Van der Cammen TJM (2007) Risk of falls after withdrawal of fall-risk-increasing drugs: a prospective cohort study. Br J Clin Pharmacol 63(2):232–237
12. Van der Velde N, Meerding WJ, Looman CW, Pols HAP, van der Cammen TJM (2008) Cost effectiveness of withdrawal of fall-risk-increasing drugs in geriatric outpatients. Drugs Aging 25(6):521–529
13. Salonoja M, Salminen M, Vahlberg T, Aarnio P, Kivelä SL (2012) Withdrawal of psychotropic drugs decreases the risk of falls requiring treatment. Arch Gerontol Geriatr 54(1):160–167
14. Chen Y, Zhu L-L, Zhou Q (2014) Effects of drug pharmacokinetic/pharmacodynamic properties, characteristics of medication use, and relevant pharmacological interventions on fall risk in elderly patients. Ther Clin Risk Manag 10:437–448
15. Zermansky AG, Alldred DP, Petty DR et al (2006) Clinical medication review by a pharmacist of elderly people living in care homes – randomised controlled trial. Age Ageing 35:586–591
16. Ferreri S, Roth MT, Casteel C, Demby KB, Blalock SJ (2008) Methodology of an ongoing, randomized controlled trial to prevent falls through enhanced pharmaceutical care. Am J Geriatr Pharmacother 6:61–81
17. Blalock SJ, Casteel C, Roth MT, Ferreri S, Demby KB, Shankar V (2010) Impact of enhanced pharmacologic care on the prevention of falls: a randomized controlled trial. Am J Geriatr Pharmacother 8:428–440
18. Haumschild MJ, Karfonta TL, Haumschild MS, Phillips SE (2003) Clinical and economic outcomes of a fall-focused pharmaceutical intervention program. Am J Health Syst Pharm 60:1029–1032
19. Sjoberg C, Wallerstedt SM (2013) Effects of medication reviews performed by a physician on treatment with fracture-preventing and fall-risk-increasing drugs in older adults with hip fracture: a randomized controlled study. J Am Geriatr Soc 61:1464–1472
20. Tamblyn R, Eguale T, Buckeridge DL et al (2012) The effectiveness of a new generation of computerized drug alerts in reducing the risk of injury from drug side effects: a cluster randomized trial. J Am Med Inform Assoc 19:635–643
21. Tzeng HM, Hu HM, Yin CY (2011) Is there a link between the hospital-acquired injurious fall rates in US acute care hospitals and these institutions' implementation levels of computerized systems? Comput Inform Nurs 29:721–729
22. Darowski A, Dwight J, Reynolds J. Medicines and falls in hospital. Oxford: John Radcliffe Hospital, 2011. www.drugsandfalls.com
23. De Groot MH, van Campen JPCM, Moek MA, Tulner LR, Beijnen JH, Lamoth CJC (2013) The effects of fall-risk-increasing drugs on postural control: a literature review. Drugs Aging 30:901–920. doi:10.1007/s40266-013-0113-9
24. Van der Velde N, Stricker BHC, Pols HAP, Van der Cammen TJM (2007) Withdrawal of fall-risk-increasing drugs in older persons: effect on mobility test outcomes. Drugs Aging 24(8): 691–699

25. Tsunoda K, Uchida H, Suzuki T, Watanabe K, Yamashima T, Kashima H (2010) Effects of discontinuing benzodiazepine-derivative hypnotics on postural sway and cognitive functions in the elderly. Int J Geriatr Psychiatr 25(12):1259–1265
26. Nurminen J, Puustinen J, Lähteenmäki R, Vahlberg T, Lyles A, Partinen M, Räihä I, Neuvonen PJ, Kivelä S-L (2014) BMC Geriatr 14:121, http://www.biomedcentral.com/1471-2318/14/121
27. Van der Velde N, van den Meiracker A, Pols HAP, Stricker BHC, van der Cammen TJM (2007) Withdrawal of fall-risk-increasing drugs in older persons: effect on tilt-table test outcomes. J Am Geriatr Soc 55:734–739
28. British National Formulary; website: http://www.bnf.org
29. Canadian Drug Formulary; website: http://www.caddac.ca/cms/CADDAC_pdf/Formulary-by-Prov-2010.pdf
30. Garfinkel D, Mangin D (2010) Feasibility study of a systematic approach for discontinuation of multiple medications in older adults: addressing polypharmacy. Arch Intern Med 170(18): 1648–1654

Chapter 18
Benzodiazepine Withdrawal in the Elderly: A Practical Approach

Louise Mallet

Abstract Benzodiazepines are widely prescribed in older patients. Studies have shown that these medications can increase the risk of falls, hip fractures, cognitive impairment, delirium, dementia, traffic accidents, drug dependence and mortality. Guidelines and expert consensus statements addressing the adverse effects of chronic benzodiazepine use have not been effective in changing prescribing practices. Different interventions have been published to decrease or stop benzodiazepines. In the elderly, benzodiazepine withdrawal under medical supervision coupled with psychotherapy has been shown to work. For pragmatic reasons (access to psychotherapy not always available), medication review coupled with patient education should be tried. There is no evidence to support a substitution of a short/intermediate half-life benzodiazepine for a long half-life benzodiazepine. Tapering a benzodiazepine should be initiated with the benzodiazepine the patient is currently taking. Using different formulations of a particular drug should also be considered to facilitate reductions in dosage. The optimal duration of withdrawal varies with each patient, and a flexible tapering schedule is suggested at a reduction rate that is acceptable for that individual. An illustration of a sample schedule to discontinue for oxazepam is presented.

Abbreviations

BZD	Benzodiazepine
CI	Confidence interval
CYP	Cytochrome P450
OR	Odds ratio

L. Mallet, BScPharm, PharmD, CGP, FESCP
Faculty of Pharmacy, University of Montréal, Montréal, QC, Canada

Department of Pharmacy, McGill University Health Center, Glen Site, Montréal, QC, Canada
e-mail: Louise.mallet@umontreal.ca

© Springer International Publishing Switzerland 2016

A.R. Huang, L. Mallet (eds.), *Medication-related falls in older people*,
DOI 10.1007/978-3-319-32304-6_18

18.1 Introduction

Benzodiazepine (BZD) usage in older patients remains a major healthcare concern. These drugs are widely prescribed around the world, with a prevalence of use in developed countries from 7 to 43 % [1]. In 2014, Olfson reported that in the United States in 2008, BZDs were prescribed primarily in older persons, mostly women and on a long-term basis [2]. Long-term use of BZDs in older patients can increase the risk of falls, hip fractures, cognitive impairment, delirium, dementia, traffic accidents, dependence and mortality [3–6]. Several guidelines and expert consensus statements have been published to avoid long-term BZD prescribing in the elderly [7, 8]. Despite these guidelines, BZDs continue to be widely prescribed. This chapter will provide a practical approach on how to discontinue BZDs in older people.

18.2 Pharmacokinetics of Benzodiazepines

Benzodiazepines are rapidly absorbed from the small intestine. The bioavailability of the different BZD molecules varies from 80 to 100 %. These drugs are also highly bound to carrier proteins such as albumin ranging from 70 % for alprazolam to 99 % for diazepam. Active drug metabolites are also highly protein bound. This property of BZDs results in a higher risk of drug toxicity in malnourished or chronically ill older patients who have low serum albumin concentrations, due to the increased levels of the unbound drug which is the pharmacologically active fraction [9–13].

BZDs enter the blood-brain barrier rapidly; the rate of diffusion is determined by its lipophilicity. These drugs are mostly distributed in fat, resulting in large volumes of distribution. With the age-related increase in proportion of body fat, the volume of distribution of BZDs may be further increased. BZDs are inactivated primarily by the liver. Long half-life BZDs such as diazepam, flurazepam and chlordiazepoxide undergo hepatic cytochrome P450 (CYP)-dependent hydroxylation, demethylation and nitroreduction (phase 1 metabolism). The CYP isoenzymes responsible for these reactions include 3A4, 3A5, 2B6, 2C9 and 2C19. Some BZDs are metabolized to active metabolites with a long half-life. For example, diazepam is metabolized to an active metabolite, desmethyldiazepam, with an elimination half-life longer than the parent compound of 36–200 h. Desmethyldiazepam undergoes glucuronidation to produce a glucuronide conjugate, which is hydroxylated to oxazepam. These metabolites are further conjugated to produce glucuronides which are renally excreted. Flurazepam by itself has a half-life of 2–3 h; an active metabolite, N-desalkylflurazepam, has a longer half-life of 40–250 h. Intermediate acting BZDs such as lorazepam, oxazepam and temazepam are metabolized via glucuronidation (phase 2 metabolism). These BZDs do not have active metabolites. Normal ageing is associated with a reduction in hepatic metabolism of medications. Decreased hepatic clearance of BZDs with advancing age can result in drug accumulation [9–13].

Table 18.1 Metabolic pathways and elimination half-lives of benzodiazepines

Benzodiazepine	Metabolism	Active metabolite	Elimination half-life (hours)
Alprazolam	Oxidation	Alprazolam	6–20
Chlordiazepoxide	Oxidation	Chlordiazepoxide	6–24
		Desmethyldiazepam	36–200
		Oxazepam	6–20
Clonazepam	Oxidation	Clobazam	10–32
		Desmethylclobazam	
Diazepam	Oxidation	Diazepam	24–48
		Desmethyldiazepam	36–200
		Oxazepam	6–20
Flurazepam	Oxidation	Flurazepam	2–3
		N-desalkylflurazepam	40–250
Lorazepam	Conjugation	Lorazepam	10–20
Lormetazepam	Conjugation	Lormetazepam	10–12
Nitrazepam	Oxidation	Nitrazepam	15–38
Oxazepam	Conjugation	Oxazepam	6–15
Temazepam	Conjugation	Temazepam	8–22

BZDs can be divided into three classes according to their elimination half-lives: short-acting BZDs (half-life less than 6 h), intermediate-acting BZDs (half-life between 6 and 24 h) and long-acting BZDs (half-life more that 24 h) [11, 14, 15]. Table 18.1 presents a summary of metabolism and elimination half-lives of selected BZDs [11, 14, 15].

18.3 Pharmacodynamics of Benzodiazepines

When compared to younger adults, elderly patients are more sensitive to the effects of BZDs. It is postulated that this increased sensitivity to BZDs by receptors in the brain is associated with increased sedation, gait impairment and memory loss [13]. Changes in postural sway have been reported after the administration of a single dose of diazepam in older patients [16, 17].

18.4 Benzodiazepine Withdrawal Strategies

18.4.1 Interventions for Reducing Benzodiazepine Use in Older People

A number of systematic reviews and meta-analyses have reported the evidence for different interventions at decreasing or stopping BZDs in different populations and settings [18–21]. However, these publications included adults of all ages and did not specifically address older patients. Recently, a meta-analysis of randomized controlled trials examined the effectiveness of different interventions for reducing BZDs in older people [22]. Ten studies discussed withdrawal strategies from BZDs and eight studies on prescribing interventions.

18.4.2 Withdrawal Interventions

The most common type of interventions described in these studies was the supervision of gradual withdrawal of BZDs. Withdrawal was combined with substitute medications or with psychotherapy in four studies. Substitute medications included the use of melatonin, carbamazepine, placebo and low-dose lormetazepam. Psychotherapy was described as cognitive behavioural therapy, relaxation behavioural therapy and psychological consulting. The duration of withdrawal interventions in these studies varied from 1 week to 12 months. Patients came from a variety of settings: community, in-patient wards, outpatient clinics and care homes. Older people were using BZDs for insomnia and/or anxiety for a time ranging from 1 to 12 months. Mean age of the participants was 74.1 years with a mean percentage of female participants of 73.4 %. Follow-up documentation was reported in only five studies, with a period ranging from 0.5 to 3 months being the most frequent follow-up evaluation period [22].

18.4.3 Prescription Interventions

Different interventions were reported, the most common being education, medication reviews and providing prescribing feedback. The length of the intervention ranged from 1 to 12 months. The interventions were conducted equally in care home and community settings. Interventions were directed primarily at physicians and/or other staff. Some studies focused on patients and some included both staff and patients. Mean age of the participants was 79.4 years and most were females (77.4 %). No follow-up assessment period was reported with respect to the use of BZDs [22].

18.4.4 What Interventions Should Be Used in Practice?

The authors of the meta-analysis reported that the odds of not using BZDs at the end of the observation period was significantly higher (OR 5.06, 95 % CI 2.68–9.52, $p<0.00001$) for the participants in the supervised withdrawal with psychotherapy group when compared with the control groups, which included treatment as usual, an education placebo, withdrawal with or without placebo or psychotherapy alone. The beneficial effects of supervised withdrawal with psychotherapy were maintained at

0.5–3 months and at 12 months follow-up. The long-term effects of discontinuation were not evaluated. Multifaceted prescribing interventions (education, medication review and audit/prescribing feedback) aimed at physicians, healthcare staff and patients improved the odds of not using BZDs (OR 1.37, 95 % CI 1.01–1.72, $p=0.006$) when compared to control interventions (treatment as usual and prescribing placebo) [22]. The authors conclude that supervision of BZD withdrawal with psychotherapy should be suggested in older adults. For pragmatic reasons, when access to psychotherapy is limited, medication review and education may be considered [22].

18.5 Eliminating Medications Through Patient Ownership of End Results (EMPOWER Trial)

The EMPOWER trial, a pharmacy-based patient education program, evaluated the effectiveness of direct patient education on drug harms on BZD cessation among community-dwelling older patients [23]. This cluster-randomized controlled trial recruited a total of 330 chronic BZD users aged 65–95 years via 30 community pharmacies in Montreal, Canada. The intervention consisted of an eight-page educational booklet on the indications for BZDs, the harmful effects of long-term BZD use and a chart describing a 20-week tapering protocol. This pamphlet was mailed to the participants in the intervention arm, and they were also advised to discuss the discontinuation of their BZD with their doctor and/or community pharmacist. Participants in the control group received usual care. The most frequent reasons reported for BZD use were insomnia and anxiety. The mean duration of use was 10 years with an average daily dose of 1.3 mg of lorazepam equivalent.

At 6 months, complete cessation of BZDs was documented in 27 % of patients in the intervention group ($n=148$) compared to 4.5 % in the control group ($n=155$). This difference was statistically significant (OR 8.33; 95 % CI 3.32–20.93) and the number needed to treat was 4.35. An additional 11 % of participants in the intervention group had a BZD dose reduction.

Withdrawal symptoms (rebound insomnia, anxiety) occurred in 42 % of participants in the intervention group. Only 13 % of patients who discontinued benzodiazepine therapy received substitutions with trazodone, amitriptyline or paroxetine. Pharmacists were less often consulted than physicians to discuss BZD discontinuation (4 % versus 35.8 %) [23]. This study showed that direct-to- patient communication was simple, feasible and effective in decreasing chronic BZD use.

18.6 Approaches to Discontinuation Benzodiazepines

Most older patients do not take more that their prescribed dose of BZDs, and they have been using them for long periods of time without having a medication review for their indication, efficacy and side effects [24]. There are no data supporting the long-term use of BZDs in older persons and guidelines caution that treatment duration should not exceed 2–4 weeks [25]. With ageing, elderly patients become more

Table 18.2 Benzodiazepine withdrawal symptoms

Physical	Headache, pain, stiffness
	Weakness, fatigue, poor balance, dizziness
	Palpitations, sweating
	Visual disturbances (blurred vision, diplopia, photophobia)
	Tinnitus, unsteadiness, light-headedness
	Tingling, numbness
	Gastrointestinal symptoms (nausea, vomiting, diarrhoea, constipation)
	Flu-like symptoms
Psychological	Insomnia, rebound anxiety
	Panic attack, nightmares
	Poor memory and concentration
	Restlessness, agitation, irritability
	Depression, paranoia, cravings

sensitive to the effect of the same dose of BZD with adverse outcomes such as memory loss, confusion, falls and fractures [25].

Discontinuation of BZDs can be safely and effectively managed in the primary care setting. A discussion should begin at the time of BZD prescription renewal with the physician or with the pharmacist during a medication review. Risks of harmful effects of long-term BZD use and benefits of discontinuation should be explained to the patient and/or caregiver. Some patients may be reluctant to stop completely. A first goal would be a reduction in the dose and further re-evaluation. Patients with alcohol, opiate or other drug addiction problems, or taking BZDs at high doses, or having mental health issues should be referred to an addiction specialist [26].

18.7 Withdrawal Symptoms

In older people, BZDs are most frequently used for insomnia. These agents are initially prescribed for a short duration but are often represcribed without being re-evaluated. Long-term usage of BZDs in the elderly can lead to dependency. Benzodiazepine withdrawal [27–29] symptoms can be divided into two categories as listed in Table 18.2. Older adults report sleep complaints, higher psychological distress and more chronic medical illnesses [27]. Onset of withdrawal symptoms in patients taking short and intermediate half-life BZDs occurs within 1–2 days compared to those taking long half-life BZDs (3–8 days or longer).

18.7.1 Switching Between Short, Intermediate and Long Half-Life Benzodiazepines

The literature does not provide universal guidelines to taper BZDs in the elderly. Different authors advocate substituting short or intermediate half-life BZDs to an

Table 18.3 Equivalent dose of benzodiazepines

Benzodiazepine	Equivalent dose (mg)
Alprazolam	0.5
Chlordiazepoxide	25
Clonazepam	0.5
Diazepam	10
Flurazepam	15–30
Lorazepam	1
Lormetazepam	1
Nitrazepam	10
Oxazepam	20
Temazepam	20

equivalent dose of long half-life diazepam [14]. It is postulated that the longer half-life BZDs may cause less withdrawal symptoms. Limited evidence exists supporting this approach, and in the elderly, the use of a long half-life BZD may increase the risk of falls, confusion and sedation. Switching a short or intermediate half-life BZD for a long half-life BZD is not supported according to a Cochrane review meta-analysis [30]. It is reported that withdrawal symptoms are equally well tolerated in older patients whether they are using a short half-life or long half-life BZD [29, 31]. In the elderly, tapering can be initiated with the BZD the patient is currently taking. For example, if the patient is using oxazepam, tapering should be initiated using oxazepam. Clinicians should be aware of the choice of formulations available for a particular medication to facilitate the decrease in dosage; for example tapering using a capsule formulation may be more difficult than the same medication in tablet form. Equivalent dose of BZDs are found in Table 18.3.

18.7.2 Duration of Drug Withdrawal

The optimal duration of withdrawal of a BZD has not been determined and will vary for each patient. No precise rule exists for the withdrawal duration. Denis et al. in their Cochrane meta-analysis proposed a progressive withdrawal over a 10-week period [30]. Some authors advocate to start with a decrease by 25 % of the dose every 1–2 weeks; others suggest a 10 % decrement of the dose every 1–2 weeks. Another strategy describes a 25 % decrease in dosage per week until 50 % of the original dose is reached followed by a subsequent 1/8 reduction in remaining dosage every 4–7 days [32]. Some authors advocate a tapering schedule over 8–12 weeks [29] and others 4–10 weeks in the ambulatory setting [26].

Tapering may not eliminate the appearance of withdrawal symptoms but will limit severe symptoms. Patients generally tolerate the early stages of BZD withdrawal better than the later stages. The rate of withdrawal should be tailored to the patients' needs, duration of use and initial dose of BZD [33]. For patients who have only been using a BZD for less than 2–4 weeks, discontinuation can be done within 2–4 weeks [33]. Long-term users should be withdrawn over a much longer period of several

Table 18.4 Key points to discuss with the patient

Discuss if it is a suitable time to discontinue the benzodiazepine
Explain the long-term negative effect of benzodiazepines
Explain that these drugs lose their efficacy and can induce dependence after a few weeks
Explain to the patient what to expect in terms of withdrawal symptoms
Agree with the patient with a start date to begin stopping the benzodiazepine and a time period to discontinue the benzodiazepine
Provide the patient with a written schedule using a calendar. This schedule may need adjustment; if symptoms are minimal, the rate of withdrawal can be increase; however, if withdrawal symptoms are bothersome, the rate of withdrawal should be reduce
Provide a written prescription with the decrease dose. Extra doses can be prescribed if patient needs an extra dose
Provide written information on the withdrawal symptoms
Physician can delegate to other health professional such as pharmacist, the follow-up/adjustment of the withdrawal plan
Schedule a clinic follow-up every week for the first 2 weeks, and then offer the patient to communicate every 2–3 weeks as needed
Provide the patient with information on sleep hygiene
Offer psychological interventions if available

months or more. In summary, a flexible tapering schedule should be used at a reduction rate acceptable for the patient with monitoring parameters. If withdrawal symptoms become disturbing for the patient, a slower tapering schedule is recommended.

18.7.3 Guidelines for Stopping Benzodiazepine

Guidelines from different countries to discontinue BZDs have previously been published [26, 29, 33, 34]. Table 18.4 presents the different points to discuss with the patient before starting a withdrawal program.

Table 18.5 illustrates an example of a schedule to discontinue oxazepam. This is an example of an 85-year-old woman who had been taking oxazepam 15 mg daily in the morning for the past 2 years. After discussion with her family physician, this patient accepted to discontinue oxazepam as suggested in Table 18.5. A reduction by 25 % for the first 2 weeks at listed in Table 18.5 was agreed upon. A tapering schedule over a 10-week period was proposed and accepted by the patient. It is often difficult to decrease exactly by 10 or 25 % per week considering the formulation of the different tablets. Adjustment need to be considered according to the different strength available.

18.8 Conclusion

Long-term prescription of benzodiazepines in the elderly is not justified. Older patients often are prescribed these medications without supervision or follow-up. Improvements in cognitive function, memory and balance have been reported when

Table 18.5 Schedule for discontinuing oxazepam

Week	Mg/oxazepam tablet	Days	Total dose (mg)/week
1	11.25 mg (3/4 of a 15 mg tablet)	7	78.75
2	11.25 mg (3/4 of a 15 mg tablet)	7	78.75
3	7.5 mg (1/2 of a 15 mg tablet)	7	52.5
4	7.5 mg (1/2 of a 15 mg tablet)	7	52.5
5	5 mg (1/2 of a 10 mg oxazepam tablet)	7	35
6	5 mg (1/2 of a 10 mg oxazepam tablet)	7	35
7	2.5 mg (1/4 of 10 mg)	7	17.5
8	2.5 mg (1/4 of 10 mg)	q 2 days	7.5
9	2.5 mg (1/4 of 10 mg)	q 3 days	5
10	2.5 mg (1/4 of 10 mg)	q 4 days	2.5
Discontinue			

these medications are withdrawn. Discontinuation should include a flexible tapering schedule along with psychotherapy where available.

References

1. Billioti de Gage S, Bégaud B, Bazin F, Verdoux H, Dartigues F, Pérès F *et al* (2012) Benzodiazepine use and risk of dementia: a prospective population based study. BMJ 345:e6231, doi:10.1136
2. Olfson M, King M, Schoenbaum M (2015) Benzodiazepine use in the United States. JAMA Psychiatry 72:136–142
3. Charlston F, Degenhardt L, McLaren J, Hall W, Lynskey M (2009) A systematic review of research examining benzodiazepine-related mortality. Pharmacoepidemiol Drug Saf 18:93–103
4. Pierfitte C, Macouillard G, Thicoipe M, Chaslerie A, Pehourcq F, Aissou M et al (2001) Benzodiazepines and hip fractures in elderly people: case-control study. BMJ 322:704–708
5. Hogan DB, Maxwell CJ, Fung TS, Ebly EM (2003) Prevalence and potential consequences of benzodiazepine use in senior citizens: results from the Canadian Study of Health and Aging. Can J Clin Pharmacol 10:72–77
6. Pariente A, Dartigues JF, Benichou J, Letenneur L, Moore N, Fourrier-Reglat A (2008) Benzodiazepines and injurious falls in community dwelling elders. Drugs Aging 25:61–70
7. American Geriatrics Society 2015 Beers Criteria Update Expert Panel. American Geriatrics Society (2015) Updated beers criteria for potentially inappropriate medication use in older adults. J Am Geriatr Soc 63:2227–2246
8. O'Mahony D, O'Sullivan D, Byrne S, O'Connor MN, Ryan C, Gallagher P (2015) STOPP/START criteria for potentially inappropriate prescribing in older people: version 2. Age Ageing 44:213–218
9. Cloyd RJ, Gates J, Collins S (2008) Benzodiazepines in epilepsy: pharmacology and pharmacokinetics. Acta Neurol Scand 118:69–86
10. Kruse WHH (1990) Problems and pitfalls in the use of benzodiazepines in the elderly. Drug Saf 5:328–4
11. Bourin M (2010) Les problèmes posés par l'utilisation des benzodiazépines chez le patient âgé. L'Encéphale 36:340–347
12. Landry P, Gervais M, O'Connor KP (2008) Mise à jour sur les considérations pharmacocinétiques, pharmacodynamiques et les interactions médicamenteuses dans le choix d'une benzodiazépine. Ann Med Psychol 166:585–594

13. Woodward M (1999) Hypnosedatives in the elderly. CNS Drugs 11:263–279
14. Ashton H (2005) The diagnosis and management of benzodiazepine dependence. Curr Opin Psychiatry 18:249–255
15. Dailly E, Bourin M (2009) The use of benzodiazepines in the aged patient: clinical and pharmacological considerations. Pak J Pharm Sci 21:144–150
16. Swift CG, Ewen JM, Clarke P, Stevenson IH (1985) Responsiveness to oral diazepam in the elderly: relationship to total and free plasma concentrations. Br J Clin Pharmacol 20:111–118
17. Ozdemir V, Fourie J, Busto U, Naranjo CA (1996) Pharmacokinetic changes in the elderly: do they contribute to drug abuse and dependence? Clin Pharmacokinet 31:372–385
18. Parr JM, Kavanagh J, Cahill L, Mitchell G, Young R (2008) Effectiveness of current treatment approaches for benzodiazepine discontinuation: a meta-analysis. Addiction 104:13–24
19. Mugunthan K, McGuire T, Glasziou P (2011) Minimal interventions to decrease long-term use of benzodiazepines in primary care: a systemic review and meta-analysis. Br J Gen Pract 61:e573–e577
20. Oude Voshaar RC, Couvée JE, Van Balkom AJLM, Mulder PGH, Zitman FG (2006) Strategies for discontinuing long-term benzodiazepine use. B J Psychiatry 189:213–220
21. Smith AJ, Tett SE (2010) Improving the use of benzodiazepines- is it possible? A non-systematic review of interventions tried in the last 20 years. BMC Health Serv Res 10:321. doi:10.1186/1472-6963-10-321
22. Gould RL, Coulson MC, Patel N, Hughton-Williamson E, Howard RJ (2014) Interventions for reducing benzodiazepine use in older people: meta-analysis of randomised controlled trials. B J Psychiatry 204:98–107
23. Tannenbaum C, Martin P, Tamblyn R, Benedetti A, Ahmed S (2014) Reduction of inappropriate benzodiazepine prescriptions among older adults through direct patient education: the EMPOWER cluster randomized trial. JAMA Int Med 174:890–898
24. Kalapatapu RK, Sullivan MA (2010) Prescription use disorders in older adults. Am J Addict 19:515–522
25. Moore N, Pariente A, Bégaud B (2014) Why are benzodiazepines not yet controlled substances? JAMA Psychiatry 2:110–111
26. Haute Autorité de Santé, Modalités d'arrêt des benzodiazépines et médicaments apparentés chez le patient âgé (2007) http://www.has-sante.fr/portail/jcms/c_601509/fr/modalites-d-arret-des-benzodiazepines-et-medicaments-apparentes-chez-le-patient-age. Accessed 15 Jan 2016
27. Authier N, Balayssac D, Sautereau M, Zangarelli A, Courty P, Somogyi AA et al (2009) Benzodiazepine dependence: focus on withdrawal syndrome. Ann Pharm Fr 67:408–413
28. Mehdi T (2012) Benzodiazepines revisited. BJMP 5:a501
29. Lader M, Tylee A, Donaghue J (2009) Withdrawing benzodiazepines in primary care. CNS Drugs 23:19–34
30. Denis C, Fatséas M, Lavie E, Auriacombe M (2006) Pharmacological interventions for benzodiazepine mono-dependence management in outpatient settings. Cochrane Database Syst Rev 3, CD005194
31. Lader M (2011) Benzodiazepines revisited—will we ever learn? Addiction 106:2086–2109
32. Melton ST, Kirkwood CK (2014) Chapter 53. Anxiety disorders I: generalized anxiety, panic, and social anxiety disorders. In: DiPiro JT, Talbert RL, Yee GC, Matzke GR, Wells BG, Posey L (eds) Pharmacotherapy: a pathophysiologic approach, 9th edn. McGraw-Hill, New York, http://accesspharmacy.mhmedical.com/content.aspx?bookid=689&Sectionid=45310504. Accessed January 22, 2016
33. British National Formulary (2013) Benzodiazepine guidance. http://benzo.org.uk/BNF.htm. Accessed 20 Jan 2016
34. Royal Australian College of General Practitioners (RACGP) Clinical guidelines (2015) Prescribing drugs of dependence in general practice Part B benzodiazepines. http://www.racgp.org.au/your-practice/guidelines/drugs-of-dependence-b/5-discontinuing-benzodiazepines/52-discontinuing-after-longer-term-use-%E2%80%93-withdrawal/. Accessed 20 Jan 2016

Chapter 19
Role of Information and Communication Technologies

Allen R. Huang

Abstract The previously predicted widespread deployment and use of information and communication technologies (ICT) in health care is still unmet. This chapter describes the promises and challenges of the use of ICT in health care. The use of ICT can improve clinician awareness of fall risk-increasing drugs. Computer-assisted prescribing can potentially exert a positive impact on drug selection. Several issues conspire against a successful utilization of ICT in health care: alert fatigue, during which users bypass or ignore the annoying computer-generated messages, the difficulty in sharing electronic health information due to a lack of standards, problems associated with data of unclear meaning, lack of training to effectively use ICT and awareness of its limitations, and impacts on workflow and high costs. Delays in knowledge transfer, which can take up to 17 years, are a trait of our current health-care systems that ICT can potentially improve. Sharing of global knowledge in a timely fashion, and reminding clinicians at the point of care of the best practices, could usher in a new era of safer health care with less falls.

Abbreviations

AFMC	Association of faculties of medicine of Canada
CI	Confidence interval
CPOE	Computerized provider (prescriber) order entry
DSS	Decision-support systems
EHR	Electronic health record
FRID	Fall risk-increasing drug
ICT	Information and communication technology
OR	Odds ratio
ROI	Return on investment/information

A.R. Huang, MDCM, FRCPC
Division of Geriatric Medicine, University of Ottawa and The Ottawa Hospital, Ottawa, ON, Canada

Adjunct Professor of Medicine, McGill University, Montréal, QC, Canada
e-mail: allenhuang@toh.ca

© Springer International Publishing Switzerland 2016

A.R. Huang, L. Mallet (eds.), *Medication-related falls in older people*,
DOI 10.1007/978-3-319-32304-6_19

"Knowing is better."
Education campaign for Canada Health Infoway, 2015.[1]

During the two decades at the end of the twentieth century, health-care system managers and thinkers repeatedly turned to information and communication technologies (ICT) as a potential answer to improving health-care quality and safety [1]. Information systems were to capitalize on computerized provider (prescriber) order entry (CPOE) and decision-support systems (DSS) to standardize processes, deliver more personalized care, and avoid adverse events. Where are we today, 35 years after the start of the personal computing era?[2] The knowledge doubling curve is a concept first proposed in the 1980s by the American architect, author, designer, and inventor, Buckminster Fuller (Jul 12, 1895–Jul 1, 1983) based on his book *Critical Path* published in 1981 [2]. Fuller described, by using all the world knowledge at year 1 Common Era (CE) as one unit, that it took 1,500 years for the first doubling, followed by an interval of 250, 150, and 50 years (up to CE 1950) for subsequent increments. Today, in 2016, the knowledge doubling time is now estimated to be 13 months! Clinicians are at a quandary: it is probably impossible to assimilate all the new knowledge in the clinical sciences without assistance from ICT. Is clinical judgment at risk of obsolescence? This chapter will present and discuss the promises and limitations of ICT in the management of medication-related falls.

If computer-assisted clinical care is better, why has it not universally taken hold? Where is the return on investment/information (ROI)? For all that a computer can do faster, for instance, make sure the global banking transactions balance perfectly at the end of each day, there are other times when computing systems unquestionably result in harm. One such case involved the Therac-25 radiation treatment machines, where a series of concurrent software programming errors which controlled the machine resulted in giving excessive radiation doses to cancer patients, some of whom died prematurely from the overdoses. Thus far clinicians have a cynical view of computer-assisted clinical care and are reluctant to embrace this technology in daily care activities. Therefore, it is more difficult to measure the benefits and the risks that the use of ICT produces. After all, computers helped launch humans into space, and no one can forget the suspense, drama, resolve, and relief as Commander James A. Lovell, aided by his crew and the NASA team, brought a crippled Apollo 13 space craft safely home to earth. Does this mean all ICT for health care is wasted?

The young man knows the rules but the old man knows the exceptions. (Oliver Wendell Holmes Sr, American writer, Aug 29, 1809-Oct 8, 1894)

Let's first look at the evidence for effectiveness of computer-assisted decision-support systems in clinical care. Since clinicians may not be aware of the presence

---

[1] Use of electronic health records in the Canadian population. Canada Health Infoway is an independent not for profit organization funded by the Canadian federal government to promote and enable the spread of digital health across Canada (https://www.infoway-inforoute.ca/en/).

[2] A term initially attributed to researchers at Xerox's Palo Alto Research Center as early as 1972 and commercialized by IBM on Aug 12, 1981, with the release of their model 5–150 personal computer

of fall risk-increasing drugs (FRIDs), the use of ICT can help correct this problem. In some cases, computer-assisted prescribing can exert a positive impact on drug selection. Using a computer-assisted reminder coupled to a clinical information system for drug order entry, a 1-year pre-post intervention study done at Yale-New Haven Hospital in Connecticut, USA, showed an 18 % reduction in prescribing for sedative-hypnotic agents (OR = 0.82 [95 % CI 0.76–0.87]) [3]. The decreased prescription rates for diphenhydramine, diazepam, and lorazepam were maintained throughout the post-intervention period, with lorazepam prescriptions decreasing 39 % during the intervention. Almost all the patients were successfully directed to a safer sedative-hypnotic drug or a nondrug sleep protocol. In the chapter describing a "Novel Personalized Fall Risk Calculator," the study by Tamblyn et al. [4] was specifically designed to answer whether computer-assisted alerts and reminders, coupled with a slick clinician-user interface would have an effect on the prescription of FRIDs and adverse events. This study was given the operational acronym Trial to Reduce Inappropriate Psychotropic Prescribing (TRIPP). The results were a convincing yes! Indeed, if clinicians are presented with the right information at the time of prescribing, they frequently made the right decisions. With the increased availability of affordable ICT, patients and their families are becoming empowered by e-health initiatives, and more people are ready to become partners in their own health decisions. Such changes can improve clinical decision-making, increase the efficiency of medical care, and strengthen communication between physicians and their patients [5]. For example, more than half of 315 people surveyed, living in urban Buffalo in New York State, USA, reported using the Web or e-mail in the past year and 68 % of those who accessed the Web used it to search for health information [6]. Information is the key, not the technology. In an elegant study by Tannenbaum and colleagues [7], a simple eight-page brochure mailed out to patients regularly taking benzodiazepines was effective in discontinuing or lowering the dose of benzodiazepines in a significant portion of people. See the chapter on "Benzodiazepines Withdrawal in the Elderly" for further details.

When computer-assisted systems save clinician time (or at least their perception of time) and provide interventions that are clinically relevant and compelling, and the alerts are designed to give pause for thinking only about an exceptional or less common scenario, then clinicians may begin to embrace new ways of doing things. In the meantime, the challenges that ICT present are not all insurmountable. Below are several issues that have been identified that can impact on the effectiveness of ICT on clinical decision-making.

19.1 The First Issue Is Alert Fatigue

When clinicians are bombarded by multiple recurrent alerts that frequently and repeatedly interrupt their task completion actions, they will be annoyed, angry, and disillusioned by the "dumbness" of the computer system. Bypassing, ignoring, and suppressing alerts then become a routine action and the important alerts are then missed (too much noise to signal) [8–10]. This limitation to computer-assisted DSS can be partly overcome, in order of complexity, by (1) assigning levels of importance to each alert – tier alerts, which can be challenging to reach consensus on with clinicians, risk management, legal experts, and financial people all vying to influence decision-making from their perspective; (2) allowing each individual clinician to decide on alert suppression parameters such as was designed for the Medical Office of the XXIst century (MOXXI) project [11], which involves additional algorithms and processing which can result in costly software customizations; and (3) an ultimate smart, learning health system [12] that combines "big data" from data warehouses of clinical systems, administrative, regulatory, licensing, and local and regional factors to generate an alert profile for each user (learner, clinician of varying experience or specialty) and implementation of new knowledge. Fear of litigation by software companies has also erected barriers to changes in alerts, but this can be managed through legislative or policy changes [13].

User-computer interface design can also affect the effectiveness of decision-support systems. User-centered design (human-factors engineering) is an emerging area with increasing importance [14]. The starkness and simplicity of the now-obsolete monochromatic 80-character-wide, 25-line-long cathode-ray tube display made for a very efficient computer-user interface. The modern high-resolution computer graphics display with 32-bit-depth color coding generating up to 16.8 million different colors, replete with un-asked for multimedia effects (sounds and animations) frequently results in distractions that diminishes the information to be conveyed [15].

19.2 A Second Issue Is the Lack of Global Standards

Even though human DNA is built from the same four nucleosides (adenine, cytosine, guanine, thymine), different clinical information systems have a hard time sharing clinically relevant information. Interoperability has been an ICT industry buzzword for years and continues to be exceptionally difficult to achieve [16]. Coding systems are required to transform digital health information from machine-readable formats (e.g., facsimile machines) to machine-interpretable formats using structured coding (e.g., LOINC, SNOMED[3]). The current ICT industry devotes a huge effort on standards as to how electronic data is reliably and securely transmitted and received between different devices and systems. These standards, defined, developed, and published by global organizations such as ISO, ANSI, IEEE, and HL7[4] deal more with the safety and reliability of communications between medical devices sold on the global market.

[3]LOINC = Logical Observation Identifiers Names and Codes (https://loinc.org); SNOMED = Systematized Nomenclature of Medicine (https://www.nlm.nih.gov/research/umls/Snomed/snomed_main.html)

[4]ISO = International Organization for Standardization (http://www.iso.org); ANSI = American National Standards Institute (https://www.ansi.org); IEEE = Institute of Electrical and Electronics

A different challenge is what the data really means. The lack of structured and coded diagnoses means a significant amount of cognitive work (involving working memory and problem-solving) has to be done by the clinician. Interruptions and other distractions that are part of the clinical work environment can impact on the completion of tasks and potentially lead to errors. Semantic persistence is a term that refers to information whose meaning and interpretation remains intact and understood by anyone anywhere and anytime. For instance, the definition of the clinical condition known as "fever" needs to be meticulously described: (1) actual temperature recording, (2) measurement unit used, (3) instrument used, (4) calibration of instrument, (5) operator of measurement instrument, (6) method of generation of digital data, (7) route of measurement, and (8) condition of measurement. Therefore, a recording of a temperature of 38.8 °C, taken by a calibrated digital thermometer orally in a patient who has not had anything by mouth for at least 10 min prior to the reading and transmitted securely into an electronic health record system, can reliably be interpreted as "low-grade fever." Semantic persistence, coupled with trust and use of clinical information systems, can help off-load some of the cognitive tasks that clinicians need to perform.

The digital representation of a fall event is therefore challenging. The increasing availability of data from accelerometer devices, which are small machines that detect movement, now embedded into smart phones and other wearable technologies, means that electrical and computer engineers have to work collaboratively with clinicians to develop algorithms that can help determine the difference between a device being dropped, a person wearing or carrying the device sustaining a fall, and a stumble or jumping down off a ledge. Much work needs to be done, and several organizations that are engaged in this work include:

- American National Standards Institute's Healthcare Informatics Standards Board (ANSI HISB)
- Joint Initiative on Standards Development Organizations Global Health Informatics Standardization (http://www.jointinitiativecouncil.org/index.asp)
- E-Health standards Australia (http://www.e-health.standards.org.au)
- Technical committee (TC) 215 dealing with health informatics within the International Organization for Standardization (http://www.iso.org/iso/iso_technical_committee?commid=54960)

19.3 A Third Issue Is Training

What training do health-care learners and practicing clinicians need to effectively use ICT to assist them in delivering safe health care? The traditional medical school undergraduate curriculum focuses on the basic and clinical science knowledge needed to equip a physician with the tools to diagnose conditions and plan for clinical management. Concerns about an education gap have been reported in 1995 [17]

Engineers (https://www.ieee.org); HL7 = Health Level Seven International (http://www.hl7.org)

and followed by a qualitative study by Buckeridge and Goel [18] in 2002 that reported the subject of medical informatics was poorly understood. A recent environmental scan and literature review in 2012 by the Association of Faculties of Medicine of Canada (AFMC) [19] describes an ongoing significant gap. Most medical schools focused on computer literacy for information searching and evaluation of evidence. Few to none actually touch upon the issue that ICT are tools, with particular strengths and limitations. Globally the situation is similar, with countries such as Germany leading the way [20]. Although the AFMC report describes e-health as an important component in modern medical education, the mandate of the report was just a review. Can we trust that medical school graduates of the "video game generation" will intuitively and correctly use ICT? This question needs to be formally evaluated.

19.4 A Fourth Issue Is a Critical Examination of How and When Tasks Are Completed During a Patient's Care Episode

Process engineering and time-motion studies are tools that can help inform and determine where ICT can assist and where it hinders [21]. As more health-care activities depend on team functioning, ICT and DSS have to be designed to enable effective interprofessional cooperation [22]. More research is needed to clarify the conditions for optimal uptake and use of ICT in clinical care.

19.5 A Fifth Issue Is Cost

Health care ICT is costly. There are at least five major cost components: (1) hardware, including redundant servers because of the mission-critical nature of e-health systems, wired and wireless network connectivity, workstations, mobile devices, peripherals and printers; (2) electronic health record (EHR) software licenses, interfaces, and maintenance contracts; (3) implementation personnel, change management, etc.; (4) training of clinicians; and (5) operating costs such as telecommunication fees, maintenance contracts, upgrades, bug fixes, data analytics, digital threat assessment, and defenses.

Several studies in the early 2000s estimated the cost of purchasing and installing an on-site EHR ranging from $15,000 to $70,000 US dollars per provider. Fleming and colleagues estimated an implementation cost of $162,000 US dollars for an average five-physician private practice, which included $85,500 in maintenance expenses during the first year. The practice implementation team needed 611 h, on average, to prepare for and implement the electronic health record system and that 134 h per end user on average were needed to prepare for use of the record system in clinical encounters [23]. Costs vary depending on whether on-site EHR deployment or Web-based (subscription) EHR deployment is selected. Subscription-based services are not necessarily less expensive. Open source software may save on software licensing fees but may be offset by the need for operations personnel who have the required knowledge and skills to maintain, modify, and customize these programs. Security and privacy concerns about sensitive health data and compliance with regulatory laws[5] add additional costs for specialized hardware, software, and professionals. Since knowledge, technology, and processes continue to advance rapidly, as well as the number and scope of malicious activities toward the systems and the stored data, a considerable investment in people and technology is required to attain and maintain the trust of users and patients that security and privacy are not compromised.

19.6 A Final Issue Is the Delay in Knowledge Transfer

A study by Morris and colleagues [24] reported that the delay between scientific discovery and uptake into clinical practice was 17 years! There should be a better and faster way to make sure that the care any person is receiving anywhere in the world is informed by the best practices and knowledge available to humankind. There has been tremendous progress and much work remains.

19.7 Moving Forward and Closing Gaps

As I have tried to illustrate in this chapter, successful small steps in the use of ICT in helping to manage medication-related falls in older people have been taken. Future work requires a significant alignment of vision, commitment, resources, and teamwork. At the highest administrative levels, policies can be developed to close gaps in interoperability and assist in securing and mandating global e-health standards. Teams whose membership must include frontline clinicians, systems managers, information technology experts, and change-management engineers are essential. We need to be vigilant about unintended consequences [25]. Individuals who are passionate about using ICT to improve clinical care, perhaps readers of this book, are needed to advance this issue. Uncharted territory and future trends will be elaborated in the final chapter of this book.

[5] PIPEDA – The Personal Information Protection and Electronic Documents Act in Canada (https://www.priv.gc.ca/leg_c/leg_c_p_e.asp); HIPPA – Health Insurance Portability and Accountability Act in the United States (http://www.hhs.gov/hipaa/); EU data protection standards Directive 95/46/EC applicable in Europe (http://ec.europa.eu/justice/data-protection/); Australian National eHealth Security and Access Framework NESAF (https://www.nehta.gov.au/implementation-resources/ehealth-foundations/national-ehealth-security-and-access-framework) as examples

References

1. Institute of Medicine (2000) To err is human: building a safer health system. The National Academies Press, Washington, DC
2. Buckminster Fuller R (1981) Critical path. St Martin's Press, New York
3. Agostini JV, Zhang Y, Inouye SK (2007) Use of a computer-based reminder to improve sedative-hypnotic prescribing in older hospitalized patients. J Am Geriatr Soc 55(1):43–48
4. Tamblyn R, Eguale T, Buckeridge DL et al (2012) The effectiveness of a new generation of computerized drug alerts in reducing the risk of injury from drug side effects: a cluster randomized trial. J Am Med Inform Assoc 19:635–643
5. Ball MJ, Lillis J (2001) E-health: transforming the physician/patient relationship. Int J Med Inf 61:1–10
6. Dickerson S, Reinhart AM, Feeley TH et al (2004) Patient internet use for health information at three urban primary care clinics. J Am Med Inform Assoc 11:499–504
7. Tannenbaum C, Martin P, Tamblyn R, Benedetti A, Ahmed S (2014) Reduction of inappropriate benzodiazepine prescriptions among older adults through direct patient education: the empower cluster randomized trial. JAMA Intern Med 174:890–898
8. Shojania KG, Jennings A, Mayhew A, Ramsay C, Eccles M, Grimshaw J (2010) Effect of point-of-care computer reminders on physician behaviour: a systematic review. Can Med Assoc J 182:E216–E225
9. Nanji KC, Slight SP, Seger DL et al (2014) Overrides of medication-related clinical decision support alerts in outpatients. J Am Med Inform Assoc 21:487–491
10. Slight SP, Seger DL, Nanji KC et al (2013) Are we heeding the warning signs? Examining Providers' overrides of computerized drug-drug interaction alerts in primary care. PLoS ONE 8:e85071
11. Tamblyn R, Huang A, Perreault R et al (2003) The medical office of the 21st century (MOXXI): effectiveness of computerized decision-making support in reducing inappropriate prescribing in primary care. CMAJ 169:549–556
12. Institute of Medicine (2011) Digital infrastructure for the learning health system: the foundation for continuous improvement in health and health care: workshop series summary. The National Academies Press, Washington, DC
13. Kesselheim AS, Cresswell K, Phansalkar S, Bates DW, Sheikh A (2011) Clinical decision support systems could be modified to reduce 'Alert Fatigue' while still minimizing the risk of litigation. Health Aff (Millwood) 30:2310–2317
14. Chan J, Shojania KG, Easty AC, Etchells EE (2011) Does user-centred design affect the efficiency, usability and safety of CPOE order sets? J Am Med Inform Assoc 18:276–281
15. Ophir E, Nass C, Wagner AD (2009) Cognitive control in media multitaskers. Proc Natl Acad Sci 106:15583–15587
16. Standards for medical identifiers, codes, and messages needed to create an efficient computer-stored medical record (1994) J Am Med Inform Assoc 1:1–7
17. Pulse: the medical student section of jama (1995) JAMA 273:1059–1065
18. Buckeridge DL, Goel V (2002) Medical informatics in an undergraduate curriculum: a qualitative study. BMC Med Inform Decis Making 2:1–5
19. AFMC (2013) Review of the Literature, competencies and standards environmental scan of e-health in undergraduate medical curriculum november 2012. Association of faculties of medicine of Canada
20. Jones R (1990) Education in medical informatics in the undergraduate medical curriculum. A review. In: O'Moore R, Bengtsson S, Bryant JR, Bryden JS (eds) Medical informatics Europe '90. Proceedings Glascow, Scotland, August 20–23, 1990. Springer, Berlin, pp 422–426
21. Meguerditchian AN, Krotneva S, Reidel K, Huang A, Tamblyn R (2013) Medication reconciliation at admission and discharge: a time and motion study. BMC Health Serv Res 13:1–11

22. Koskela T, Sandstr+Âm S, M+ñkinen J, Liira H (2016) User perspectives on an electronic decision-support tool performing comprehensive medication reviews – a focus group study with physicians and nurses. BMC Med Inform Decis Making 16:1–9
23. Fleming NS, Culler SD, McCorkle R, Becker ER, Ballard DJ (2011) The financial and nonfinancial costs of implementing electronic health records in primary care practices. Health Aff (Millwood) 30:481–489
24. Morris ZS, Wooding S, Grant J (2011) The answer is 17 years, what is the question: understanding time lags in translational research. J R Soc Med 104:510–520
25. Ash JS, Sittig DF, Poon EG, Guappone K, Campbell E, Dykstra RH (2007) The extent and importance of unintended consequences related to computerized provider order entry. J Am Med Inform Assoc 14:415–423

Chapter 20
A Novel Personalized Fall Risk Calculator: A Prototype for Improving the Safety of Prescribing Through Computerized Decision Support

Robyn Tamblyn

Abstract It is widely accepted that electronic prescribing and integrated drug information systems can reduce avoidable errors in prescribing and dispensing. An optimal system that both enhances the uptake by clinicians and improves the safety of prescribing would have features and functionality that includes the integration of patient demographic information, retrieval of all currently active drugs, automated alerts for relevant prescribing problems, integration of electronic prescriptions and drug discontinuation orders into pharmacy systems, and monitoring of patient adherence. Targeted alerts about the overuse of psychotropic drugs in the elderly would be particularly relevant since this situation represents a potentially preventable cause of injuries. This chapter describes the results of a cluster randomized trial using a cutting-edge custom-designed computer-assisted alert for the detection and management of psychotropic drug use. The results showed that physicians who were exposed to the personalized patient alerts were more likely to reduce drugs that were shown to contribute to fall risk, with greater changes occurring when greater risk was displayed. These positive findings are promising, since prescribers will do the right thing when given the information in an easily understandable format. Computerized decision support is a powerful tool to deliver value-added information to consumers and clinicians at the point of care. The next steps involve establishing the standards for delivering evidence into practice, determining what data is needed for personalized predictions, and determining how to deploy decision-support systems across multiple platforms.

R. Tamblyn, BScN, MSc, PhD
Department of Medicine and Department of Epidemiology, Biostatistics and Occupational Health, Clinical and Health Informatics Research Group, McGill University, Montreal, QC, Canada

Institute for Health Services and Policy Research, Canadian Institutes for Health Research, Ottawa, ON, Canada
e-mail: robyn.tamblyn@mcgill.ca

© Springer International Publishing Switzerland 2016

A.R. Huang, L. Mallet (eds.), *Medication-related falls in older people*,
DOI 10.1007/978-3-319-32304-6_20

Abbreviations

ADE Adverse drug event
CIHR Canadian Institutes for Health Research
RR Relative risk

20.1 Prescription Drug Use and Drug-Related Illness

Drug expenditures are responsible for an increasing proportion of health costs, accounting for $1.4 trillion US dollars in annual expenditure worldwide by 2020 and increasing at a rate of 4–7 % per year [1, 2].

While improvement in health status should result from the appropriate use of prescription drugs, the potential benefits of drug treatment are compromised by avoidable errors in the drug, dose, and duration of therapy prescribed, inadequate drug monitoring, and patient nonadherence.

Drug-related illness accounts for 5–25 % of hospital admissions [3–8] and is now claimed to be among one of the top leading causes of mortality [9–11]. Hospital-based studies of adverse events systematically identify errors in prescribing and drug management among the leading causes of preventable injury or death [12–20]. Preventable adverse drug events (ADE) in ambulatory practice, where the vast majority of prescriptions are generated, are estimated to occur in 2–3 % of patients treated per year, of which 58 % are related to prescribing errors [21–24]. Indeed, an Australian study found that 40 % of avoidable adverse events among hospitalized patients arose because of problems initiated in community-based practice [25].

A variety of potential causes of ambulatory prescribing problems have been identified. The rapid increase in the number of drugs, contraindications, interactions, and side effects makes it difficult for any physician to keep up-to-date on potential prescribing problems [26, 27]. Multiple prescribing physicians and dispensing pharmacies increase the risk of avoidable prescribing errors [28, 29], likely because of the inability to readily access accurate information on all current prescriptions. Transcription errors, mistakes made in transcribing the written prescription into the appropriate drug dispensed, are estimated to occur in 15 % of prescriptions dispensed in community pharmacies [30]. Indeed, there is sufficient concern over this avoidable source of error that the US Medicare Prescription Drug and Modernization Act of 2003 required the nationwide implementation of an electronic prescription drug program by January 1, 2006 [31].

20.2 Improving Drug Safety by Computerized Prescribing and Drug Management Systems

It is widely accepted that electronic prescribing and integrated drug information systems can reduce avoidable errors in prescribing and dispensing [22, 26, 32–43].

Systematic reviews of the effect of computer-based decision-support systems on physician decision-making have identified three types of systems [44, 45]: (1) stand-alone computer-based registries that track information on patient care, such as preventive screening, and generate reminders for follow-up care that are inserted into the patient chart, (2) stand-alone, interactive computer programs that can be used to generate disease risk and/or treatment recommendations after the clinician has entered relevant patient information, and (3) integrated clinical information systems that retrieve electronically stored patient information (e.g., labs, pathology, drugs) and generate recommendations for screening or treatment that are presented to the clinician through an order-entry system or full electronic health record. The provision of decision support through integrated clinical information systems has produced the most substantial improvements in reducing treatment errors [46–48] and increasing adherence to evidence-based treatment recommendations [44, 48–53]. This is likely because integrated systems have the capacity to fit into the workflow of physicians and provide value-added benefits with minimal effort. Integrated systems provide patient-specific treatment recommendations at the time decisions are being made, without the requirement that extensive patient information be entered by the clinician before receiving treatment advice. Integrated drug information systems that retrieve information from community pharmacies are also considered to be essential for widespread use of electronic prescribing systems [22, 40, 54].

In the case of drug management, the specific functionalities needed for an integrated system to improve the safety and quality of drug management have been defined [22, 38] based on an analysis of the causes of preventable adverse drug events. These include the (1) integration of and display of patient demographic information from office management systems; (2) retrieval and display of all currently active drugs from community pharmacy systems; (3) automated alerts for relevant prescribing problems (therapeutic duplication; excess dose; dose-adjustment for weight and renal impairment; drug-disease, drug-drug, drug-age, and drug-allergy contraindications), prioritized by importance; (4) integration of electronic prescriptions (e-Rx) into pharmacy software to avoid transcriptions errors; (5) transmission of orders to discontinue medication to dispensing pharmacies; and (6) monitoring of patient adherence and treatment outcomes.

However, the vast majority of prescribing system do not provide these critical functions [40, 44, 55–63]. To obtain these value-added benefits in community-based electronic prescribing, there is consensus that an electronic infrastructure is needed so that physicians can obtain information on dispensed prescriptions from community-based pharmacists, transmit prescriptions electronically, and manage refill requests efficiently [40]. Unlike the hospital environment where a single pharmacy is involved in dispensing prescriptions for hospital patients, the ambulatory setting is more complex as up to 40 % of patients may obtain their prescriptions from a variety of retail pharmacies and 60–80 % obtain prescriptions from different physicians [29]. Thus, an information infrastructure is mandatory to facilitate information sharing needed for safe prescribing. In the last decade, progress has been made in establishing the infrastructure for data exchange in ambulatory care [40], with nationwide efforts to build the legal framework and regional clinical repositories to facilitate the implementation of community-based computerized drug management [39, 64, 65]. Primary care physicians using an early Canadian prototype of an integrated drug management system were less likely to prescribe inappropriate medications, and physicians used the system most frequently for patients with multiple medications and lower socioeconomic status [33, 66, 67].

20.3 Computerized Alert Systems for Drug Safety Problems

One of the benefits of computerizing prescribing and drug management is the opportunity to automatically screen for potential drug safety problems such as drug interactions, therapy duplications, incorrect dose, and drug-disease and drug-allergy contraindications. In a recent review of decision-support systems, four additional factors were identified that were associated with successful change in behavior: (1) computerization of decision-support alerts, (2) automated provision of decision support as part of clinician workflow, (3) provision of decision support at the time of clinical decision-making, and (4) provision of recommendations rather than just assessment [45].

Drug interaction detection is the domain of most alert systems [68, 69]; however, a substantially greater risk of adverse drug events is associated with drug-allergy, drug-disease, and drug dose contraindications [70, 71]. This may be why 22 % of physicians surveyed indicate that they often override alerts because they are not clinically relevant [68, 72–75]. However, analysis of actual behavior in primary care practice indicates that overriding alerts is more common as 91.2 % of drug-allergy alerts, and 89.4 % of high severity drug interaction alerts were overridden [72, 75]. Two-thirds of these alerts were judged to be clinically significant, and three preventable ADEs occurred as a result of alerts being overridden. Physicians do appear to be more likely to respond to alerts in patients who may be at greater risk, those with multiple allergies, renal impairment, or new prescriptions [72, 76]. But to date, no system has been developed to categorize prescription drug alerts by level of risk for individual patients.

20.4 A New Generation of Clinically Relevant Drug Safety Alerts

In order to develop clinically relevant drug alerts, patient-specific risks and recommendations for improved treatment need to be developed. To do so, new generations of clinically relevant alerts need to be developed within a defined subpopulation of drugs, patients, and treatment indications so that problem-specific recommendations can be developed that are tailored to patients at highest risk.

20.4.1 Targeting Prescribing Alerts to Psychotropic Medication and to Patients at High Risk of Fall-Related Injury

One area where targeted alerts would be particularly relevant is in injury prevention in relationship to the overuse of psychotropic drugs (anxiolytics, antidepressants, antipsychotics) in the elderly. Injuries are a common cause of morbidity and mortality in older adults [77, 78]. The majority of injuries are fall related, and 5–10 % are fatal [79–81]. A further 9–27 % lead to a permanent loss of capacity for independent living [78, 82].

Psychotropic drug use is a potentially preventable cause of injury [83–89]. These drugs are commonly used in older adults, often for indications such as insomnia or pain, where strong evidence of efficacy is lacking [90–92]. Based on systematic reviews, the risk of injury is increased by 39 %, 59 %, and 50 % with the use of benzodiazepines, antidepressants, and antipsychotics, respectively [83]. Risks are dose dependent, particularly for antipsychotics and opioids where the most rapid increase in use is seen for older adults [83, 90, 91, 93, 94].

Effective management of psychotropic medication is challenging. In older adults, 21–33 % are prescribed drugs that are contraindicated [95–97], and 29 % in doses that exceed those recommended [97]. Moreover, 20 % of older adults use more than one psychotropic drug concurrently, and 69 % have more than one physician prescribing treatment, increasing the risk of undetected cumulative toxicity [29]. Unfortunately, the majority of safety alerts for psychotropic drugs are overridden [72–75] even when drug alert systems are customized to present only clinically important interactions.

20.4.2 An Analysis of Psychotropic Drugs in Primary Care: Opportunities for Reducing the Risk of Fall-Related Injuries in Canada

For example, in a 4-month period, 8.1 % of the 3774 patients seen by primary care physicians in the *M*edical *O*ffice of the *XXI*st century (MOXXI) trial had at least one alert related to psychotropic medication (Table 20.1). Therapy duplication (e.g., multiple benzodiazepines), drug-age contraindications, and cumulative toxicity from multiple medications with the same side effects (e.g., antidepressant, antihistamine, antiemetic) were the main problems identified. The adverse effects associated with these prescribing problems are a dose-related increase in the risk of sedation, confusion, and psychomotor instability which in turn increase the risk of fall-related injuries [93, 98–100]. Use of psychotropic medications in elderly persons is associated with a 2- to 29-fold increase in the risk of falls [98–100] and a two to fivefold increase in the risk of hip fracture [98, 99, 101].

At particular risk are individuals over the age of 70, those with a prior history of falls, cognitive impairment, stroke, Parkinson's disease, or other conditions that

Table 20.1 Proportion of patients seen in primary care in a 4-month period with one or more psychotropic drug problem alerts

	Psychotropic drug alert		Women ($n=2114$)		Men ($n=1335$)	
Psychotropic prescribing alert	Yes % (n)	No % (n)	Yes % (n)	No % (n)	Yes % (n)	No % (n)
Any problem	8.1 % (280)	91.9 % (3169)	8.8 % (186)	91.2 % (1928)	7.1 % (95)	92.9 % (1240)
Drug-age contraindication	5.1 % (176)	94.9 % (3273)	5.7 % (120)	94.3 % (1994)	4.2 % (56)	95.8 % (1279)
Cumulative toxicity	5.0 % (172)	95.0 % (3277)	5.8 % (122)	94.2 % (1992)	3.7 % (50)	96.3 % (1285)
Therapy duplication	3.5 % (120)	96.5 % (3329)	3.9 % (82)	96.1 % (2032)	2.8 % (38)	97.2 % (1297)
Dose too high	0.2 % (8)	99.8 % (3441)	0.2 % (4)	99.8 % (2110)	0.3 % (4)	99.7 % (1331)

Table 20.2 Proportion of patients seen in primary care in a 4-month period with one or more psychotropic drug problem alerts and the proportion of patients who had other risk factors for fall-related injuries

	Any psychotropic drug alert		Any psychotropic drug alert		Any psychotropic drug alert	
			Women		Men	
Risk profile	Yes ($n=280$)	No ($n=3169$)	Yes ($n=185$)	No ($n=1929$)	Yes ($n=95$)	No ($n=1240$)
Any risk factor	67.5 % (189)	56.5 % (1790)	70.3 % (130)	53.1 % (1025)	62.1 % (59)	61.7 % (765)
Recent fall injury	7.1 % (20)	6.2 % (196)	9.2 % (17)	5.7 % (110)	3.2 % (3)	7.0 % (89)
>70 years	63.6 % (178)	52.9 % (1677)	66.5 % (123)	50 % (964)	57.9 % (55)	57.5 % (713)
Stroke	4.6 % (13)	3.2 % (102)	4.9 % (9)	2.7 % (53)	4.2 % (4)	4.0 % (49)
Dementia	1.8 % (5)	1.5 % (47)	1.6 % (3)	1.4 % (27)	2.1 % (2)	1.6 % (20)
Parkinson's	2.1 % (6)	1.3 % (42)	1.6 % (3)	1.3 % (26)	3.2% (3)	1.3 % (16)

would impair balance or gait. In the MOXXI study population (Table 20.2), 67.5 % of persons with a psychotropic drug safety alert had at least one additional risk factor for fall-related injuries. This was particularly true for women who not only were more likely to have a psychotropic drug prescribing alerts than men but were also more likely to have other risk factors. 70.3 % of women who had a psychotropic prescribing alert had other risk factors in comparison to 62.1 % of men, particularly as it is related to older age and a history of a fall-related fracture or soft-tissue injury in the past 12 months.

Physicians revised their treatment plans because of alerts for a slightly higher proportion of patients with at least one other risk factor (10.7 %) compared to persons with no risk factor (8.7 %), but for the vast majority of patients, the alerts were ignored. A recent in-hospital study showed that providing physicians with patient-specific recommendations for changes in high-risk psychotropic therapy through a computerized order-entry system reduced the prescription of non-recommended drugs and doses by 10 %, which in turn was associated with a significant twofold reduction in the in-hospital fall rate [101]. If even a 5 % reduction (annual prevalence 16.1–11.1 %) could be achieved in primary care through targeted recommendations for high-risk patients with psychotropic drug prescribing alerts, it could conservatively reduce the number of falls among Canadian elderly (assuming the lowest risk of RR = 1.66) from 116,064 to 82,212 and the number of fall-related injuries from 11,606 to 8221. Based on the average costs (in 1998 dollars) of treating fall-related injuries of $20,000 US dollars/injury [102], a reduction in adverse events of this magnitude would be associated with an annual savings of $67,708,000 Canadian dollars in direct care costs (Table 20.3).

The main reasons for overriding safety alerts for psychotropic drugs are that the alert is not clinically relevant for a particular patient, and/or the benefit of drug therapy is believed to exceed the risk [72–74, 103, 104]. Perception of risk and benefit is known to be inaccurate by both physicians and patients—with a systematic trend to overestimate benefit and underestimate risk [105–107]. Indeed, the patient-specific risk is rarely known for drug safety alerts. However, this can be estimated by incorporating predictive models of adverse events into drug alert systems [108]. Although these forms of risk calculators, developed on the basis of epidemiological models, are increasingly available for calculating risks of mortality and morbidity such as cardiovascular disease [109, 110], they have not been used in drug safety alerts. A golden opportunity exists to incorporate the risk assessment of adverse events from a substantial universe of pharmacoepidemiological studies into a new generation of personalized alerts. The computing power available in today's electronic medical record systems and the focus on individualized medicine provides an unprecedented opportunity to integrate detailed patient data into complex predictive models for estimating individual patient risk and benefit.

20.5 Drug Safety Alerts for Reducing Fall-Related Injuries Attributable to Psychotropic Drugs: Developing the First Prototype

There is abundant literature on the risks of fall-related injuries with the use of psychotropic drugs [111–115]. Ideally, a meta-analysis of estimated risks from different studies could be used to provide the most informative prediction of the risk of fall-related injuries for a personalized drug safety alert system. However, there were fundamental and surprising limitations in existing studies [116]. The most important limitation was that drug dose was rarely modeled, even though this is highly clinically relevant as the risk of adverse events as well as benefit is typically dose related. Second, patients are often prescribed different therapeutic classes of psychotropic drugs together such as anxiolytics and antidepressants [117–119].To provide

Table 20.3 Estimated number and cost of fall-related injuries attributable to psychotropic drug use among the 4,030,000 Canadian elderly: status quo versus targeted intervention effect of a 5 % reduction in inappropriate psychotropic drug use

Status	# falls /year [99]	Prevalence (%) inappropriate psychotropic drug	Relative risk of falls with any psychotropic drug use [100, 101]	% of falls attributable to psychotropic drugs (PAR) (%)	# falls due to psychotropic drugs	# fall-related injuries/ year due to psychotropic drugs [142]	Cost of fall-related injuries/year due to psychotropic drugs [142]
Status quo	1,209,000	16.1	1.66	9.6	116,064	11,606	$232,128,000
		16.1	3.0	24.5	296,205	29,621	$592,420,000
		16.1	5.0	39.2	473,928	47,393	$947,860,000
Expected	1,209,000	11.1	1.66	6.8	82,212	8221	$164,420,000
Effect of intervention		11.1	3.0	18.2	220,038	22,004	$440,080,000
		11.1	5.0	30.7	371,163	37,116	$742,320,000

clinically useful information for risk reduction, clinicians need to know the relative and independent contribution to the risk of adverse events among all drugs prescribed. In this manner, better decisions can be made about which drugs to target for discontinuation or dose reductions among all drugs prescribed with central nervous system sedating side effects for individual patients. To provide this type of clinically relevant information, all drugs that can increase the risk of fall-related injuries through sedation side effects need to be included in predictive models to provide the independent assessment of risk associated with a specific drug or therapeutic class. For these reasons, an available cohort of 460,000 Quebec seniors was used to estimate the risk of fall-related injuries in relationship to all therapeutic classes of drugs with central nervous system sedating side effects [116]. The resulting predictive model was used to create personalized risk predictions that could be integrated into computerized prescribing and drug management software.

20.6 The Prototype: Making Decisions About How to Present Personalized Patient-Specific Risk Estimates Within a Computerized Prescribing and Drug Management System

Based on the principles and requirements of effective computerized clinical decision-support systems, the following decisions were made about the requirements for prototype development:

1. *Fit with Workflow*: Personalized information about patient risk should be provided at the time decisions are being made about their drug treatment.
2. *Eliminate Data Entry Requirements*: Retrieve all data needed for risk assessment from the electronic health record.
3. *Identify Risks that Are Modifiable*: Separate and display the magnitude of drug-related risks and those related to non-modifiable parameters such as age, sex, prior injury history, and comorbidities, and identify the offending drugs within the patient's current medication list.
4. *Provide Evidence of Immediate Feedback on the Change in Risk with Drug and Dose Changes*: Dynamically display the risk for modifiable and non-modifiable determinants of fall-related injury and the absolute and relative change in risk with newly prescribed medication, drug discontinuations, and dose changes.
5. *Display Risk Information in a Understandable Form for Numerate and Innumerate Users*: Provide graphical and quantitative information about risk by showing an easily understood display.
6. *Allow for Clinical Justification for Overriding Alerts*: Having users indicate the reason for ignoring alerts is one factor that increased the likelihood of modifying drug treatment for safety concerns.

On the basis of these principles, we designed a fall risk thermometer that would appear when a patient's electronic medical record was opened (Fig. 20.1).

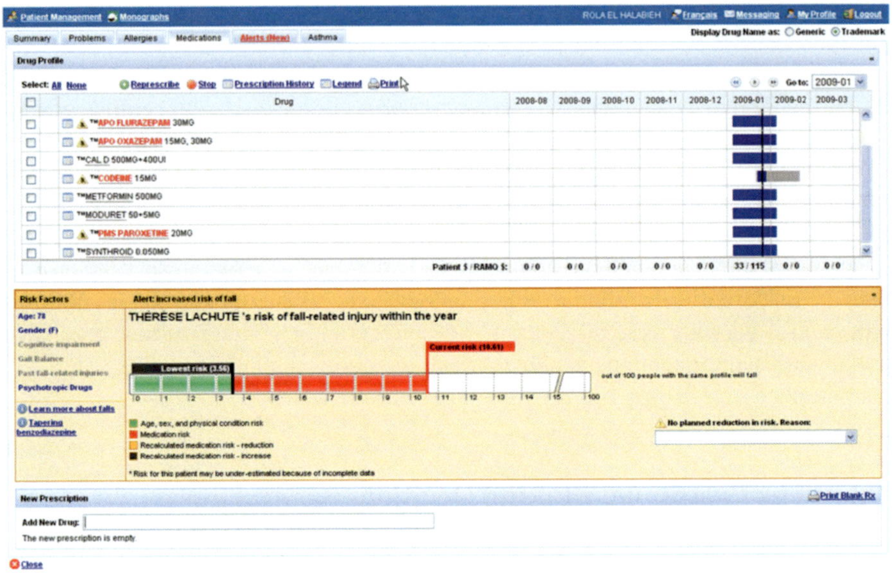

Fig. 20.1 The personalized fall risk calculator (illustrating a fictitious case) (Reproduced with permission from Tamblyn et al. [111])

It presents the probability of injury for a given patient in the next year based on age, sex, prior injury history, comorbid conditions, and use of drugs with central nervous system sedating side effects (opiates, psychotropic drugs, first-generation antihistamines). The portion of the risk that is non-modifiable (e.g., age, sex) is colored in green, and modifiable risks due to drug therapy is displayed in red.

Drugs that are implicated in the calculation of modifiable risk in the patient's drug profile are highlighted in red text with the appearance of a "fall icon" alongside. Review papers of risk factors for fall-related injuries and tapering schedules for discontinuing benzodiazepines are hyperlinked to the alert so that they can be quickly accessed by the clinician.

If the clinician decides to discontinue or reduce the dose of one or more of the drugs implicated in the alert, the fall risk is automatically recalculated and displayed as both an absolute and relative reduction in risk (Figs. 20.2 and 20.3).

Similarly if the clinician decides to prescribe a new drug that increases the risk, the additional risk will be calculated and shown both in absolute and relative risk increase. Increases in risk are displayed in black.

20.7 The Effectiveness of Personalized Risk Assessment for Fall-Related Injury

The impact of this form of decision support was tested in a cluster randomized trial, where physicians were randomized to receiving personalized fall risk injury alerts versus standard alerts for drug and disease contraindications, therapy duplications, dosing errors, drug-allergy problems, and cumulative side effect problems [111].

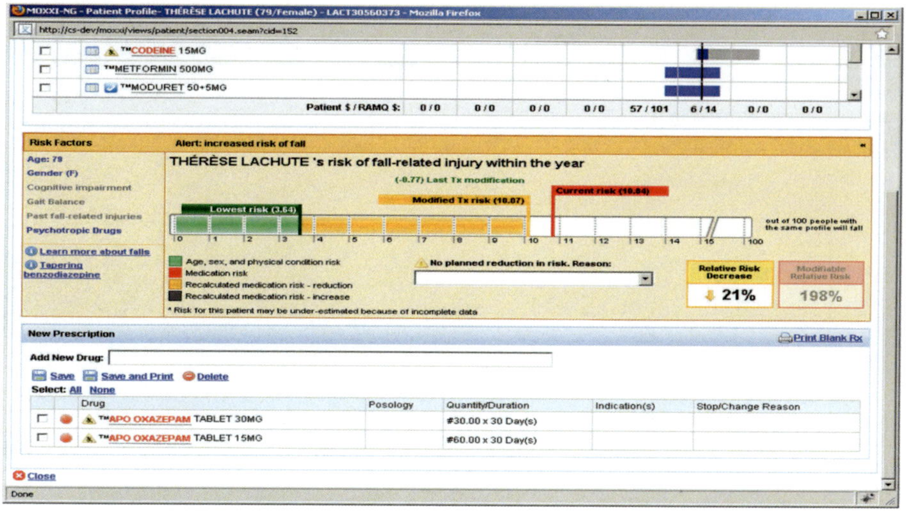

Fig. 20.2 Personalized risk calculator showing immediate feedback on risk reduction by discontinuing or decreasing the dose of a psychotropic drug (Reproduced with permission from Tamblyn et al. [111])

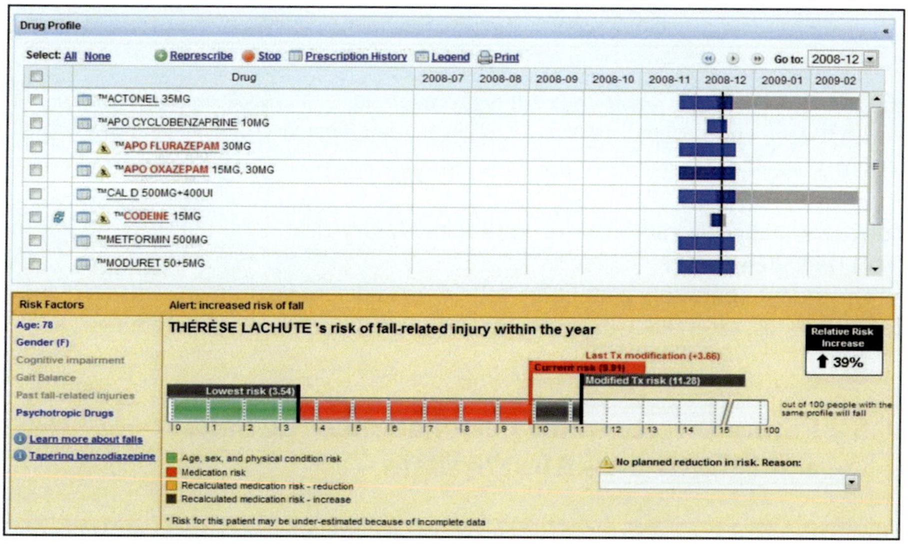

Fig. 20.3 Personalized risk calculator showing immediate feedback on risk increase by adding or increasing the dose of a psychotropic drug (Reproduced with permission from Tamblyn et al. [111])

The investigators found that physicians were more likely to reduce the risk of drug-related contributors to fall-related injury with the personalized patient alerts. Moreover, there was a significant interaction between the magnitude of the risk and the intervention. As the overall risk of fall-related injury increased, so did the effect of the intervention. Physicians were more likely to modify drug treatment for

	Control N=2741		Intervention N=2887		Cluster adjusted reduction in the risk of injury per 1000	
	Mean	**SD**	**Mean**	**SD**	**Reduction**	**95% CI (p Value)**
Number of days of follow-up	467	178	452	181		
Risk of injury at the end of follow-up	3.77	1.73	3.58	1.31	−0.17	−0.32, −0.02 (0.02)

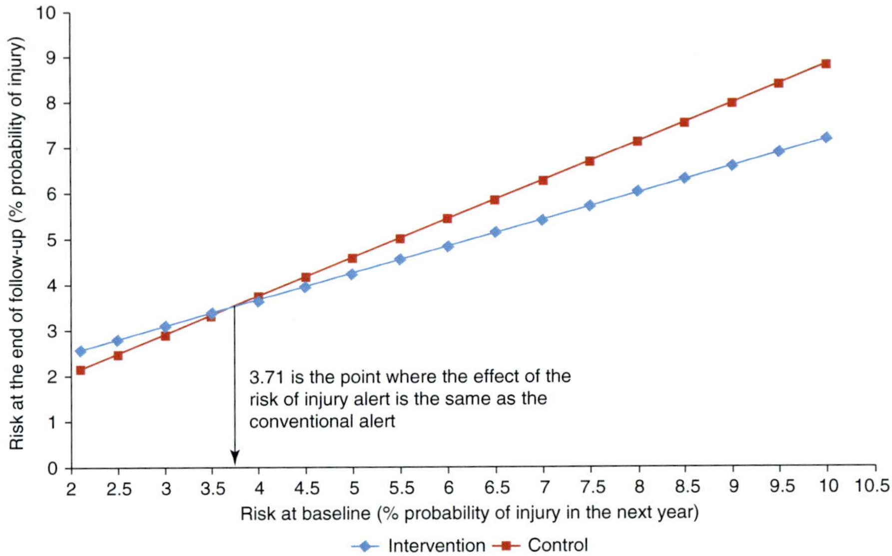

Fig. 20.4 The effect of a personalized fall injury alert compared to standard drug alert systems on the risk of injury among patients in primary care (Reproduced with permission from Tamblyn et al. [111])

patients at higher overall levels of fall-related injury risk in the intervention group [111] (Fig. 20.4).

This study is currently continuing follow-up to determine if there is also a reduction in injuries, emergency department visits, hospitalizations, and mortality.

20.8 Future Directions for Personalized Drug Safety and Effectiveness Alert Systems

In the future, in the era of big data, there will be a proliferation of personalized prediction systems that would alert consumers, patients, and providers with information that could influence their decision-making [120, 121]. The interest in having information about personalized health risk is reflected in the many "health apps" that have been created and are downloaded daily by consumers and patients [122–124] to obtain feedback on risk and benefit [125–128]. Predictive models to guide behavior is already well advanced in the consumer marketing field where marketing agencies are fully exploiting "big data" from Internet audits of consumer behavior to influence decision-making. For example, Walmart has been using data to determine consumer behavior

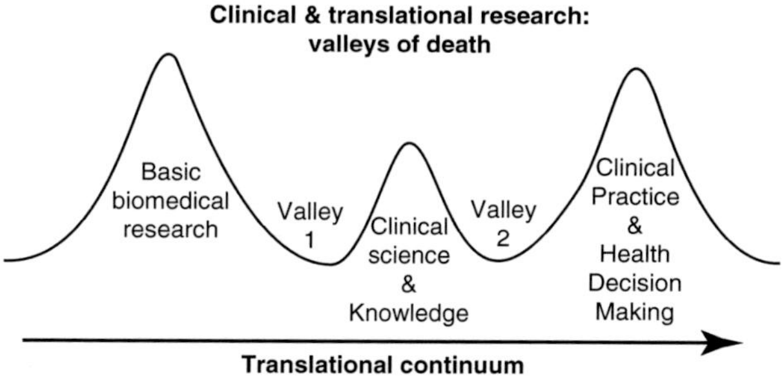

Fig. 20.5 Bridging the valleys of death (Source: http://www.ncbi.nlm.nih.gov/pmc/articles/PMC2635103/pdf/nihms64943.pdf)

since 2004, when they analyzed the sales data after Hurricane Charley to help predict what items would be needed to respond to the upcoming Hurricane Frances [129]. As expected, flashlights and emergency equipment were high-priority items for customers and that information allowed Walmart to pre-stock their stores as needed.

In the area of drug management, strategic analysis of big data will be particularly pertinent. First, in social health care systems such as that found in Canada, comprehensive health services utilization and medication use information is constantly collected on the population. These data have been extensively used to characterize the population risks of various drug treatments [130–133], as well as their benefits. Augmentation of these data with information from population genomics and metabolomics as well as clinical data on effectiveness of drug treatment from electronic health records and patient reported outcomes [121, 133, 134] are creating a vast science to support better implementation of personalized risk and benefit assessment at multiple levels: consumers, patients, clinicians, and policy-makers. The emergence of computerized decision-support systems to support the implementation of these personalized risk/benefit systems at the point of care is lagging behind the data available. The gap between knowledge and implementation has been generically characterized by the Canadian Institutes for Health Research (CIHR) and other granting agencies as "valleys of death" for knowledge translation, representing failures or delays in putting into clinical practice what is known in clinical, health services, and population health research [135–138] (Fig. 20.5).

Computerized decision support is a powerful tool to deliver value-added information to consumers and clinicians at the point of care when they are making decisions about health care management [139–141].

To optimize the capacity for this new world of opportunities, we need to do the following:

1. Establish the standards for delivering evidence into practice—what studies matter for clinical decision-making, how to use these decision points to identify what studies should be included and how they should be synthesized, and how to represent the findings of these studies in personalized prediction models.
2. Determine what data is needed for personalized prediction (e.g., genomic, clinical, personal preferences) and how to incorporate these data into personalized

assessment of risk and benefit to optimize decision-making about the risk and benefit of drug therapy.
3. Establish standards for data documentation and harmonization to enable decision-support systems to be used in multiple platforms. Minimizing the costs of software systems customization and encouraging the deployment of interoperability platforms such as Smart systems (http://www.smarthealthit.org) can enable rapid scale-up.

Harnessing the power of data to optimize drug management will change the paradigm for science and clinical care by empowering patients and clinicians with the best, most timely, and customized evidence for individualized decision-making.

References

1. IMS Institute for Healthcare Informatics (2013) The global use of medicines: outlook through 2017. IMS Institute, Parsippany, New Jersey, USA
2. IMS Institute (2015) Global medicines use in 2020: outlook and implications. IMS Institute, Parsippany, New Jersey, USA
3. Grymonpre RE, Mitenko PA, Sitar DS, Aoki FY, Montgomery PR (1988) Drug-associated hospital admissions in older medical patients. J Am Geriatr Soc 36:1092–1098
4. Ives TJ, Bentz EJ, Gwyther RE (1987) Drug-related admissions to a family medicine inpatient service. Arch Intern Med 147:1117–1120
5. Hurwitz N (1969) Predisposing factors in adverse reactions to drugs. Br Med J 1:536–539
6. May FE, Stewart RB, Cluff LE (1977) Drug interactions and multiple drug administration. Clin Pharmocol Ther 22:322
7. Samoy LJ, Zed PJ, Wilbur K, Balen RM, Abu-Laban RB, Roberts M (2006) Drug-related hospitalizations in a tertiary care internal medicine service of a Canadian hospital: a prospective study. Pharmacotherapy 26:1578–1586
8. Wilbur K, Hazi H, El-Bedawi A (2013) Drug-related hospital visits and admissions associated with laboratory or physiologic abnormalities-a systematic-review. PLoS One 8:e66803
9. Lazarou J, Pomeranz BH, Corey PN (1998) Incidence of adverse drug reactions in hospitalized patients: a meta-analysis of prospective studies. JAMA 279:1200–1205
10. Ohta Y, Sakuma M, Koike K, Bates DW, Morimoto T (2014) Influence of adverse drug events on morbidity and mortality in intensive care units: the JADE study. Int J Qual Health Care 26:573–578
11. Page RL, Ruscin JM (2006) The risk of adverse drug events and hospital-related morbidity and mortality among older adults with potentially inappropriate medication use. Am J Geriatr Pharmacother 4:297–305
12. Baker GR, Norton PG, Flintoft V et al (2004) The Canadian adverse events study: the incidence of adverse events among hospital patients in Canada. CMAJ 170:1678–1686
13. Leape LL, Bates DW, Cullen DJ et al (1995) Systems analysis of adverse drug events. ADE Prev Study Group JAMA 274:35–43
14. Bates DW, Cullen DJ, Laird N et al (1995) Incidence of adverse drug events and potential adverse drug events. Implications for prevention. ADE Prevention Study Group. JAMA 274:29–34
15. Forster AJ, Clark HD, Menard A et al (2004) Adverse events among medical patients after discharge from hospital. CMAJ 170:345–349
16. Neale G, Woloshynowych M, Vincent C (2001) Exploring the causes of adverse events in NHS hospital practice. J R Soc Med 94:322–330
17. Vincent C, Neale G, Woloshynowych M (2001) Adverse events in British hospitals: preliminary retrospective record review. Br Med J 322:517–519

18. Thomas EJ, Studdert DM, Burstin HR et al (2000) Incidence and types of adverse events and negligent care in Utah and Colorado. Med Care 38:261–271
19. Leape LL, Brennan TA, Laird N et al (1991) The nature of adverse events in hospitalized patients. Results of the Harvard Medical Practice Study II. N Engl J Med 324:377–384
20. Brennan TA, Leape LL, Laird NM et al (1991) Incidence of adverse events and negligence in hospitalized patients. Results of the Harvard Medical Practice Study I. N Engl J Med 324: 370–376
21. Gurwitz JH, Field TS, Harrold LR et al (2003) Incidence and preventability of adverse drug events among older persons in the ambulatory setting. JAMA 289:1107–1116
22. Bell DS, Cretin S, Marken RS, Landman AB (2004) A conceptual framework for evaluating outpatient electronic prescribing systems based on their functional capabilities. J Am Med Inform Assoc 11:60–70
23. Gandhi TK, Weingart SN, Borus J et al (2003) Adverse drug events in ambulatory care. N Engl J Med 348:1556–1564
24. Forster AJ, Murff HJ, Peterson JF, Gandhi TK, Bates DW (2003) The incidence and severity of adverse events affecting patients after discharge from the hospital. Ann Intern Med 138:161–167
25. Wilson RM, Runciman WB, Gibberd RW, Harrison BT, Newby L, Hamilton JD (1995) The quality in Australian Health Care study. Med J Aust 163:458–471
26. eHealth Initiative (2004) Electronic prescribing: toward maximum value and rapid adoption. eHealth Initiative, Washington, DC
27. Lesar TS, Briceland L, Stein DS (1997) Factors related to errors in medication prescribing [see comments]. JAMA 277:312–317
28. Mackinnon NJ, Helper CD (2003) Indicators of preventable drug-related morbidity in older adults 2. Use within a managed care organization. J Manag Care Pharm 9:134–141
29. Tamblyn RM, McLeod PJ, Abrahamowicz M, Laprise R (1996) Do too many cooks spoil the broth? Multiple physician involvement in medical management and inappropriate prescribing in the elderly. Can Med Assoc J 154:1177–1184
30. Kistner UA, Keith MR, Sergeant KA, Hokanson JA (1994) Accuracy of dispensing in a high-volume, hospital-based outpatient pharmacy. Am J Hosp Pharm 51:2793–2797
31. Blendon RJ, DesRoches CM, Brodie M et al (2002) Views of practicing physicians and the public on medical errors. N Engl J Med 347:1933–1940
32. Shane R (2002) Computerized physician order entry: challenges and opportunities. Am J Health Syst Pharm 59:286–288
33. Tamblyn R, Huang A, Perreault R et al (2003) The medical office of the 21st century (MOXXI): effectiveness of computerized decision-making support in reducing inappropriate prescribing in primary care. CMAJ 169:549–556
34. Maslakowski C (1996) Cut adverse drug reactions with clinical decision support. Health Manag Technol 17:28–30
35. Hume M (1999) Computer-aided drug selection can sharply cut adverse events. Qual Lett Healthc Leadersh 11:10–12
36. Karow HS (2002) Creating a culture of medication administration safety: laying the foundation for computerized provider order entry. Joint Comm J Qual Improv 28:396–402
37. Teich JM, Osheroff JA, Pifer EA, Sittig DF, Jenders RA, Panel TC (2005) Clinical decision support in electronic prescribing: recommendations and an action plan. J Am Med Inform Assoc 12:365–376
38. Bell DS, Marken RS, Meili RC, Wang CJ, Rosen M, Brook RH (2004) Recommendations for comparing electronic prescribing systems: results of an expert consensus process. Health Aff (Millwood) Suppl Web Exclusives:W4–17
39. Institute of Medicine (2001) Crossing the quality chasm: a new health system for the 21st century. National Academy Press, Washington, DC
40. Lipton HL, Miller RH, Wimbush JJ (2003) Electronic prescribing: ready for prime time? J Healthc Inf Manag 17(4):72–79

41. Porterfield A, Engelbert K, Coustasse A (2014) Electronic prescribing: improving the efficiency and accuracy of prescribing in the ambulatory care setting. Perspect Health Inf Manag 11:1g
42. Tamblyn R (2004) Improving patient safety through computerized drug management: the devil is in the details. Healthc Pap 5:52–68
43. Kaushal R, Kern LM, Barron Y, Quaresimo J, Abramson EL (2010) Electronic prescribing improves medication safety in community-based office practices. J Gen Intern Med 25:530–536
44. Hunt DL, Haynes B, Hanna SE, Smith K (1998) Effects of computer-based clinical decision support systems on physician performance and patient outcomes. A Syst Rev JAMA 280: 1339–1346
45. Kawamoto K, Houlihan CA, Balas EA, Lobach DF (2005) Improving clinical practice using clinical decision support systems: a systematic review of trials to identify features critical to success. Br Med J 330:765
46. Bates DW, Leape L, Cullen DJ et al (1998) Effect of computerized physician order entry and a team intervention on prevention of Serious medication errors. JAMA 280(15):1311–1316
47. Teich JM, Merchia PR, Schmiz JL, Kuperman GJ, Spurr CD, Bates DW (2000) Effects of computerized physician order entry on prescribing practices. Arch Intern Med 160: 2741–2747
48. Bates DW, Cohen M, Leape LL, Overhage JM, Shabot MM, Sheridan T (2001) Reducing the frequency of errors in medicine using information technology. J Am Med Inform Assoc 8:299–308
49. Tierney WM (1988) Computer predictions of abnormal test results. JAMA 259:1194–1198
50. Overhage JM, Tierney WM, Zhou XH, McDonald CJ (1997) A randomized trial of "corollary orders" to prevent errors of omission. J Am Med Inform Assoc 4(5):364–375
51. Evans RS, Pestotnik sL, Classen DC et al (1998) A computer-assisted management program for antibiotics and other anti-infective agents. N Engl J Med 338(4):232–238
52. Dexter PR, Wolinsky FD, Gramelspacher GP et al (1998) Effectiveness of computer-generated reminders for increasing discussions about advance directives and completion of advance directive forms. A randomized, controlled trial. Ann Intern Med 128(2):102–110
53. Pestotnik SL, Classen DC, Evans S, Burke JP (1996) Implementing antibiotic practice guidelines through computer-assisted decision support: clinical and financial outcomes. Ann Intern Med 124:884–890
54. Williams RB (2002) Successful computerized physician order entry system implementation. Tools to support physician-driven design and adoption. Healthc Leadersh Manag Rep 10:1–13
55. Fox GN, Weidmann E, Diamond DE, Korbey AA (2001) Hand-held electronic prescribing. J Fam Pract 50:449–454
56. Gibson PG, Powell H, Coughlan J et al (2002) Limited (information only) patient education programs for adults with asthma. Cochrane Database Syst Rev (4):CD001005
57. Gibson PG, Coughlan J, Wilson AJ et al (2000) Self-management education and regular practitioner review for adults with asthma. [Review] [30 refs]. Cochrane Database Syst Rev (1):CD001117.
58. Turner RC, Peden JG Jr, O'Brien K (1994) Patient-carried card prompts vs computer-generated prompts to remind private practice physicians to perform health maintenance measures. Arch Intern Med 154:1957–1960
59. Eccles M, McColl E, Steen N et al (2002) Effect of computerised evidence based guidelines on management of asthma and angina in primary care: cluster randomised controlled trial. Br Med J 325:941–947
60. Montgomery AA, Fahey T, Peters TJ, MacIntosh C, Sharp DJ (2000) Evaluation of computer based clinical decision support system and risk chart for management of hypertension in primary care: randomised controlled trial. Br Med J 320:686–690
61. Frame PS, Zimmer JG, Werth PL, Hall WJ, Eberly SW (1994) Computer-based vs manual health maintenance tracking. A controlled trial. Arch Fam Med 3:581–588

62. McPhee SJ, Bird JA, Fordham D, Rodnick JE, Osborn EH (1991) Promoting cancer prevention activities by primary care physicians. Results of a randomized, controlled trial. JAMA 266:538–544
63. Bates DW, Ebell M, Gotlieb E, Zapp J, Mullins HC (2003) A proposal for electronic medical records in U.S. primary care. J Am Med Inform Assoc 10:1–10
64. Papshev D, Peterson AM (2001) Electronic prescribing in ambulatory practice: promises, pitfalls, and potential solutions. Am J Manag Care 7(7):725–736
65. Kilbridge P, Gladysheva K, First Consulting Group (2001) E-prescribing. 1–43. California HealthCare Foundation, Oakland
66. Kawasumi Y, Tamblyn R, Platt R, Ernst P, Abrahamowicz M, Taylor L (2008) Evaluation of the use of an integrated drug information system by primary care physicians for vulnerable population. Int J Med Inform 77:98–106
67. Tamblyn R, Huang A, Kawasumi Y et al (2006) The development and evaluation of an integrated electronic prescribing and drug management system for primary care. J Am Med Inform Assoc 13:148–159
68. Magnus D, Rodgers S, Avery AJ (2002) GPs' views on computerized drug interaction alerts: questionnaire survey. J Clin Pharm Ther 27:377–382
69. Ashworth M (2002) Re: GPs' views on computerized drug interaction alerts. J Clin Pharm Ther 27:311–312
70. Bates DW, Boyle DL, Vander VM, Schneider J, Leape L (1995) Relationship between medication errors and adverse drug events. J Gen Intern Med 10:199–205
71. Lindley CM, Tully MP, Paramsothy V, Tallis RC (1992) Inappropriate medication is a major cause of adverse drug reactions in elderly patients. Age Ageing 21:294–300
72. Weingart SN, Toth M, Sands DZ, Aronson MD, Davis RB, Phillips RS (2003) Physicians' decisions to override computerized drug alerts in primary care. Arch Intern Med 163:2625–2631
73. van der Sijs H, Aarts J, Vulto A, Berg M (2006) Overriding of drug safety alerts in computerized physician order entry. J Am Med Inform Assoc 13:138–147
74. Taylor LK, Kawasumi Y, Bartlett G, Tamblyn R (2005) Inappropriate prescribing practices: the challenge and opportunity for patient safety. Healthcare Q 8 Spec No:81–85
75. Tamblyn R, Huang A, Taylor L et al (2008) A randomized trial of the effectiveness of on-demand versus computer-triggered drug decision support in primary care. J Am Med Inform Assoc 15:430–438
76. Bates DW, Teich JM, Lee J et al (1999) The impact of computerized physician order entry on medication error prevention. J Am Med Inform Assoc 6:313–321
77. Jemal A, Ward E, Hao Y, Thun M (2005) Trends in the leading causes of death in the United States, 1970–2002. JAMA 294:1255–1259
78. Tinetti ME, Williams CS (1997) Falls, injuries due to falls, and the risk of admission to a nursing home. N Engl J Med 337:1279–1284
79. Centers for Disease Control and Prevention (CDC) (2003) Public health and aging: nonfatal injuries among older adults treated in hospital emergency departments—United States, 2001. MMWR Morb Mortal Wkly Rep 52:1019–1022
80. Rubenstein LZ, Josephson KR (2002) The epidemiology of falls and syncope. Clin Geriatr Med 18:141–158
81. Tinetti ME, Doucette J, Claus E, Marottoli R (1995) Risk factors for serious injury during falls by older persons in the community. J Am Geriatr Soc 43:1214–1221
82. Scuffham P, Chaplin S, Legood R (2003) Incidence and costs of unintentional falls in older people in the United Kingdom. J Epidemiol Community Health 57:740–744
83. Bloch F, Thibaud M, Dugue B, Breque C, Rigaud AS, Kemoun G (2011) Psychotropic drugs and falls in the elderly people: updated literature review and meta-analysis. J Aging Health 23:329–346
84. Liu B, Anderson G, Mittmann N, To T, Axcell T, Shear N (1998) Use of selective serotonin-reuptake inhibitors or tricyclic antidepressants and risk of hip fractures in elderly people. Lancet 351:1303–1307

85. Nurminen J, Puustinen J, Piirtola M, Vahlberg T, Kivela SL (2010) Psychotropic drugs and the risk of fractures in old age: a prospective population-based study. BMC Public Health 10:396
86. Moden B, Merlo J, Ohlsson H, Rosvall M (2010) Psychotropic drugs and falling accidents among the elderly: a nested case control study in the whole population of Scania, Sweden. J Epidemiol Community Health 64:440–446
87. Kragh A, Elmstahl S, Atroshi I (2011) Older adults' medication use 6 months before and after hip fracture: a population-based cohort study. J Am Geriatr Soc 59:863–868
88. Gill SS, Bronskill SE, Normand SL et al (2007) Antipsychotic drug use and mortality in older adults with dementia. Ann Intern Med 146:775–786
89. Vitry AI, Hoile AP, Gilbert AL, Esterman A, Luszcz MA (2010) The risk of falls and fractures associated with persistent use of psychotropic medications in elderly people. Arch Gerontol Geriatr 50:e1–e4
90. Sullivan MD, Edlund MJ, Fan MY, Devries A, Brennan BJ, Martin BC (2008) Trends in use of opioids for non-cancer pain conditions 2000–2005 in commercial and Medicaid insurance plans: the TROUP study. Pain 138:440–449
91. Vestergaard P, Rejnmark L, Mosekilde L (2006) Fracture risk associated with the use of morphine and opiates. J Intern Med 260:76–87
92. Holbrook AM, Crowther R, Lotter A, Cheng C, King D (2000) Meta-analysis of benzodiazepine use in the treatment of insomnia. CMAJ 162:225–233
93. Tamblyn R, Abrahamowicz M, du Berger R, McLeod P, Bartlett G (2005) A 5-year prospective assessment of the risk associated with individual benzodiazepines and doses in new elderly users. J Am Geriatr Soc 53:233–241
94. Simoni-Wastila L (2008) Increases in opioid medication use: balancing the good with the bad. Pain 138:245–246
95. Mort JR, Aparasu RR (2000) Prescribing potentially inappropriate medications to the ambulatory elderly. Arch Intern Med 160:2825–2831
96. Curtis LH, Ostbye T, Sendersky V et al (2004) Inappropriate prescribing for elderly Americans in a large outpatient population. Arch Intern Med 164:1621–1625
97. Pugh MJ, Fincke BG, Bierman AS et al (2005) Potentially inappropriate prescribing in elderly veterans: are we using the wrong drug, wrong dose, or wrong duration? J Am Geriatr Soc 53:1282–1289
98. King MB, Tinetti ME (1995) Falls in community-dwelling older persons. J Am Geriatr Soc 43:1146–1154
99. Leipzig RM, Cumming RG, Tinetti ME (1999) Drugs and falls in older people: a systematic review and meta-analysis: I. Psychotropic drugs. J Am Geriatr Soc 47:30–39
100. Souchet E, Lapeyre-Mestre M, Montastruc JL (2005) Drug related falls: a study in the French Pharmacovigilance database. Pharmacoepidemiol Drug Saf 14:11–16
101. Peterson JF, Kuperman GJ, Minalkumar P, Avorn J, Bates DW (2005) Guided prescription of psychotropic medications for geriatric inpatients. Arch Intern Med 165:802–807
102. Rizzo JA, Friedkin R, Williams CS, Nabors J, Acampora D, Tinetti ME (1998) Health care utilization and costs in a Medicare population by fall status. Med Care 36:1174–1188
103. Grizzle AJ, Mahmood MH, Ko Y et al (2007) Reasons provided by prescribers when overriding drug-drug interaction alerts. Am J Manag Care 13:573–578
104. Kuperman GJ, Reichley RM, Bailey TC (2006) Using commercial knowledge bases for clinical decision support: opportunities, hurdles, and recommendations. J Am Med Inform Assoc 13:369–371
105. Hoffmann TC, Del Mar CB, Strong J, Mai J (2013) Patients' expectations of acute low back pain management: implications for evidence uptake. BMC Fam Pract 14:7
106. Siegel CA, Levy LC, MacKenzie TA, Sands BE (2008) Patient perceptions of the risks and benefits of infliximab for the treatment of inflammatory bowel disease. Inflamm Bowel Dis 14:1–6
107. Roberts E, Delgado N, V, Buckner S et al (2015) Paracetamol: not as safe as we thought? A systematic literature review of observational studies. Ann Rheum Dis 75:552–559

108. Julien M, Hanley JA (2008) Profile-specific survival estimates: making reports of clinical trials more patient-relevant. Clin Trials 5:107–115
109. Matheny M, McPheeters ML, Glasser A, Mercaldo N, Weaver RB, Jerome RN et al (2011) Systematic review of cardiovascular disease risk assessment tools. 85. Agency for Healthcare Research and Quality, Rockville
110. Paredes S, Rocha T, de Carvalho P, Henriques J, Morais J, Ferreira J (2015) Integration of different risk assessment tools to improve stratification of patients with coronary artery disease. Med Biol Eng Comput 53:1069–1083
111. Tamblyn R, Eguale T, Buckeridge DL et al (2012) The effectiveness of a new generation of computerized drug alerts in reducing the risk of injury from drug side effects: a cluster randomized trial. J Am Med Inform Assoc 19:635–643
112. de Jong MR, Van der Elst M, Hartholt KA (2013) Drug-related falls in older patients: implicated drugs, consequences, and possible prevention strategies. Ther Adv Drug Saf 4: 147–154
113. Huang AR, Mallet L, Rochefort CM, Eguale T, Buckeridge DL, Tamblyn R (2012) Medication-related falls in the elderly: causative factors and preventive strategies. Drugs Aging 29:359–376
114. Chen Y, Zhu LL, Zhou Q (2014) Effects of drug pharmacokinetic/pharmacodynamic properties, characteristics of medication use, and relevant pharmacological interventions on fall risk in elderly patients. Ther Clin Risk Manag 10:437–448
115. Hill KD, Wee R (2012) Psychotropic drug-induced falls in older people: a review of interventions aimed at reducing the problem. Drugs Aging 29:15–30
116. Buckeridge D, Huang A, Hanley J et al (2010) Risk of injury associated with opioid use in older adults. J Am Geriatr Soc 58:1664–1670
117. Christensen AN (2015) Concomitant use of psychotropic drugs in patients with dementia—a Nationwide Study [abstract]Ane Norgaard Christensen. Alzheimer's Association International Conference 2015
118. Mojtabai R, Olfson M (2010) National trends in psychotropic medication polypharmacy in office-based psychiatry. Arch Gen Psychiatry 67:26–36
119. Vasudev A, Shariff SZ, Liu K et al (2015) Trends in psychotropic dispensing among older adults with dementia living in long-term care facilities: 2004–2013. Am J Geriatr Psychiatry 23:1259–1269
120. Alyass A, Turcotte M, Meyre D (2015) From big data analysis to personalized medicine for all: challenges and opportunities. BMC Med Genomics 8:33
121. Panahiazar M, Taslimitehrani V, Jadhav A, Pathak J (2014) Empowering personalized medicine with big data and semantic web technology: promises, challenges, and use cases. Proc IEEE Int Conf Big Data 2014:790–795
122. Fisher J, Clayton M (2012) Who gives a tweet: assessing patients' interest in the use of social media for health care. Worldviews Evid Based Nurs 9:100–108
123. Pennic F 6 mobile health apps for Healthcare professionals or patients. 5-3-2013. HIT Consultant. 1-7-2016. Ref Type: Online Source
124. Ho K (2013) Health-e-Apps: a project to encourage effective use of mobile health applications. BMCJ 55:458–460
125. O'Neill S, Brady RR (2012) Colorectal smartphone apps: opportunities and risks. Colorectal Dis 14:e530–e534
126. Luxton DD, McCann RA, Bush NE, Mishkind MC, Reger GM (2011) mHealth for mental health: integrating smartphone technology in behavioral healthcare. Prof Psychol: Res Pract 42:505–512
127. Dayer L, Heldenbrand S, Anderson P, Gubbins PO, Martin BC (2003) Smartphone medication adherence apps: potential benefits to patients and providers. J Am Pharm Assoc 53:172–181
128. Goldzweig CL, Towfigh A, Maglione M, Shekelle PG (2009) Costs and benefits of health information technology: new trends from the literature. Health Aff (Millwood) 28:w282–w293
129. Marr B Big data, Walmart and the future of retail. 2-19-2015. LinkedIn. 1-8-2016
130. Kepes B (2016) Better health risk analysis powered by big data. 1-7-2016

131. Raghupathi W, Raghupathi V (2014) Big data analytics in healthcare: promise and potential. Health Inf Sci Syst 2:3
132. Sarker A, Ginn R, Nikfarjam A et al (2015) Utilizing social media data for pharmacovigilance: a review. J Biomed Inform 54:202–212
133. Shah NH, LePendu P, Bauer-Mehren A et al (2015) Proton pump inhibitor usage and the risk of myocardial infarction in the general population. PLoS One 10:e0124653
134. Sacristan JA, Dilla T (2015) No big data without small data: learning health care systems begin and end with the individual patient. J Eval Clin Pract 21:1014
135. Grimshaw JM, Eccles MP, Lavis JN, Hill SJ, Squires JE (2012) Knowledge translation of research findings. Implement Sci 7:50
136. Lavis JN, Robertson D, Woodside JM, McLeod CB, Abelson J (2003) How can research organizations more effectively transfer research knowledge to decision makers? Milbank Q 81:221–222
137. Holmes B, Scarrow G, Schellenberg M (2012) Translating evidence into practice: the role of health research funders. Implement Sci 7:39
138. Reis SE, McDonald MC, Byers SJ (2008) Crossing the research valleys of death: the University of Pittsburgh approach. Clin Transl Sci 1:9–10
139. Roshanov PS, Fernandes N, Wilczynski JM et al (2013) Features of effective computerised clinical decision support systems: meta-regression of 162 randomised trials. Br Med J 346:f657
140. Institute of Medicine (2000) To err is human: building a safer health system. National Academy Press, Washington, DC
141. Hunt DL, Haynes RB, Hanna SE, Smith K (1998) Effects of computer-based clinical decision support systems on physician performance and patient outcomes: a systematic review. JAMA 280:1339–1346
142. CMS Media Affairs (2005) HHS proposes new Medicare E-prescribing rules process will improve quality, accuracy. U S Department of Health & Human Services [serial online]

Chapter 21
Future Directions

Allen R. Huang

Abstract Falling is part of human life. It is unlikely that medical science can completely prevent humans from falling. However, we can manage risk better and minimize the consequences of falls. The Haddon matrix is a framework used in the injury prevention field and has been adapted to help researchers to systematically assess events and identify methods of fall prevention. The use of medications with strong anticholinergic activity has been associated with impaired cognitive and physical functioning in older patients and possibly increase fall risk. Patient sitters have been used as a substitute for chemical or physical restraints for agitated hospitalized patients. A study showed that the use of antipsychotics and drugs with high anticholinergic activity was associated with sitter use. Therefore, modifying the use of these drugs can impact on patient safety, use of sitters, and hospital costs. Some predictions for the future include personalized medications, applications for wearable technology, and altering ourselves through the convergence of genomics, nanotechnology, and robotics that can eventually "fix" our own DNA. Improved interoperability between computer systems can enable innovation and patient-centered care and support a learning health-care system. Leveraging social media can help spread the knowledge about fall risk-increasing drugs. Leading countries and academic organizations have to continue to spread the message that medication-related falls in older people are important to recognize and manage. Each time our decisions and actions can help avoid an adverse event, we have succeeded in improving the care given to an individual person. After all, wouldn't each of us want this kind of sophisticated, safe, appropriate care for ourselves and our loved ones?

Abbreviations

CI	Confidence interval
FRID	Fall risk-increasing drug
OR	Odds ratio
PRO	Patient-reported outcome

A.R. Huang, MDCM, FRCPC
Division of Geriatric Medicine, University of Ottawa and The Ottawa Hospital, Ottawa, ON, Canada

Adjunct Professor of Medicine, McGill University, Montréal, QC, Canada
e-mail: allenhuang@toh.ca

© Springer International Publishing Switzerland 2016

A.R. Huang, L. Mallet (eds.), *Medication-related falls in older people*,
DOI 10.1007/978-3-319-32304-6_21

Predicting the future has always been a fascinating phenomenon and sometimes fraught with peril. In the "Dark Ages" (the period between the decline of the Roman Empire and the emergence of the Renaissance, roughly sixth to thirteenth centuries in European history), rock crystal, or quartz, held such mystical qualities that spheres of the material were considered capable of showing the future. People who possessed such objects were imbued with clairvoyance (clear view) of future events. I do not claim to possess any algorithm with clairvoyant properties. In this chapter, I wish to engage the reader in an analysis of trends. I trust that readers by now agree with me that medication-related falls in older people is an important clinical issue which deserves a collective health-care system and clinician response to manage risk so that the safety and quality of the lives of our patients are optimized.

> Yesterday's the past, tomorrow's the future, but today is a gift. That's why it's called the present. Bil Keane, Oct 5, 1922-Nov 8, 2011; American cartoonist, "Family Circus"

21.1 The Past as It Predicts the Future

Since humans began to walk upright, falling has been an inevitable consequence. An older person who falls once has at least a 30 % chance to fall again in the next year. Can medical science prevent humans from falling? I think this is highly unlikely within my lifetime. Can we minimize the consequences of falls or manage risk? I think these are achievable goals.

21.2 Some Unexplored Corners

21.2.1 The Haddon Matrix

Are falls in older people "accidents"? Should we consider using a different tool to manage this important health problem? The Haddon matrix is a framework used in the injury prevention field [1] and was originally developed to apply basic principles of public health to the problem of car crashes and traffic safety. This framework has been adapted to help researchers to systematically assess injury and identify methods of prevention [2–4]. Injuries are described in terms of causal factors and contributing factors. The Haddon matrix helps to analyze an injury event based on the person who has been injured (host), what caused the injury (the agent), and the environment (the physical and social context in which the injury occurred). These factors are identified and grouped into the pre-injury phase (primary prevention), the injury phase (secondary prevention), and post-injury phase (tertiary prevention). Table 21.1 illustrates an example of the Haddon matrix as applied to falls. The key areas involving clinicians that have potential impact on falls prevention are changing medication use, modifying prescribing practices, and performing medication

Table 21.1 Haddon matrix example as applied to falls (n.b. the cell contents are not comprehensive but illustrative)

	Factors		
Event period	Personal	Physical	Socioeconomic
Pre-event: risk of fall	*Intrinsic*: age, comorbidities (e.g., diabetes, stroke, Parkinson's), dizziness, muscular weakness, sarcopenia, cognitive impairment, and visual and auditory impairments Behavioral: sedentary, excessive alcohol intake, malnutrition, poor medication adherence, risk-taking polypharmacy	*Extrinsic*: environment (insufficient lighting, slippery surfaces, clutter, loose objects; water, ice, snow) cracks and uneven surfaces in public areas, lack of rest areas	Inappropriate prescribing, medication reconciliation not done at discharge from hospital Social isolation, lack of continuity of health-care services Safety code standards nonexistent or not enforced, inadequate infrastructure maintenance Inadequate living conditions: income, housing, food
Event: risk of injury	Low bone mass and osteoporosis, low body weight, low muscle strength, insufficient protective reactions to falling	Energy-absorbing flooring materials Non-age-friendly infrastructure (e.g., sidewalks without ramps)	
Post-event: complications of injuries	Inability to arise following a fall Fracture, fear of falling, muscular deconditioning, death	Absence of telephone or emergency response device, distance to nearest medical care facility	Insufficient services for trauma/accident, rehabilitation, community, home support

Table is adapted from Huang et al. [27]

reconciliation at care transitions, such as during discharge from hospital. The Haddon matrix is a useful construct since it can be used to engage others outside of health care, such as civil and social engineers, industry, and policy-makers.

21.2.2 Anticholinergic Burden

The use of medications with strong anticholinergic activity has been associated with impaired cognitive and physical functioning in older patients [5–7]. Even though clues point to adverse events associated with these drugs, little is known about the direct evidence between the use of these medications and falls. In Cao's study of 932 participants in the Women's Health and Aging Study I, users of these drugs had balance difficulty OR = 4.9 (95 % CI 2.0, 12.00), mobility difficulty OR = 3.2 (95 % CI 1.5, 6.9), slow gait OR = 3.6 (95 % CI 1.6, 8.0), difficulty rising OR = 4.2 (95 % CI 2.0, 8.7), and difficulty in performing activities of daily living

OR = 3.4 (95 % CI 1.7, 6.9) [8]. Hilmer and colleagues developed the Drug Burden Index to study the effects of sedatives and medications with strong anticholinergic activity and their association with falls [9, 10]. A small case-control study of older mental health patients found that a higher "anticholinergic burden score" (an additive score based on the quantitative anticholinergic effect of all drugs taken) was associated with fallers [11]. Salahudeen and colleagues reported in their systematic review that although there is not one standardized risk tool in use, the use of these drugs remains consistently associated with cognitive and functional impairments [12–14]. The evidence that discontinuation of these drugs completely reverses its deleterious effects is even less certain [12]. The difficulty in studying these drugs is that they comprise of nonprescription, prescription, and herbal products. For example, the commonly available over-the-counter drugs diphenhydramine (antihistamine) and dimenhydrinate (anti-nausea) and the prescription antidepressant drug amitriptyline and the herbal products of henbane, jimson weed [15], and belladonna all fall into the group of high anticholinergic activity medications. A definitive answer to the association between the use of these medications and falls in older patients awaits the results of future studies, including a well-designed intervention trial.

21.2.3 Hospital Sitters for Agitated Patients

In response to hospitalized patients who are physically agitated and are at risk for falls, a substitute for chemical or physical restraints has been the increasing use of patient sitters [16].

Patient sitters are unlicensed health-care providers, whose functions are to provide close surveillance of "at-risk" patients and give an early warning signal to other hospital health-care providers when the behavior of these patients deteriorates. One monitored behavior is patient attempts at mobilization with a high risk of falling and sustaining fall-related injuries [16–20]. The use of sitters is expensive, with some US hospitals reporting an annual cost in 2009 of $1.3 million US dollars and their effectiveness is questionable [20, 21]. Rochefort and colleagues reported the results of a nested case-control study done in an urban teaching hospital in Montreal, Canada, which showed that the use of antipsychotics (OR = 1.26 [95 % CI 1.07, 1.49]), intermediate-acting benzodiazepines (OR = 1.28 [95 % CI 1.08, 1.51]), long-acting benzodiazepines (OR = 2.85 [95 % CI 2.02, 4.01]), and short-acting benzodiazepines (OR = 3.70 [95 % CI 2.93, 4.69]) was each independently associated with greater sitter use [22, 23]. A further case-control study among medical patients aged 65 years and older showed that the risk of sitter use increased by 40 % (OR = 1.4 [95 % CI 1.1, 1.7; $p = 0.005$]) for each drug with an anticholinergic load of one added to the patient medication profile during the antecedent exposure [24]. These findings suggest that a reduction in the use of psychotropic drugs and minimizing the anticholinergic load in older hospitalized patients may not only reduce falls but also the use of patient sitters as well as their costs.

21.3 Looking to the Future

Futurists, or futurologists, whose membership contains over 100 people from around the world at the time of this writing, have thought that predictions for health-care advancements were easy pickings. They see the obvious increase in the number of older people in the world and those that present with illnesses and conditions needing health-care services. Technology and innovation are then combined into that scenario. Some of the futurists aim for a short horizon of 5–10 years. I too propose to project my thoughts within that timeframe. Technological advances continue to accelerate dramatically such that a 5-year horizon may be reaching too far. The British author, inventor, and futurist Arthur C. Clarke (Dec 16, 1917–Mar 18, 2008) wrote “Any sufficiently advanced technology is indistinguishable from magic.” This phrase has now been embodied as Clarke’s Third Law. Maybe in the next 5 years if any of the developments described below are operationalized, then it will seem like “magic” that medication-related falls will be better managed or even reduced.

21.4 Technologies and Developments Promising to the Management of Falls in Older Adults

21.4.1 Personalized Medications

A disruptive technology could appear where medications are custom-made to the needs of an individual patient, based on their unique pharmacokinetic and pharmacodynamic response to drugs. The analysis of individual genomic data could also be used to increase the precision of traditional drug dosing. For example, an 85-year-old woman, based on a detailed physiologic, genomic, and proteomic analysis, may be dispensed a combination tablet consisting of 1.05 mg of enalapril +72 mg of aspirin +742 mg of metformin as her morning pill, followed by another pill made of metformin 812 mg + bisoprolol 0.7 mg to be taken in the afternoon. These two pills would be sufficient to manage her diabetes, hypertension, and stroke risks. This concept would resemble the customized compounding that pharmacists did in bygone days or the dispensing of traditional herbal medicines. Medications in liquid form already partly offer such flexibility in dosage. Perhaps advances in three-dimensional printing technologies may catalyze another way forward.

21.4.2 Wearable Technologies

Mobile and ubiquitous electronically enabled wireless health care is already past the prototype phase. Micro-robotics, with devices integrated into clothing, along with the appropriate accompanying smart analytics software, can help detect conditions, for example, worsening sway, or gait ataxia, that places the individual at higher risk for falls. A wireless voice message delivered directly to a person's hearing aid can alert that person to stop and sit down or to remind them to use a walking aid. In the event that a fall has already occurred, these smart devices can automatically initiate a call for assistance for the distressed individual. Other sensing devices, for heart rate, blood pressure, blood glucose, etc., can also be used to detect risky situations and proactively suggest to the individual person to sit down or to take some glucose. People who suffer from orthostatic hypotension may avail themselves of clothing that can dynamically constrict, perhaps similar to military antishock trousers with embedded inflatable air bladders or electrically controlled compression fibers. Automatic deployment of these devices may increase the standing blood pressure and avoid a pre-syncopal event and a subsequent fall. What about a personal "air bag" that can deploy on sensing a fall in progress and help mitigate a serious injury to a person's hip or head? Other wearable exoskeletal machines can multiply the existing strength of an individual, correcting for present sarcopenia and improving balance so that individual people can regain the ability to stay safely upright and avoid falls. Creative thinking and tinkering with currently available technologies can potentially lead to new applications.

21.4.3 Altering Ourselves

Ray Kurzweil, an American futurist, inventor, computer scientist, and author, has written about the "Singularity"[1] which is the convergence of genetics, nanotechnologies, and robotics. Continued miniaturization of technology will lead to machines that act at the molecular, atomic, and perhaps even at the subatomic levels. Mr Kurzweil's prediction is that nanorobotics can eventually "fix" our actual DNA, thereby eliminating many diseases. These nanobots could conceivably reverse sarcopenia by growing new muscle fibers. Others could supplant failing neurons and improve neurologic functioning. Engineering at the molecular level would greatly expand the field of therapeutics.

21.4.4 Interoperability

The next-generation electronic health record systems will be able to foster innovation, support patient-centered care delivery, and support a learning health-care system when it is successfully linked to big data and analytics. The time lag in translating knowledge to practice will continue to shrink. More clinicians will embrace intuitive, clinician-friendly computing systems based on human factors design. The Internet of Things (IOT) holds both promises of smart environments (maybe even age-friendly) and perils of when machines break through the

[1]The Singularity is Near. *When Humans Transcend Biology*. Ray Kurzweil. Viking USA, New York, New York. Aug 18, 2005, ISBN-13: 978-0670033843.

boundaries of control or are subservient to malicious intent. Trust in the security and privacy of health information systems has to be universally accepted to enable ubiquitous use. The current process of securing privacy by using RSA[2] keys will need to be re-engineered since these keys will eventually be broken with the relentless increases in computing power.

> The Information Age offers much to mankind, and I would like to think that we will rise to the challenges it presents. *But it is vital to remember that information — in the sense of raw data — is not knowledge, that knowledge is not wisdom, and that wisdom is not foresight.* But information is the first essential step to all of these. Sir Arthur C. Clarke in OneWorld South Asia, December 5, 2003

21.4.5 Leveraging Social Media

Spreading knowledge about fall risk-increasing drugs (FRIDs) to patients and their families can be enabled through social media channels. Academic organizations, such as those supporting Geriatric Medicine specialists around the world, may be well placed to broadcast knowledge about medication-related falls and various management approaches to the blogosphere[3] or reach out to the Twitterati.[4] Perhaps a benzodiazepine user self-help and tapering support group could be created. Reasonable and rational oversight and editing would ensure that the information is accurate and free of unsolicited ideologies.

21.5 Continuing Research

More high-quality research needs to be conducted to clarify which specific drugs, or different dosage thresholds, or cumulative exposure duration cause harm. Different environments offer different opportunities to modify, monitor, and manage medications and potential falls. Hospital processes need to be changed to make it difficult to prescribe FRIDs. Patients are already at higher risk for immobility and loss of function [25] when hospitalized. People living in the community and in long-stay institutions can also be the targets of a public health initiative to decrease FRID use. Research on the tools and methods for optimal interventions needs to continue. The use of modern information technologies in patient co-management of fall risks, including appropriate medication use, introduces a new area of investigation. An additional trend is the inclusion of patient-reported outcomes (PROs) in studies. For example, participant patients in a drug trial may decide that avoidance of falls is a more important outcome to them than an investigator-driven target blood pressure measurement.

---

[2] Cryptographic public-key encryption system devised by Ron Rivest, Adi Shamir, and Leonard Adleman, in 1977. This system is based on the product of two large prime numbers.

[3] Pertaining to all blogs and their interconnections.

[4] Avid or frequent users of the social media website Twitter.

21.6 Leading Countries

What leadership responsibilities lie with the developed countries? Perhaps they can enable emerging frameworks that are coming from academic organizations, from health care, and from informatics and health service delivery research to align private sector businesses through governmental coaxing or legislation when necessary. An increased involvement in public health activities can result in improved well-being for everyone. Advertisements to encourage smoking cessation, to encourage physical activity, and perhaps even to educate the public about making informed health-care choices could be effective tools. For example, the Choosing Wisely initiative was led by the American Board of Internal Medicine Foundation (http://www.choosingwisely.org/) and has gained international acceptance in twelve countries around the world including the United States, Australia, Canada, Denmark, England, Germany, Italy, Japan, the Netherlands, New Zealand, Switzerland, and Wales [26]. One of the recommendations is: "Don't use benzodiazepines or other sedative-hypnotics in older adults as first choice for insomnia, agitation or delirium." In my opinion, the shared knowledge of people, their families and caregivers, and clinicians will definitely have an impact on reducing medication-related falls.

21.7 Conclusions

As closing comments for this book, I wish to leave the reader with several thoughts. Because you chose to read this book, either selected chapters or its entirety, you are interested in learning about and perhaps wanting to help advance the knowledge on the effects of medications in older people and the risk for falls. I want to welcome you to the club. Whenever our actions can help avoid an adverse event, we have succeeded in improving the care given to an individual person. Despite the focus of many health industries on the continued chase for material gain, I believe a balance can be reached where a knowledgeable person can choose wisely for him or herself the outcomes they wish for maintaining their function, utility, and happiness. After all, wouldn't each of us want this kind of sophisticated, safe, appropriate care for ourselves and our loved ones?

References

1. Baker SP, Haddon W Jr (1974) Reducing injuries and their results: the scientific approach. Milbank Mem Fund Q Health Soc 52:377–389
2. Haddon J (1980) Options for the prevention of motor vehicle crash injury. Isr J Med Sci 16(1):45–65, *Date of Publication*: *1980*:1980
3. Haddon W Jr (1970) On the escape of tigers: an ecologic note. Am J Publ Health Nation's Health 60:2229–2234

4. Runyan CW (1998) Using the Haddon matrix: introducing the third dimension. Inj Prev: J Int Soc Child Adolesc Inj Prev 4(4):302–307, *Date of Publication*: *Dec 1998*: Dec
5. Campbell N, Boustani M, Limbil T et al (2009) The cognitive impact of anticholinergics: a clinical review. Clin Interv Aging 4:225–233
6. Minzenberg MJ, Poole JH, Benton C, Vinogradov S (2004) Association of anticholinergic load with impairment of complex attention and memory in schizophrenia. Am J Psychiatry 161:116–124
7. Landi F, Russo A, Liperoti R et al (2007) Anticholinergic drugs and physical function among frail elderly population. Clin Pharmacol Ther 81:235–241
8. Cao YJ, Mager DE, Simonsick EM et al (2008) Physical and cognitive performance and burden of anticholinergics, sedatives, and ACE inhibitors in older women. Clin Pharmacol Ther 83:422–429
9. Hilmer SN, Mager DE, Simonsick EM (2007) A drug burden index to define the functional burden of medications in older people. Arch Intern Med 167:781–787
10. Wilson NM, Hilmer SN, March LM et al (2011) Associations between drug burden index and falls in older people in residential aged care. J Am Geriatr Soc 59:875–880
11. Aizenberg D, Sigler M, Weizman A, Barak Y (2002) Anticholinergic burden and the risk of falls among elderly psychiatric inpatients: a 4-year case-control study. Int Psychogeriatr 14:307–310
12. Salahudeen M, Duffull S, Nishtala P (2014) Impact of anticholinergic discontinuation on cognitive outcomes in older people: a systematic review. Drugs Aging 31:185–192
13. Salahudeen MS, Hilmer SN, Nishtala PS (2015) Comparison of anticholinergic risk scales and associations with adverse health outcomes in older people. J Am Geriatr Soc 63:85–90
14. Salahudeen MS, Duffull SB, Nishtala PS (2015) Anticholinergic burden quantified by anticholinergic risk scales and adverse outcomes in older people: a systematic review. BMC Geriatr 15:31
15. Alagiakrishnan K, Wiens CA (2004) An approach to drug induced delirium in the elderly. Postgrad Med J 80:388–393
16. Tzeng HM, Yin CY, Grunawalt J (2008) Effective assessment of use of sitters by nurses in inpatient care settings. J Adv Nurs 64:176–183
17. Jaworowski S, Raveh D, Lobel E, Fuer A, Gropp C, Mergui J (2008) Constant observation in the general hospital: a review. Isr J Psychiatry Relat Sci 45:278–284
18. Rausch DL, Bjorklund P (2010) Decreasing the costs of constant observation. J Nurs Adm 40:75–81
19. Donoghue J, Graham J, Mitten-Lewis S, Murphy M, Gibbs J (2005) A volunteer companion-observer intervention reduces falls on an acute aged care ward. Int J Health Care Qual Assur Inc Leadersh Health Serv 18:24–31
20. Worley LL, Kunkel EJ, Gitlin DF, Menefee LA, Conway G (2000) Constant observation practices in the general hospital setting: a national survey. Psychosomatics 41:301–310
21. Torkelson DJ, Dobal MT (1999) Constant observation in medical-surgical settings: a multihospital study. Nurs Econ 17:149–155
22. Rochefort CM, Ward L, Ritchie JA, Girard N, Tamblyn RM (2011) Registered nurses' job demands in relation to sitter use: nested case-control study. Nurs Res 60:221–230
23. Rochefort CM, Ward L, Ritchie JA, Girard N, Tamblyn RM (2012) Patient and nurse staffing characteristics associated with high sitter use costs. J Adv Nurs 68:1758–1767
24. Charbonneau-Allard A-M, Fluet J, Lessard A, Rochefort CM, Tamblyn RM, Mallet L (2011) Mécanismes pharmacologiques comme facteurs modifiables de la prescription de sitters. Faculté de pharmacie, Université de Montréal
25. Creditor MC (1993) Hazards of hospitalization of the elderly. Ann Intern Med 118:219–223
26. Levinson W, Kallewaard M, Bhatia RS, Wolfson D, Shortt S, Kerr EA (2015) Choosing wisely: a growing international campaign. BMJ Qual Saf 24:167–174
27. Huang AR et al (2012) Medication-related falls in the elderly: causative factors and preventive strategies. Drugs Aging 29(5):359–376